Isokinetics

To Miki, who struggled and won, with endless love

For Churchill Livingstone

Editorial Director, Health Professions: Mary Law
Project Development Manager: Dinah Thom
Project Manager: Jane Dingwall
Design direction: Judith Wright

Isokinetics

Muscle Testing, Interpretation and Clinical Applications

Zeevi Dvir PhD(BioEng) LLB
Department of Physical Therapy, Sackler Faculty of Medicine, Tel-Aviv University, Israel

SECOND EDITION

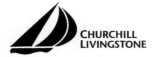

CHURCHILL
LIVINGSTONE

EDINBURGH LONDON NEW YORK OXFORD PHILADELPHIA ST LOUIS SYDNEY TORONTO 2004

CHURCHILL LIVINGSTONE
An imprint of Elsevier Limited

First edition 1995
Second edition 2004

ISBN 0443 07199 3

British Library Cataloguing in Publication Data
A catalogue record for this book is available from the British Library

Library of Congress Cataloging in Publication Data
A catalog record for this book is available from the Library of Congress

Note
Medical knowledge is constantly changing. Standard safety precautions must be followed, but as new research and clinical experience broaden our knowledge, changes in treatment and drug therapy may become necessary or appropriate. Readers are advised to check the most current product information provided by the manufacturer of each drug to be administered to verify the recommended dose, the method and duration of administration, and contraindications. It is the responsibility of the practitioner, relying on experience and knowledge of the patient, to determine dosages and the best treatment for each individual patient. Neither the Publisher nor the author assumes any liability for any injury and/or damage to persons or property arising from this publication.

The Publisher

 your source for books,
journals and multimedia
in the health sciences
www.elsevierhealth.com

The
publisher's
policy is to use
**paper manufactured
from sustainable forests**

Transferred to digital print 2008
Printed and bound by CPI Antony Rowe, Eastbourne

Contents

Preface to the second edition

When the first edition of this book was published in 1995 the scientific basis of isokinetic dynamometry (ISD) consisted of about 1000 papers. Since 1993, when the final draft of the first edition was submitted to the publisher, more than 1500 new papers, all listed in the major electronic databases, were added. This is a serious indication for the importance attributed to ISD among researchers coming from a multitude of disciplines.

The structure of the second edition does not deviate significantly from the first. However there are a number of changes that are worth mentioning.

Three new chapters have been added relating to reproducibility of findings, medicolegal applications and isokinetics of elbow, wrist and hand muscles. In the previous edition reproducibility and validity were presented as independent entities within the same chapter. However, I have become increasingly convinced that the main methodological issue facing ISD (as well as many other clinical methods/tools) is the reproducibility of the findings derived from this method. The errors associated with the employment of various statistical tools and the advantages offered by others, have therefore been presented and applied to isokinetic findings in this new chapter.

On the other hand, the issue of validity seems to have receded and quite justifiably so. The relentless drive to prove that ISD provides valid findings may be an erroneous one. Isokinetic findings inform the examiner about the strength, or its mechanical derivatives, and about the endurance of muscles: no more, no less. The clinical (in the wide sense) significance of these findings must be assessed in combination with other factors, not least the psychological. Clearly when a muscle is directly compromised, ISD *is* the standard tool for its assessment. Moreover, hundreds of clinical papers that have used ISD to judge the outcomes of various interventions are the best indication for the validity of this method.

The issue of medicolegal applications of ISD has been divorced from the original chapter on reproducibility and validity and made into an individual chapter. Although of a more limited usage, medicolegal applications require profound understanding of the issues and careful consideration of the chronic status of muscular insufficiency. Finally, a chapter was dedicated to the distal muscles of the upper extremity, an emerging application of ISD.

The other general chapters (1, 2 and 4) as well as the joint-related chapters were all updated with the exception of the chapter dedicated to knee muscles. Surprisingly, no major breakthroughs seem to have taken place with respect to the quadriceps and hamstrings although many of the new papers use these muscles for modeling or proving the efficacy of some interventions. Perhaps isokinetics of knee muscles deserves a special contribution.

This book is dedicated to my beloved wife and best friend, Miki, without whose wonderful support and absolute patience, this second edition would have remained a plain wish.

Tel Aviv 2003   Zeevi Dvir

Preface to the first edition

It is now slightly over 25 years since isokinetic dynamometry was first introduced into clinical practice and exercise science. Physical therapy, in particular, has benefited significantly from this technology, which rapidly became the tool of choice in hundreds of research papers as well as the cornerstone of quantitative muscle performance assessment in the clinical setting. About a decade ago, the technology behind isokinetic dynamometry made considerable progress when computers were incorporated to control the hardware, that is the integral power sources and the on-line processing of mechanical signals. This enabled users to establish a common basis for carrying out eccentric contractions and to obtain comprehensive information on muscle strength immediately.

My own experience of isokinetic dynamometry did not start when I first switched on the system my department acquired in 1986. For a period of about 2 years from 1980 I approached a number of independent manufacturers of high-tech medical equipment in my country with a proposal for constructing an active dynamometer, based on a design I then had. The result was disappointing, and as a result I abandoned the idea. Thus, although the advent of active dynamometry, at a later date, did not surprise me, the feeling of having missed an exclusive opportunity was very acute.

Hence, when the next opportunity in isokinetics arose years later – to write a book about isokinetic dynamometry – I decided to be more tenacious. The need for such a reference source was very obvious. In spite of the fact that there

were thousands of users of isokinetic dynamometers in the US alone, the number of books whose main subject was isokinetics could be counted on the fingers of one hand. Moreover, I felt that there was a conspicuous lack of texts defining the main methodological and procedural problems surrounding this technology. This book does not pretend to cover all the topics that have been examined under isokinetics. Nor is it intended to be a quick and superficial introduction to clinical applications. Rather, it is aimed at those who have at least some experience and are at a stage where they are beginning to ask some very serious questions, and would not necessarily be happy with very simple answers.

In this book I have attempted to draw an unbiased picture of isokinetics. The source material used throughout the book is based exclusively on papers which appeared in peer review journals. Published abstracts are referred to in only a few cases. The first four chapters cover relevant biomechanical and physiological issues, aspects of operation, measurement, validity and reproducibility, and isokinetically-based muscle conditioning methods. The other five chapters describe the use of isokinetics on the major joint systems of the body: the hip, knee, ankle, spine and shoulder. I decided not to deal with the elbow and wrist joints in separate chapters as the database was insufficiently comprehensive.

The section on the medicolegal applications of isokinetics, perhaps the most involved and fascinating aspect of this technology, is not based exclusively on published material. I decided to include this topic, not only because of its increasing importance, but also because it reflects my personal experience with a wide spectrum of legal cases.

Finally, I would like to thank Mr Angus Strover FRCS of the Droitwich Knee Clinic, UK, for his thoughtful reflections on the chapter on the knee, and Mr Asher Pinchasoff from the Sackler Faculty of Medicine, Tel-Aviv University, for the photographic work. However, this book is first and foremost a tribute to the exquisite patience, encouragement and love shown and given to me by my beloved ones throughout the long period of writing.

Tel Aviv 1995   Zeevi Dvir

1

Physiological and biomechanical aspects of isokinetics

This book deals with the measurement and conditioning of isokinetic muscle performance, primarily in the clinical setting. The term 'isokinetic' refers to a specific situation in which a muscle or muscle group contracts against a *controlled accommodating resistance*, which causes a limb segment to move at a *constant angular* or *linear velocity* within a prescribed sector of its range of motion. Isokinetic dynamometry is concerned with the provision of this resistance and its measurement. In this chapter some independent physiological and biomechanical issues concerning the use of isokinetic systems are discussed.

Before turning to the main issues of this chapter, the need for such measurements should be highlighted. Muscle *strength* which is the principal factor in the general muscle performance domain has been assessed for close to a century using the manual muscle testing (MMT) technique. Of particular relevance to isokinetics are the MMT grades 3, 4 and 5 which are defined as the ability of a muscle (group) to overcome gravitational resistance (grade 3), to overcome gravitational resistance and *some* resistance (grade 4) and to exert maximal resistance (grade 5). These grades also refer largely to static (isometric) rather than dynamic capacity.

It should be realized that whereas grade 3 is an objective measure, grades 4 and 5 are assessed by the clinician and thus in fact reflect sensory acuity in judging the degree of effort exerted by the examinee. However, the human capacity to accurately judge the amount of resistance in both absolute and relative terms is especially poor

(Sapega 1990). For instance, differences in strength of less than 25% are generally non-detectable. Consequently deciding for example whether muscles in the involved side have reached parity with the reference (uninvolved) side or a given percentage of its strength cannot, by definition, be reliably derived from MMT. Moreover, progression in muscle performance cannot be effectively estimated.

This problem is further and seriously complicated by the fact that grade 4 accounts for some 60–90% of the muscular strength range. This figure derives from an analysis of the (maximal) strength of extremity muscles as indicated by isokinetic measurements versus the strength required to resist the gravitational demands, namely grade 5 versus grade 3, respectively (Dvir 1997a). Table 1.1 outlines the range of values which, for grade 3, were computed based on the position of the segment where maximal gravitational demand is expected. Grade 5 scores were based on various published sources. Clearly, with the exception of hip abductors and flexors which in the side-lying and supine position are required to balance the sizeable moment exerted by the weight of the lower extremity, in all other instances the gravitational resistance is equivalent to 4–20% of the maximal moment (strength) that the respective muscles can exert. Consequently, almost all muscular potential is embedded in one grade: 4. Although this led inevitably to subdivisions (e.g. 3+, 5−) the application of these subcategories is neither reproducible nor valid. By virtue of their sensitive load cells and the associated technological innovations, isokinetic dynamometers can effectively and accurately measure the true maximal capacity of muscles as well as subtle differences between performance levels. They can do so under both dynamic and static exertions and provide information that far exceeds that which is obtained using all other techniques, manual or instrumental.

BASIC PRINCIPLES

LENGTH–TENSION RELATIONSHIP

Voluntary and involuntary muscle performance

Isokinetic dynamometry has been employed almost exclusively for assessing the performance of voluntarily contracting muscles. This means that besides the physiological and mechanical factors, psychological factors are also involved.

Table 1.1 Maximal gravitational moment (MGM) vs maximal isokinetic moment (MIM) in Nm and their corresponding percentage ratios

Joint	Muscles	MGM		MIM		MGM/MIM (%)	
		Women	Men	Women	Men	Women	Men
Shoulder[1]	Abductors	7.46	11.7	28	57	27	21
	Flexors	7.46	11.7	36	62	21	19
	Extensors	7.46	11.7	39	85	19	14
	Int. Rot.	1.78	2.99	27	42	7	7
	Ext. Rot.	1.78	2.99	16	25	11	12
Elbow[1,m]	Flexors	1.78	2.99	26	39	7	8
	Extensors	1.78	2.99	25	31	7	10
Hip[2]	Abductors	42.6	45.1	66	103	65	44
	Flexors	28.8	33.9	91	152	32	22
	Extensors	42.6	45.1	110	177	39	25
	Int. Rot.	4.4	5.7	87	139	5	4
	Ext. Rot.	4.4	5.7	53	84	8	7
Knee[3]	Flexors	8.8	11.35	89	147	10	8
	Extensors	8.8	11.35	166	250	5	5

[1] age range, 20–30; [2] age range, 20–40; [3] average age, 30; [m] based predominantly on male subjects.

Indeed, motivation and cooperation are essential components in isokinetic testing. However, it is also possible to use isokinetic dynamometers for measuring muscle performance which may be initiated involuntarily, for instance in patients suffering from spastic paresis following stroke.

The fundamental relationship

The most basic relationship governing muscle performance is perceived as the association between the length of the muscle and the magnitude of the corresponding tension. Our understanding of this relationship is almost exclusively based on animal preparations. In those few instances where human experimentation has been allowed, the findings, in volunteers who underwent cineplastic amputation (Ralston et al 1949), proved to be in close agreement with the principles established from animal experiments.

Principles of isometric contractions

Investigation of isometric contractions is based on an experimental set-up in which the length of the muscle is set by the experimenter ('the independent variable') and the tension under passive pull or electrical stimulation ('the dependent variable') is recorded by a force-measuring device (Hill 1953).

Starting in a slack position so that the distance between the ends of the muscle is shorter than its total length, the muscle is tetanized using electrical stimulation. The tension developed is measured by a load cell connected in series with the muscle. The distance between the ends of the muscle is then increased by small amounts and at a certain point, passive resistance is recorded by the load cell even before stimulation. The process is repeated until no increase in tension is apparent.

The tension recorded by the dynamometer reflects two independent sources (Fig. 1.1):

1. the active tension produced by the contractile elements in the muscle
2. the passive tension produced by the non-contractile elements.

As the two components are physically intertwined it is impossible to simultaneously measure their independent contributions. However the active tension is found by subtracting the value of the passive tension, as recorded before stimulation, from the corresponding value of the total tension. The curve describing the active component then has an almost perfectly symmetrical inverted 'U' shape (Fig. 1.1).

The muscle length corresponding to the maximal active tension is known as the 'resting length' which should not be confused with the length of the muscle at the 'anatomical position'. Furthermore, the strength (see below) developed by the muscle at the resting length is unlikely to be its maximal.

The length–tension relationship of the whole muscle reflects the mechanical behavior of the muscle fiber (Gordon et al 1966). The amount of tension developed is related to the number of cross-bridges between the actin and myosin filaments in the fibers, which in turn is related to their degree of overlap.

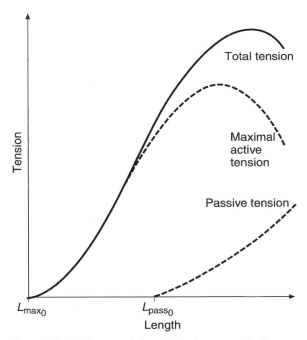

Figure 1.1 In vitro muscle length–tension curve. The lower dotted line represents the resistance to stretch contributed by the passive elastic elements of a denervated muscle. The solid line represents the total tension contributed by active and passive elements during stimulation which produces maximal tetanic tension. (From Kandel et al 1991, with permission.)

STRENGTH IN LIVE SUBJECTS

The maximal moment

The techniques, be they isometric, isokinetic or other, employed to measure muscle 'force' in live subjects, are based on a different method. Instead of force, which is basically a linear entity, the appropriate term is strength. This is defined as *the rotational effect of the force*, generated by a single muscle or a muscle group, about the joint under consideration, and is also called the *moment*. Although strength is defined with respect to any point along the joint range of motion (ROM) in which the muscle(s) exert this effect, the common meaning of strength is the point in the ROM where strength reaches its maximum. Hence the term peak moment or peak torque (see below). Strength also involves the concept of synergy, reference being made, where applicable, to the combined action of a number of muscles rather than of a single muscle (Herzog et al 1991).

Disregarding for a moment the effect of gravity (see below), strength is measured by recording the force exerted on the sensor of the dynamometer by the body segment distal to the joint, and multiplying the value obtained by the length of the force sensor's lever-arm (Fig. 1.2) to give a moment, M. In other words the mechanical potential of the muscle is only inferred rather than measured directly. Moreover, simple mechanical considerations indicate that the amount of force exerted on the force sensor is inversely proportional to the distance between the joint axis and the point of force application. Since the length of body segments is generally small, a deviation of even 1 cm from the original placement of the sensor may, upon retesting, introduce errors of approximately 2.5–5% with a corresponding effect on the reproducibility of the test findings.

Total force and measurable force

There is however another fundamental difference between the direct and the common methods namely that in the latter only a fraction of the total muscle force is measurable. For instance consider Figure 1.3, a schematic, planar view of the elbow joint. The force, F, developed by the brachialis, which here represents the total flexor force, is a vector with two components, the transarticular, F_{ta} and the rotatory, F_r. The transarticular component acts to stabilize the joint but does not contribute to generating the moment about the elbow.

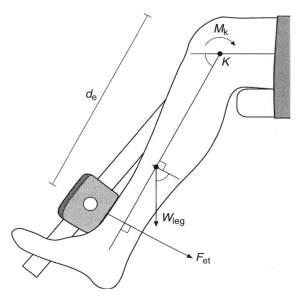

Figure 1.2 In an isometric or isokinetic gravity-free situation the moment M_k, generated by the muscle (the quadriceps femoris in this case) would be equal to the distance between the force resistance pad and the instantaneous center of rotation of the knee, d_e, times the force recorded by the sensor, F_{et}. W_{leg}, weight of leg (shank + foot). (Adapted from Nisell et al 1989, with permission.)

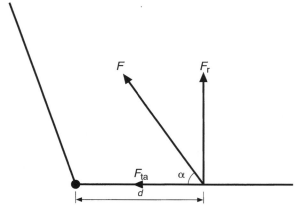

Figure 1.3 The total muscle force, F, is a vector with two components: F_r, the rotatory component and F_{ta}, the transarticular component. α, angle of application (AOA); d, lever of F_r.

In dynamic situations, this function of flexing or controlling the extension of the forearm is performed by the rotatory component of the brachialis force. The value of the moment, M, is obtained through multiplying the rotational component, F_r (Fig. 1.3) by the length of the lever, d, which is the perpendicular distance from F_r to the center of rotation (the elbow joint).

$$M = F_r d$$

From trigonometry:

$$F_r = F \sin \alpha$$

where α is the direction in which F is being applied or the 'angle of application' (AOA) (Fig. 1.3). It follows that:

$$M = dF \sin \alpha$$

The moment–angular position curve

Therefore, as well as increasing with the length, d, the muscular moment depends on two factors: the muscle force and the sine of its angle of application ($\sin \alpha$). These variables behave in a somewhat opposite manner. When the muscle is at its most stretched position the AOA is very small and hence the sine of the angle is minimal, tending to reduce the value of M. As the muscle becomes shorter, its tension generating capacity diminishes, i.e. F decreases, but the corresponding AOA, and hence $\sin \alpha$, becomes greater.

Since during the initial sector of the total ROM the rate of increase of $\sin \alpha$ is much faster than the corresponding rate of decrease in the muscle force, F, the moment, M, generated by the muscle tends to increase in this sector. This is the reason for the observed rise in muscle strength from the so-called 'outer end' to the 'middle range' position. The opposite may generally prevail in the later sector, from the 'middle range' to 'inner end position', leading to a decrease in the moment, M. The shape of the resulting moment–angular position curve is illustrated in Figure 1.4 which is based on an isokinetic test of the elbow supinators and pronators.

The gravitational correction

In dynamic contractions, the external moment, namely the moment which has to be overcome by the muscle, is normally generated by three distinct elements:

1. the individual weight of the segment(s) distal to the joint
2. the load against which one acts, for instance lifting an object
3. the inertial resistance of the segment ($I\alpha$).

As soon as the isokinetic condition is reached, namely the lever-arm proceeds at a constant angular velocity, the accelerational components are negligible. Therefore in order to determine the net muscle force it is necessary to account for the effect of weight. Consider Figure 1.5 which refers to the

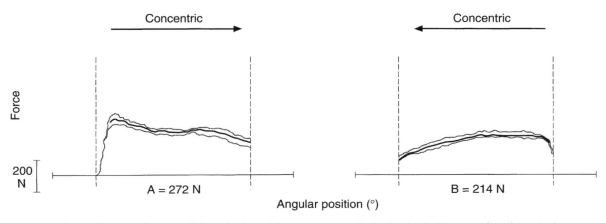

Figure 1.4 Isokinetic strength curves: left, supinators; right, pronators; multiplication by the lever-arm length results in moment rather than force units. A and B are the average force (in N).

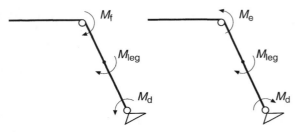

Figure 1.5 Moment configuration simulated during isokinetic testing of flexors (M_f) and extensors (M_e). M_d, moment generated by the dynamometer's lever-arm; M_{leg}, gravitational moment of the leg.

isometric measurement of the strength of the knee extensors and flexors in the seated position.

The extensors act in the opposite direction to the weight of the leg and the resistance of the dynamometer. The moment exerted by the extensors, M_e (anticlockwise in Fig. 1.5), must be equal to the moment of weight of the leg (shank and foot), M_{leg} plus the moment exerted by the resistance of the dynamometer, M_d (both clockwise in Fig. 1.5). This relationship is given by the equation:

$$M_e = M_d + M_{leg}$$

On the other hand, when the flexors contract isometrically, the moment they generate, M_f, and the moment exerted by the weight of the leg act in the same direction (clockwise in Fig. 1.5), and hence the equation is:

$$M_f + M_{leg} = M_d$$

Or by rearranging:

$$M_f = M_d - M_{leg}$$

Thus, in the 'gravitational position' the strength of the extensors may be underestimated and that of the flexors overestimated by an amount equal to the gravitational moment.

In isokinetic testing the above argument is valid for the analogous case of extensor and flexor concentric (see below) contractions, i.e. where the muscle is overcoming the weight of the limb and the resistance of the dynamometer. In order to obtain the true value of the muscle strength it is therefore necessary to perform the so-called 'gravity correction' procedure which is incorporated in commercially available isokinetic systems. The procedure is based on 'weighing' of the

segment at a given recorded position (normally as close to the horizontal as possible) which is performed by the system's load cell and a simple trigonometric calculation which is incorporated in the force or moment data processing by the computer. However as indicated by a number of recent papers (Bygott et al 2001a,b; see Chapter 9 for a detailed exposition) gravity correction procedures are error prone. This error is primarily due to two factors:

1. Biological joints cannot be simulated by a perfect hinge-type joint which serves as the basic assumption of the software procedure.
2. There is a measure of active and passive resistance in addition to the gravitational that must be accounted for (and is not).

The active element is contributed by surrounding muscles that may fire even though when the measurement is done subjects are required to relax completely. The passive element results from the stretch of ligaments, tendons and capsule. Therefore instead of a sinusoidal component, the resistance assumes a different pattern. An effective example is depicted in Wessel et al (1992) where testing of trunk flexor strength and the 'gravitational' component of the trunk were measured. Although the alternative solution – moving the tested segment *passively* through the ROM and subtracting the obtained resistance from the active strength in order to derive the *net* strength – partially solves the first difficulty (non-axial movement), it certainly suffers from the same problems regarding the passive/active components. As a result, isokinetic tests should have been done in the non-gravitational position. However this is not only non-functional in many instances but requires awkward subject positioning and special attachments.

Gravity correction is admittedly less of a problem in extremity testing since for deriving the percentage deficiency, the contralateral (uninvolved) segment serves as the basis for comparison. Unless indicated otherwise, the weight of symmetrical segments is considered equal. On the other hand, where no collateral segment exists, such as the case with the trunk, the poor accuracy of the commonly employed procedures for correcting this effect or abstaining from using it, has significant ramifications in terms of the correct clinical interpretation.

The agonist/antagonist strength ratio

Clearly failure to account for gravitation in calculating the net moment developed by tested muscles is particularly conspicuous in terms of agonist/antagonist moment (strength) ratio. This statement is generally valid in the case of those muscles which move the limbs in the frontal and sagittal planes but not in rotations.

Consider for instance the case of the strength ratio between the hip extensors and flexors, Ext/Flx, where Ext and Flx are the respective muscular moments. Let us assume that the weight of the limb exerts, at a certain point in the tested ROM, a moment of 20 Nm, and that each muscle exerts a maximal 'uncorrected' moment of 60 Nm at this point. (For a detailed discussion of units of measurement see Chapter 2.) Based on these 'uncorrected' values:

$$\frac{Ext}{Flx} = \frac{60}{60} = 1.0$$

If however the gravitational moment is added to the extensors and subtracted from the flexors the result is:

$$\frac{Ext}{Flx} = \frac{(60 + 20)}{(60 - 20)} = 2.0$$

This is a very significant difference which in the case of trunk flexor/extensor strength ratio may reach much higher values.

THE MOMENT–ANGULAR VELOCITY RELATIONSHIP IN DYNAMIC CONTRACTIONS

MUSCLE TENSION AND SPEED OF CONTRACTION

If the relationship between force and length (moment–angular position) is the most basic physiological parameter of skeletal muscle, the other basic parameter is the relationship between the force, or tension, developed within the muscle and its velocity or speed of contraction. Dynamic muscle performance may be measured by:

1. controlling the external load and measuring and/or calculating the resulting velocities and accelerations, or
2. controlling the velocity and measuring the force (moment) output.

The second approach, for which isokinetic dynamometers are particularly suitable, has been adopted for quantifying muscle performance since the late 1960s.

In discussing the tension–velocity of contraction relationship, findings based on isolated muscle preparations and those based on live subject experiments should be distinguished. In the latter instance, the term 'moment–angular velocity relationship' should be used.

Mathematical description

A formula which describes the force–velocity relationship has been proposed by Hill (1953):

$$(T + a)(v + b) = \frac{(T_0 + a)}{b}$$

where T is the tension, T_0 is the isometric tension, v is the speed of shortening, and a and b are constants, such that $v_{max} = bT_0/a$, where v_{max} is the speed of shortening with no load.

This equation may also be expressed in a normalized form, namely:

$$v' = (1 - T')\left(1 + \frac{T'}{k}\right)$$

where $v' = v/v_{max}$, $T' = T/T_0$, and $k = a/T_0 = b/v_{max}$.

Power output

The power output, P, available from the muscle is given by (McMahon 1984):

Power = Tension × speed of shortening

or

$$P = Tv$$

Using Hill's formula, this may be expressed as:

$$P = \frac{v(bT_0 - av)}{(v + b)}$$

Its maximal value is reached when the speed of shortening is 25–33% of v_{max}.

The above equations are depicted graphically in Figure 1.6 (McMahon 1984), which is based on $k = 0.25$. It should be noted that the force–velocity equation allows for active lengthening (where 'active' refers to a contractile state). In this case the rise in muscle tension as a function of the imposed active stretching velocity is dramatically steeper than in the corresponding case of shortening.

MUSCLE MOMENT AND ANGULAR VELOCITY

In studies based on live subjects the terms 'force' and (linear) 'velocity' are no longer appropriate. The former is replaced by the moment (also widely known by the term torque) whereas the latter is replaced by the angular velocity (ω) of the lever-arm which represents (but is not equal to) the angular velocity of the joint. It should also be emphasized that this statement is valid for angular motion testing which is also known by the erroneous term open kinetic chain (see below) but should not be applied to so-called closed kinetic chain testing. In addition, the terms shortening and (active) lengthening are replaced by 'concentric' and 'eccentric contractions' (see Box 1.1).

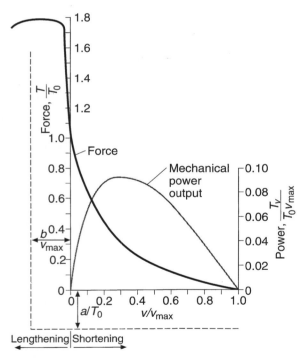

Figure 1.6 Hill's force–velocity curve. The shortening part of the curve was calculated with $k = 0.25$. The asymptotes for Hill's hyperbola (broken lines) are parallel to the T/T_0 and v/v_{max} axes. Near zero shortening velocity, the lengthening part of the curve has a negative slope approximately six times steeper than the shortening part. The externally delivered power was calculated from the product of tension and shortening velocity. (From McMahon T A Muscles, reflexes and locomotion. Copyright © 1984 by PUP. Reproduced by permission of Princeton University Press.)

Box 1.1   Concentric and eccentric contractions

- Concentric contraction occurs when active muscle undergoes shortening while overcoming external resistance
- Eccentric contraction occurs when active muscle undergoes lengthening while being overcome by an external resistance

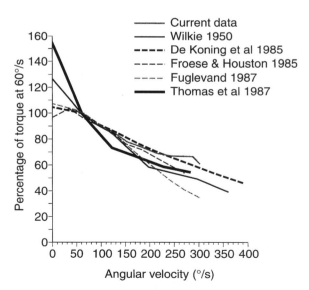

Figure 1.7 Gravity-corrected, normalized angle-specific moment–velocity relationships for arm flexion, ankle plantar flexion and knee extension. 'Moment' here is referred to as 'torque'. (From Taylor et al 1991 copyright © Springer-Verlag.)

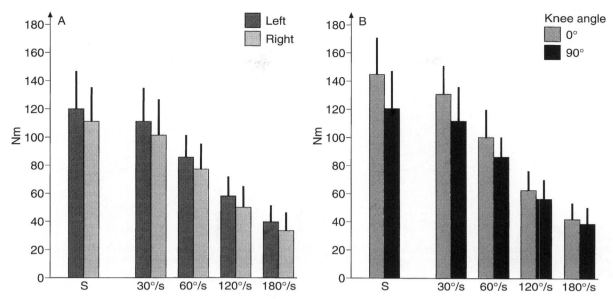

Figure 1.8 Moment–angular velocity relationship in ankle plantar flexion. (A) Right and left knees flexed at 90°. (B) Knee at either 90° or 0° flexion. (From Fugl-Meyer et al 1979.)

Applicability of in vitro muscle behavior

Studies based on isokinetic measurements of various muscle groups have indicated that the principles governing in vitro muscle behavior – namely the force–velocity relationships – are only partially reflected in their in vivo counterparts. There are some exceptions mainly with regard to concentric activity at very low velocities (Perrine & Edgerton 1978, Froese & Houston 1985) and in eccentric contractions (see below).

When the imposed test velocity is increased:

1. For concentric contractions, there is a decrease in the maximal moment developed by the muscle/muscle group (Figs 1.7–1.9). This inverse relationship is not confined to the case of a single joint. It is valid for two-joint muscles like the hamstring and, in a more global form, to multijoint systems such as the extensors of the trunk (Timm 1988).
2. For eccentric contractions, the maximal moment may rise initially but at higher velocities it remains stable or even decreases (Figs 1.10–1.14).

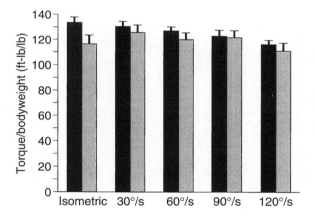

Figure 1.9 Isometric and multispeed isokinetic extensor moment/bodyweight ratios for 18–29 (dark bars) and 30–44 (light bars) year-old male subjects. (From Smith et al 1985.)

Additionally,

1. For the same velocity, the eccentric strength is greater than the concentric strength.
2. According to the principle proposed by Elftman (1966), the order of strength, dependent on contraction mode, is: eccentric > isometric > concentric. This order is

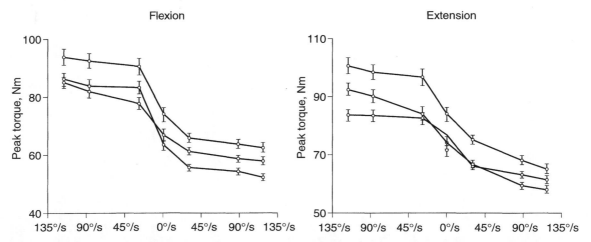

Figure 1.10   Moment–angular velocity curves for concentric and eccentric forearm flexion and extension. Moment is referred to as 'torque' and angular velocity is in radians/second. (From Hortobágyi & Katch 1990 copyright © Springer-Verlag.)

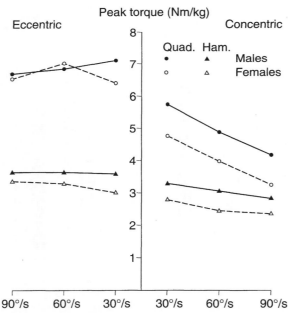

Figure 1.11   Bodyweight-normalized moment–angular velocity curves for concentric and eccentric contractions of the quadriceps (circles) and hamstring (triangles) in males (solid symbols) and females (open symbols). (From Colliander & Tesch 1989 copyright © Springer-Verlag.)

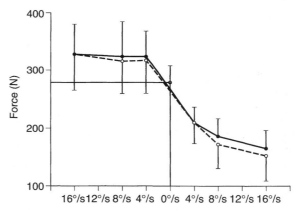

Figure 1.12   The in vivo force–velocity (F–ω) curve of isokinetic grip. On the X axis 4, 8 and 16 refer to the angular velocity of the lever-arm when the fingers are concentrically flexing (dynamic grip) whereas the parallel negative values correspond to the forced extension of the fingers, i.e. the eccentric component. (After Dvir 1997b.)

The moment during eccentric contractions

The behavior of the eccentric branch of the moment–angular velocity (M–ω) curve deviates from both the theoretical model and the in vitro findings. It is characterized by the leveling off of the curve which takes place even at relatively low velocities. This finding has been confirmed in a number of studies including those of the elbow

graphically depicted in Figure 1.12 with respect to grip strength (Dvir 1997b). (See Table 11.9 for peak and average force values of grip strength from this study.)

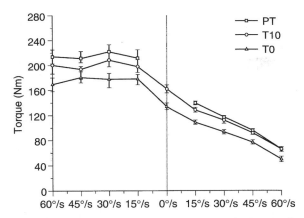

Figure 1.13 Moment–angular velocity curves for concentric and eccentric trunk lateral flexion. PT, peak torque; T10, torque at 10°; T0, 0° lateral flexion. (From Huang & Thorstensson 2000.)

(Griffin 1987, Hortobágyi & Katch 1990), the shoulder (Shklar & Dvir 1995), the knee (Rizzardo et al 1988, Colliander & Tesch 1989, Ghena et al 1991) and the trunk (Dvir & Keating 2001, 2003).

The explanation for this phenomenon which probably has the widest acceptance posits a negative feedback loop which involves peripheral and spinal regulation in order to avoid excessive stresses on the muscle itself (Stauber 1989). According to this explanation the central nervous system monitors total tension over the time concerned (the tension–time integral, or impulse), and limits the eccentric potential of the muscle which could exceed the isometric strength by about 100% (Edman et al 1979). Indeed, when this loop fails to operate properly, as might occur in sudden

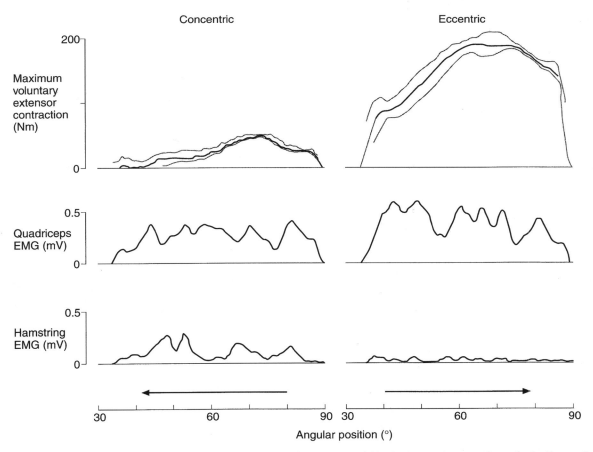

Figure 1.14 Abnormal eccentric/concentric strength ratio (test velocity, 180°/s) in the knee extensors of a patient with spastic paraparesis. (From Knutsson 1987.)

and vigorous stretching of an active muscle, tear of the musculotendinous unit could result. A typical example is the rupture of the Achilles tendon during an unexpected forward fall.

THE ECCENTRIC TO CONCENTRIC (E/C) STRENGTH RATIO

The E/C ratio occupies an important niche in isokinetic studies. Commonly this ratio has been defined with respect to the same velocity (e.g. E/C at 30 or 120°/s). The 'strength' to which this ratio refers may be either the peak moment (PM) or the average moment (AM). Since under normal conditions and maximal performance the eccentric strength is invariably greater than the respective concentric strength, the resulting ratio should be greater than 1. This general principle has been challenged in only a single study (Trudelle-Jackson et al 1989) with respect to the low end of the velocity spectrum, claiming that 35–54% of normal subjects had an E/C ratio of less than 0.85. On the other hand, in a large number of papers this proposition has been shown to be valid, sometimes even in the presence of a pathology (Conway et al 1992). Additionally considering the M–ω curve, the E/C ratio should increase proportionately with the test velocity. Current knowledge regarding the range of this ratio refers mostly to the low–medium sector of the velocity spectrum. Table 1.2 shows the consistent findings for the E/C ratio in normal individuals. Some exceptions have been noted, with a general tendency towards higher values, but the upper limit has remained by and large at 2.0.

These typical figures of the E/C ratio may not necessarily be confined to single joint instances. Muscle performance in concentric and eccentric simultaneous extension of the hip and knee (legpress) has been studied with a particular focus on variations of the ratio (Dvir 1996). Measurement was performed in the supine position with the hip and knee initially at 100° and the foot supported by a special attachment. The lever-arm moved through an arc of about 30°. The return movement of the lever-arm to the initial position was resisted eccentrically. The overall ratios between the forces exerted against the foot attachment were 1.56 and 1.68 for the velocities of 8 and 15°/s respectively. Although these values are relatively high for such very low velocities, it should first be borne in mind that force rather than moment was measured as the latter is largely irrelevant in terms of individual joint–muscle configurations.

Pathological increases in the E/C ratio

Deviations from the above range, related to pathological conditions have been reported. A particularly low E/C (less than 0.85) was proposed as a potential source in patellofemoral problems by Bennett & Stauber (1986). This proposition, which was based on 'an error in the neuromotor control' of the quadriceps, is discussed at length in Chapter 6. An alternative explanation proposes

Table 1.2 The range of the maximal eccentric moment/maximal concentric moment (E/C) ratio

Joint	E/C range	Angular velocity range (degrees/sec)	Author(s)
Knee	1.1–1.5	45–180	Kramer & McDermid 1989 (based on data in the text)
	1.3–1.7	60–180	Rizzardo et al 1988
	1.2–1.6	30–150	Colliander & Tesch 1989
Elbow	1.1–1.3	30–120	Griffin 1987
	1.4–1.7	30–120	Hortobágyi & Katch 1990
Shoulder (all six common motions tested independently)			Shklar & Dvir 1995
Minimal (internal rotation)	1.1–1.2	60–180	
Maximal (adduction)	1.2–1.7	60–180	

a selective inhibition of eccentric performance due to pain. This theory relies on the high stresses produced during eccentric contractions as well as the opposite motion of the patella (see also Chapter 6). On the other hand, exceedingly high values were reported based on performance of chronic low-back dysfunction patients (Shirado et al 1995). In this case a plausible explanation lies in intentionally limiting the concentric strength output due to either apprehension or 'cultural factors' (Shirado et al 1995).

Other examples of rather extreme values of the E/C ratio may be found in cases of spastic paresis and β-thalassemia major. The previous pathology is neurophysiologically mediated. Quadriceps performance has been studied in patients suffering from spastic paresis. In these patients, eccentric contractions are not supposed to trigger antagonistic spastic responses, since the resulting motion works to relax the antagonists rather than stretch them. Furthermore, there is probably an increased output from the primary endings of the spindles in the agonist (Knutsson 1987).

Figure 1.14 depicts the concentric and eccentric strength curves of the quadriceps in a patient with spastic paresis. There is a very sharp decrease in the concentric strength (the paresis) to about 10% of normal (for the appropriate gender and age). On the other hand, the eccentric strength is within the normal range. The E/C ratio is therefore strikingly high: between 4 and 5.

The phenomenon of a sharp increase in the E/C ratio has also been demonstrated in another clinical group, where there may be no neurological involvement. Patients suffering from β-thalassemia major (a severe form of hereditary anemia which leads, among other complications, to scarring and degeneration of muscle tissue) have been tested using concentric and eccentric exertions of the quadriceps. These patients who have an acute concentric strength deficiency retain an eccentric strength which, although not on a par with the norm, leads to a ratio which is far in excess of the normal (Fig. 1.15). The excessive connective tissue component may be the reason for this phenomenon.

THE DYNAMIC CONTROL RATIO

Although the E/C ratio has traditionally been used as an internal muscle performance parameter (i.e. within the same muscle or muscle group) information is accumulating indicating that it may be equally applicable in describing inter-muscle relationships. Specifically dividing the eccentric moment of the antagonist by the concentric moment of the agonist results in what has been termed the dynamic control ratio (DCR; Dvir et al 1989). Aagaard et al (1998) have suggested that this ratio be termed 'functional' as opposed to the conventional (concentric/concentric) ratio. The DCR is of particular significance in those

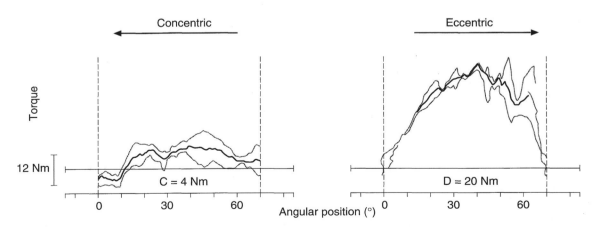

Figure 1.15 Abnormal eccentric/concentric strength ratio (test velocity, 30°/s) in a patient with β-thalassemia major. C and D are the average moment (in Nm).

situations where the agonist and antagonist are working simultaneously to avert potential jeopardy to the joint. Such instances are typical in joints like the knee (Dvir et al 1989) and shoulder (Bak & Magnusson 1997) where either forceful activities or inherent instability characterizes the joint. Consider for instance the shoulder in fast adduction and internal rotation. Such an activity may be brought about by the concentric agonistic activity of the pectoralis major coupled with that of subscapularis (Glousman et al 1988). Unless the external rotators are acting simultaneously to restrain the forward moving humeral head, there is a tangible likelihood for anterior subluxation. Since the agonists ultimately overcome the antagonists the latter are undergoing elongation meaning that they contract eccentrically. Obviously the active DCR – namely the moment relationships between the agonist and antagonist during the actual execution of the movement – cannot exceed 1 otherwise motion will not proceed. On the other hand the isokinetic DCR depends on the relative strength of the agonist and antagonist.

Dynamic versus static bilateral differences

Measurement findings of muscle performance (strength and/or other mechanical parameters) may be expressed in absolute or relative terms, the latter being commonly employed when unilateral compromise is evident. Specifically, assuming that dominance has a negligible effect on gross muscle performance, the mechanical parameter of choice, invariably strength, is compared between the involved and uninvolved side and the deficiency is expressed as a percentage using the following formula:

$$\% \text{ deficiency} = \frac{100(SU - SI)}{SU}$$

where SU and SI stand for the strength of the uninvolved and the contralateral involved muscle(s). One of the major questions facing clinicians which even today remains elusive, although not unchallenged, relates to the mode of contraction that should serve for calculating the deficiency.

Traditionally the isometric mode has served as the criterion not only in the context of the MMT technique but also as the definitive criterion in hand impairment. The reason for the latter's role is the availability of a simple and accurate instrument – the Jamar hand dynamometer – which effectively accommodates the major gross function of hand musculature: static grip. However, other than the hand whose special morphological and functional characteristics enable such measurement, all other major muscle groups necessitate a different measurement approach which is effectively provided by isokinetic dynamometry. But in spite of their widespread use, no large scale isokinetic study involving diverse pathologies has provided a clear-cut answer to the question whether unilateral deficiency was singularly represented by each of the three contraction types. In other words, if a muscular deficiency exists, is it likely to be greater using isometric, concentric or eccentric representation?

This question concerns intermodal comparison: static (isometric) versus dynamic (isokinetic) based deficiencies as well as intramodal: concentric versus eccentric based deficiency. At the very core of these comparisons lies the question: is strength a unitary construct or is it mode and condition dependent? It should also be emphasized that even if a definitive answer to the above question was available, the more relevant question regarding the relationship between the specific strength deficit (isometric, concentric or eccentric) and the resulting reduction in function would still be left unanswered.

Intermodal comparison

Concerning first the intermodal issue, the evidence points to a higher strength deficit when calculations are based on the isokinetic compared to the isometric method. In a study relating to quadriceps function in women suffering from gonarthrosis, the reduction in strength relative to a matched control group was 15% using isometric measurement and 40% using the isokinetic method (Madsen et al 1995). Besides mentioning the acceptable reliability of isokinetic knee strength tests, it was also suggested that compared to isometric strength, the level of isokinetic strength was a better predictor of pain and pain disability. This conclusion is a significant factor in deciding which type of strength reduction should serve as the criterion. In another study, Carter et al (1995) tested patients suffering from hereditary motor and sensory neuropathy types I and II and compared their muscular performance to gender and age matched control groups. Findings indicated that the reduction in strength based on isometric measurement was similar to that derived from isokinetic measurements amounting to approximately 30% when averaged across different muscle groups. Findings based on a study of patients with unilateral limb injury indicate that isometric strength of the quadriceps was very slightly lower than either concentric or eccentric strength (Holder-Powell & Rutherford 1999).

Intramodal comparison

Regarding the intramodal comparison, in the same study by Carter et al (1995) it was indicated that eccentric reductions were invariably smaller than concentric reductions. Likewise in the study of Holder-Powell & Rutherford (1999) no discernible bilateral differences were recorded between the concentric and eccentric strength scores. Yet unpublished results of a large group of patients presenting with unilateral isokinetic strength deficiency in the knee, shoulder, ankle and hand (grip) seem however to reveal a higher deficiency rate in concentric compared to eccentric contractions (Dvir 2003). This variation has been attributed to the more limited control of muscle tension production. Consequently, it is possible that the commonly employed practice of expressing deficiency by mainly referring to the concentric modality will have to change so as to include the eccentric component. Moreover, given the central functional role of eccentric contractions, an average concentric–eccentric score will probably be more appropriate.

Controlling eccentric contractions

Perhaps the most significant contribution of isokinetic dynamometry to the study of muscle performance, besides making accurate measurement of concentric activity possible, was the introduction and incorporation of the means for the performance and measurement of eccentric contractions. The in vivo parameters of truly eccentric exertions – namely those that cannot be arrested volitionally, for example the ability to stop forward bending, an eccentric activity of the trunk extensors – was largely neglected until the advent of the first active dynamometers at the mid-1980s. The study of eccentric exertions was pursued by several disciplines, among them neurophysiology. One of the most fascinating issues studied using neurophysiological techniques relates to the question as to whether the nervous system issues a specific command for an eccentric contraction. In his excellent review Enoka (1996) offers the following hints that lead to a positive answer to this question:

1. It was indicated that normal subjects could not achieve a level of even 90% of the maximal eccentric voluntary contraction compared with a level of 100% which was obtained using electrical stimulation (Westing et al 1990).

2. When subjects expected to produce a concentric contraction but were forced eccentrically, the EMG excitation increased significantly indicating that the intended mode of contraction was centrally modulated (Grabiner et al 1995).

3. The age-related decline in strength is less conspicuous in eccentric contractions, a phenomenon that was related to neural adaptation (Hortobágyi et al 1995).

4. The reduced EMG excitation seen in maximal eccentric contraction is probably related to the activation of a subset of the neuronal pool rather than homogenous reduction across the population (Laidlaw et al 1994).

5. Recruitment order of motor units is altered during eccentric, compared to concentric, contractions (Nardone et al 1989) and is probably mediated by descending signals from the brain (Tax et al 1990).

6. Fatigue studies have indicated that eccentric performance was substantially different from concentric performance, i.e. the decline in mechanical

output was minimal in the former (Tesch et al 1990). It was also indicated that the fatigue curve resulting from eccentric contractions undertook a different shape from that which resulted from concentric contractions (Binder-Macleod & Lee 1996).

7. In addition to the above, whereas feigned muscle weakness as expressed by concentric strength output is highly adjustable, the ability to modulate feigned eccentric output is seriously limited (see Chapter 5). This phenomenon is highly indicative of central involvement in modulating eccentric strength.

Put together, these findings support the existence of a unique neural activation strategy. The implications of such a mechanism are far reaching in terms of defining what exactly strength is, in interpreting strength test findings and in considering optimal approaches for its restitution following trauma or pathology.

THE MOMENT–ANGULAR VELOCITY RELATIONSHIP IN PASSIVE MOTION

Passive stretching in healthy individuals

When a limb segment of a healthy individual is moved passively in such a way that a gravitational component acts on the segment, the resisting moment may be attributed to the force of gravity, and also to the viscoelastic characteristics of the muscle and its associated connective tissues. However, since the second element starts to exert an appreciable force only after the resting length has been reached, a position well into the far ROM of the joint, it is unlikely to play a decisive role in mediating the moment.

Another factor is the reflex contraction in some muscles which normally move the segment in the opposite direction ('antagonist activation'). This phenomenon seldom occurs in normal subjects, and then only when passive motion is performed at the highest velocities (Thilmann et al 1991).

Restraint of antagonist activation

Indeed, one characteristic of a well coordinated neuromuscular system is its ability to perform smoothly even in extremely high velocities, by virtue of restraining antagonist activation. For instance in a highly trained baseball pitcher, concentric contraction of the glenohumeral depressors may proceed from late cocking to acceleration (Glousman et al 1988) at maximal force, resulting in arm angular velocities in the order of thousands of degrees per second without provoking appreciable antagonist activity. (*Cocking* means the pull back of the arm before its forceful forward movement, a concept based on the action of the cock of a gun.)

One of the reasons an untrained athlete, with equivalent dynamic performance of the former muscles, may find it difficult to generate the same arm angular velocity, is the reciprocal activation of the latter muscles. This 'deactivation' of antagonists is acquired following intensive specific training.

SPASTICITY AND PARESIS
Antagonist activity

Without elaborating on the complex mechanisms which underlie the phenomenon of spasticity, antagonist muscle performance is clearly impaired in some patients with neurological involvement. It is most conspicuous in those presenting with spastic paresis following a lesion in the central nervous system. Spasticity is described as 'a motor disorder characterized by a velocity-dependent increase in tonic stretch reflexes (muscle tone) with exaggerated tendon jerks, resulting from hyperexcitability of the stretch reflex, as one component of the upper motor neuron syndrome' (Lance 1980).

The component of paresis or weakness is evident in the voluntary, as well as in the automatic or semiautomatic, movements of daily living such as walking (Knutsson 1987). One source for this weakness may be the spastic restraint exerted by the antagonist activity mentioned earlier. In such a case, agonist performance may be intact but the countermoment may result in an overall reduction in strength.

Evaluation using isokinetic dynamometers

The exact evaluation of spasticity and paresis is essential for the determination of the patient's clinical and disability status. Common methods are based on clinical scales (manual), and electro-physiological and mechanical instruments (Katz & Rymer 1989). In the latter, the role of isokinetic dynamometers is unique. These instruments are also capable of passively moving a limb segment at a predetermined velocity and consequently enable a systematic measurement of involuntary muscular resistance. Indeed, this was one of the first applications of the KinCom system, which was the prototype of active systems.

Although the velocity dependence of spasticity has been challenged (Katz & Rymer 1989), the ability of these dynamometers to accurately measure the 'spastic resistance' with regard to the angular position in the total available ROM, render them an important tool in this field.

Demonstration of abnormal antagonist activity

Active isokinetic systems have been used in the pioneering studies of Knutsson and his colleagues, at the Karolinska Institute in Sweden, to demonstrate the effect of abnormal antagonist activity (Knutsson & Martensson 1980, Knutsson 1987). Figure 1.16 depicts the flexor strength curve during a voluntary contraction of the hamstring in a patient with spastic paresis. The sharp decrease in the moment at 120°/s was associated with greatly increased electromyographic activity in the quadriceps. Activity of this magnitude does not occur in normal subjects at such a relatively low velocity. In the opposite motion, the

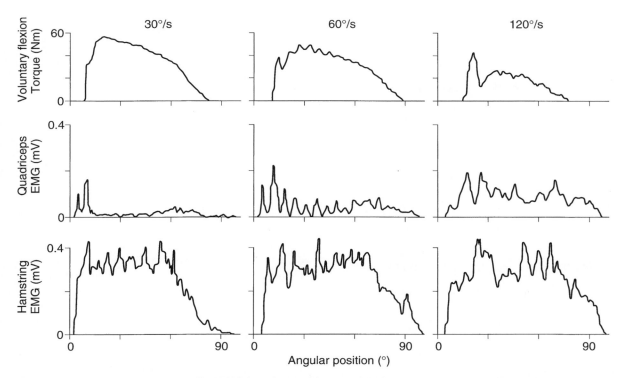

Figure 1.16 Strength curves and rectified EMG from the quadriceps and the hamstring in a patient with spastic paraparesis at angular velocities of 30, 60 and 120°/s. (From Knutsson 1987.)

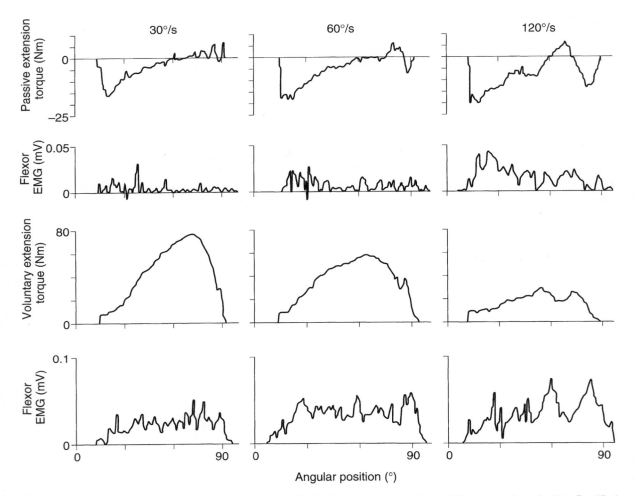

Figure 1.17   Passive extension and strength curves in isokinetic knee extensions at three different angular velocities. Rectified EMG traces from knee flexors stretched during extensions. (From Knutsson 1987.)

hamstrings are activated both in passive and active extension of the knee (Fig. 1.17).

Variability of spasticity measurement

Though the application of isokinetic dynamometers to measuring spasticity is obvious, studies using them have generally confirmed the agreement that this condition is highly variable among, and often within subjects (Knutsson 1987, Dvir & Panturin 1993). Moreover, although spastic restraint may be clinically felt by the examiner, isokinetic measurements have failed

to corroborate this impression in one group of paraplegic patients (Zelig 1992).

Whether this finding reflects a different source of spasticity, i.e. predominantly from a spinal or a higher CNS lesion, or a residual drug effect even after wash-out, or an improper test velocity range, is at present difficult to determine. For instance, Thilmann et al (1991) have suggested that in moderately involved patients, the critical velocity required to elicit enhanced stretch reflex was around $100°/s$. Nevertheless, in some of our patients, a velocity of even $180°/s$ was not sufficient to elicit the expected response.

TYPES OF TESTING

MULTIJOINT MOTION

The design of almost all commercially available isokinetic dynamometers is based on *angular motion (AM)* of the lever-arm. Since the force sensor is attached (in most systems) to the lever-arm, this means that the measured forces are exerted in a substantially *perpendicular* fashion to the moving segment. This configuration is particularly suitable for assessing 'hinge' movements, whose typical example is the knee. Thus when the shank moves against the lever-arm, either concentrically or eccentrically, the counterforce exerted by the motor operates approximately at a right angle to the tibia. This principle is generally valid for all AM testing and thus constitutes the bulk of isokinetic practice. It is also the case that the number of muscles involved in executing such motion is normally minimal.

However function-oriented motion rarely involves a single joint. Rather it normally consists of several joints moving in concert. Not only may such a motion not necessarily be planar, it invariably involves a well coordinated activity pattern of a larger number of muscles compared to the abovementioned 'hinge' type activity. Moreover, although the total moment output may be isokinetically measurable, the individual contributions of the muscle groups responsible for executing the motion cannot for the larger part be experimentally determined, or at least not in the way possible for planar, single-joint motion.

The analysis and practical use of multijoint motion are of considerable interest in rehabilitation, because of the growing awareness of the need to integrate motions and emphasize the whole rather than the part. Isokinetic dynamometers can play an important role in this respect but the advantages and limitations must be clearly stated. For this purpose it is necessary to redefine and describe the concepts of 'closed' and 'open' kinetic chains. Although both are well established in the physical rehabilitation literature, it seems that this use has been impaired by some basic misunderstanding.

Open kinetic chain (OKC)   This is defined as a sequence of articulated segments: the 'tail' of the nth segment is connected to the $(n - 1)$th and its 'head' is connected to the $(n + 1)$th segment. The first segment is commonly regarded as stationary, and is called the 'frame' whereas the end segment is free to move. A classical example for an OKC is the upper limb, where the frame is the ribcage and the distal link is the hand.

Closed kinetic chain (CKC)   This is an arrangement of sequentially articulated segments in which the distal segment and the frame are also articulated, thus closing the otherwise open chain. While the motion of the end segment in a true OKC is not constrained, any segment in a CKC may be considered 'end' or 'tail'. Thus OKC and CKC are frequently described as distal-end-free or distal-end-fixed (or in fact distal-end-bound) respectively. An example of a CKC is the configuration of the whole body in a hand-assisted rise from a seat. As long as the hands grip the forearm rests, the chain consists of the 'articulation' between the floor and the feet, the other body articulations leading to the hands, and back to the floor via the chair.

OKC or CKC?

The human body presents an intricate array of OKCs and CKCs. For instance although bringing the hand to a specific location may be an OKC activity, a function such as pinching an object, performed by two fingers, is typically characterized as a CKC activity. The swing phase of gait finds the foot of the swinging leg in an OKC state but once ground contact is established (double support) a CKC is formed. Likewise, during stair climbing or descending, the 'swing' phase (namely transferring the lower extremity from one step to the next) finds the thigh, leg and foot freely moving in space, and therefore motion is taking place in an OKC mode. However, as soon as contact is made with the step, and before the contralateral extremity disengages from the step, i.e. during the weight acceptance phase, motion of all joints becomes interdependent as both feet are 'connected' to the step which constitutes a common segment in this CKC. The same reasoning applies in seat rise, bicycle pedalling, lifting of objects, etc.

Thus, when the distal segment is constrained to move in a certain fashion (and so are the other segments) the system behaves like a CKC, while when the distal segment is unconstrained the movement is characteristic of OKC. It is therefore the temporary set-up of the joints/segments rather than their anatomical articulations that decides whether the configuration is OKC or CKC.

Angular versus linear motion testing

Common isokinetic testing is erroneously understood to be conducted in a true OKC mode. In, for instance, the measurement of internal–external rotation of the shoulder, assuming that the forearm–hand complex is 'free' to move ignores their firm harnessing to the lever-arm, which in turn is part of the dynamometer. Since the trunk is also stabilized, the configuration is a CKC rather than an OKC. However, it should be borne in mind that the vector of counterforce operating against the forearm is directed *perpendicular* to the forearm.

What is commonly perceived as isokinetic CKC testing is based on the use of dynamometers like the Liftask. The subject is asked to exert effort while using a number of joints where the resulting motion of the end-segment pattern is substantially linear rather than angular. For instance, in performing an isokinetic leg-press, an activity which involves simultaneous extension of the knee and hip (and a likely plantarflexor component) the foot typically undergoes linear motion away from the pelvis. In this case the vector of the counterforce is directed across the foot and therefore in a substantially *non-perpendicular* fashion relative to the shank. *Thus linear motion (LM) of the end segment is associated with non-perpendicular forces much as angular motion of the end segment is associated with perpendicular forces.* Therefore the true flavor of the so-called CKC testing actually relates to the direction of the major force component throughout the movement.

To put these nuances in full perspective consider another instance where AM ('OKC') and LM ('CKC') testing are employed in the same territory: the trunk. In the AM set-up, there is ostensibly a single joint about which the trunk rotates when performing flexion or extension. The counterforce is assumed to operate at a right angle to the 'rigid' trunk and therefore the moment developed by the extensor apparatus is equal to the force recorded by the force sensor multiplied by the distance to the mechanical axis. In the LM configuration the measurement portrays mainly the combined strength of the trunk and knee extensors. Clearly the counterforce does not form a right angle with either the thigh or trunk segments. Consequently the recorded strength is a global (multijoint) rather than a local ('single' joint) measure.

Physiological demands

Compared to AM configuration which rarely simulates physiological demands, testing and conditioning using multijoint (LM) set-ups has increasingly attracted the attention of practitioners. The advantage of using this approach has been particularly highlighted in relation to anterior cruciate ligament (ACL) surgery and rehabilitation (Shelbourne & Nitz 1990). In this case full activation of the quadriceps need not result in considerable tibiofemoral shear forces. Rather, due to coactivation of the hamstring (posterior shear) and larger compressive forces, the strain of the reconstructed ACL is kept at a lower level.

MULTIJOINT PERFORMANCE AND ISOKINETIC TESTING
Limitations

The measurements of muscle performance in LM mode using AM dynamometers is not as straightforward as it is in the single-joint-testing mode. This is because the lever-arm turns about a fixed axis whereas motion is simultaneously taking place in a number of joints. To simulate a linear motion of the force pad when the lever-arm moves radially, the preferred solution is both to remove the pad as far away as possible from the motor's axis while maintaining a particularly short ROM of the lever-arm. For instance if the ROM is 10°

and the force pad is located about 45 cm away from the axis, the arc of motion drawn by the force pad is substantially linear. The measured strength may then be expressed by force (N) rather than moment (Nm) units since the only true axis is that of the motor rather than the biological (Dvir 1996).

It should also be borne in mind that in those dynamometers where the force transducer is attached to the lever-arm it is sensitive to stresses acting at a right angle to the lever-arm. Thus if the multijoint activity is one of leg-press, and assuming a fixed neutral ankle joint position, there is only one angular position in the test ROM at which the recorded force reliably represents the combined moments generated by the acting muscles. Therefore, reference to moment values recorded elsewhere in the test ROM is irrelevant. This, incidentally, does not deny acceptable reproducibility for this test (Levine et al 1991).

JOINT LOADING DURING DYNAMIC EXERTIONS

It is one of the basic tenets of isokinetics that the muscular force level generated during a maximal contraction isokinetic test performed in an 'OKC' (single-joint-testing) mode is the maximum possible. This, apart from the rate at which the joint moves, is basically what distinguishes isokinetic from the so-called isotonic or isoinertial contractions.

Even in the absence of any external load, i.e. during pure antigravity motions, the force generated by muscle is much larger than the weight (which is also a force) of the relevant segment(s). This situation is due to the conspicuous mechanical disadvantage of muscles which derives from their comparatively very short levers. For example if the weight of the upper limb is 60 N (9.81 N = 1 kgf), the deltoid force needed to maintain the limb in 90° elevation could reasonably exceed 600 N. Ultimately, only a relatively small percentage of the muscle force is used to counteract the external load, the rest is transmitted through the joint articular surfaces or taken up by anatomical structures such as the ligaments and capsule.

Magnitude of forces in isokinetic exercise

Obviously when loads are to be moved, supported or resisted, the muscular forces increase both in proportion to the magnitude of the load and its distance from the instantaneous joint axis. Hence, it is expected that exertions under isokinetic conditions will result in considerable joint forces.

It should be emphasized that these forces are not necessarily the largest that a particular joint may be called on to support. These may occur in the course of strong impact loading, due to force absorption in the course of landing, or during simultaneous contraction of antagonistic muscles.

Also if different models are used for prediction of joint forces, significantly different results may be obtained. Nevertheless, those models which have been applied in the case of the knee, give an idea of the magnitude of the relevant forces. Kaufman et al (1991) have used a complex isokinetic set-up in order to study the tibiofemoral and patellofemoral forces that act on the knee during maximal isokinetic exercise. Their findings indicated that the average tibiofemoral force was four times bodyweight (4 bw), approximately equal to that obtained during walking except that it was reached at a different, and much higher, knee angle. The anterior and posterior shear forces (resisting the anterior and posterior drawer forces respectively) were on average 0.3 and 1.7 bw. The anterior shear force was larger than what would be expected during walking, whereas the posterior shear force was much larger than in walking but on a par with the posterior shear in stair climbing.

Very high patellofemoral forces, reaching 5.1 bw at 60°/s, were calculated as acting during isokinetic exercise. This force should be compared with only 0.5 bw during walking and 3.3 bw in ascending or descending stairs, but 7.6 bw in squat descent (Dahlqvist et al 1987) or 20 bw during jumping (Smith 1975).

Nisell and colleagues (1989, 1992) have used other models in their analysis of the knee joint and have obtained much higher forces: 9 bw and 12 bw in the tibiofemoral and patellofemoral joints respectively.

Implications of high isokinetic forces

Notwithstanding the large differences in the above findings, it is clear that *maximal* isokinetic exertions may result in considerable knee joint forces. The significance of such high forces hardly needs further elaboration especially where pain, articular surface derangement or recent surgical intervention are involved.

Though analogous forces have not so far been calculated for other joint systems, it would not be unreasonable to assume that equivalent conditions prevail. An indication of this may be found, for example, with the shoulder, where maximal isokinetic exertions are not tolerated in many patients who suffer from some joint dysfunction. Thus although isokinetically related joint forces may not be comparable to those obtained during specific athletic activities, their magnitude must be allowed for in the planning of testing and muscle conditioning of normal subjects and especially patients.

REFERENCES

Aagaard P, Simonsen E B, Magnusson S P, Larsson B, Dyhre-Poulsen P 1998 A new concept for isokinetic hamstring: quadriceps muscle strength ratio. American Journal of Sports Medicine 26: 231–237

Bak K, Magnusson P 1997 Shoulder strength and range of notion in symptomatic and pain-free elite swimmers. American Journal of Sports Medicine 25: 454–459

Bennett G, Stauber W T 1986 Evaluation and treatment of anterior knee pain using eccentric exercise. Medicine and Science in Sports and Exercise 18: 526–530

Binder-Macleod S A, Lee S C 1996 Catchlike property of human muscle during isovelocity movements. Journal of Applied Physiology 80: 2051–2059

Bygott I L, McMeeken J, Carroll S 2001a Gravity correction in trunk dynamometry: is it reliable? Isokinetics and Exercise Science 9: 1–9

Bygott I L, McMeeken J, Carroll S, Story I 2001b A preliminary analysis of the gravity correction procedures applied in trunk dynamometry. Isokinetics and Exercise Science 9: 53–64

Carter G T, Abresch R T, Fowler W M et al 1995 Profiles of neuromuscular diseases: hereditary motor and sensory neuropathy types I and II. American Journal of Physical Medicine and Rehabilitation 74(suppl 1): 40–149

Colliander E B, Tesch P 1989 Bilateral eccentric and concentric torque of quadriceps and hamstring muscles in females and males. European Journal of Applied Physiology 59: 227–232

Conway A, Malone T R, Conway P 1992 Patellar alignment/tracking: effect on force output and perceived pain. Isokinetics and Exercise Science 2: 9–17

Dahlqvist N J, Mayo P, Seedhom B B 1987 Forces during squatting and rising from a deep squat. Engineering in Medicine 11: 69–76

De Koning F L, Blinkhorst R A, Vos J A, van't Hof M A 1985 The force velocity relationship of arm flexion in untrained males and females and arm-trained athletes. European Journal of Applied Physiology 54: 89–94

Dvir Z 1996 An isokinetic study of combined activity of hip and knee extensors. Clinical Biomechanics 11: 135–138

Dvir Z 1997a Grade 4 in manual muscle testing: the problem with submaximal strength assessment. Clinical Rehabilitation 11: 36–41

Dvir Z 1997b The measurement of isokinetic fingers flexion strength. Clinical Biomechanics 12: 472–481

Dvir Z 2003 Concentric vs. eccentric strength deficiencies. An isokinetic study of patients with chronic knee, shoulder, ankle, hand and trunk compromise. Submitted.

Dvir Z, Keating J 2001 The reproducibility of isokinetic trunk extension: a study using very short range of motion. Clinical Biomechanics 16: 627–630

Dvir Z, Keating J 2003 Trunk extension strength and validation of trunk extension effort in chronic low-back dysfunction patients. Spine 28: 685–692

Dvir Z, Panturin E 1993 Measurement of spasticity and associated reactions in stroke patients before and after physiotherapeutic intervention. Clinical Rehabilitation 7: 15–21

Dvir Z, Eger G, Halperin N, Shklar A 1989 Thigh muscles activity and anterior cruciate ligament insufficiency. Clinical Biomechanics 4: 87–91

Edman K A, Elizinga G, Noble M I 1979 The effect of stretch on contracting skeletal muscle fibers. In: Sugi H, Pollack G H (eds) Cross bridge mechanism in muscle contraction. University Park Press, Baltimore, pp 297–309

Elftman H 1966 Biomechanics of muscle. Journal of Bone and Joint Surgery 48A: 363–373

Enoka R M 1996 Eccentric contractions require unique activation strategies by the nervous system. Journal of Applied Physiology 81: 2339–2346

Froese E A, Houston M E 1985 Torque–velocity characteristics and muscle fiber type in human vastus lateralis. Journal of Applied Physiology 59: 309–314

Fuglevand A J 1987 Resultant muscle torque, angular velocity and joint angle relationships and activation patterns in maximal knee extension. In: Johnsson B (ed) Biomechanics X-A. International series on biomechanics. Human Kinetics, Champaign, Illinois, pp 559–565

Fugl-Meyer A R, Sjostrom M, Wahlby L 1979 Human plantar flexion strength and structure. Acta Physiologica Scandinavica 107: 47–56

Ghena D G, Kurth A L, Thomas M, Mayhew J 1991 Torque characteristics of the quadriceps and hamstring muscles during concentric and eccentric loading. Journal of Orthopaedic and Sports Physical Therapy 14: 149–154

Glousman R E, Jobe F W, Tibone J E et al 1988 Dynamic electromyographic analysis of the throwing shoulder with glenohumeral instability. Journal of Bone and Joint Surgery 70A: 220–226

Gordon A M, Huxley A F, Julian F T 1966 The variations in isometric tension with sarcomere length in vertebrate muscle fibers. Journal of Physiology 1984: 170–192

Grabiner M D, Owings T M, George M R, Enoka R M 1995 Eccentric contractions are specified a-priori by the CNS. Proceedings of the 15th Congress of the International Society of Biomechanics, Jyväskylä, Finland, pp 338–339

Griffin J W 1987 Differences in elbow flexion torque measured concentrically, eccentrically and isometrically. Physical Therapy 67: 1205–1208

Herzog W, Hasler E, Abrahamse S 1991 A comparison of knee extensor strength curves obtained theoretically and experimentally. Medicine and Science in Sports and Exercise 23: 108–114

Hill A V 1953 The mechanics of active muscle. Proceedings of the Royal Society 141B: 104–117

Holder-Powell H M, Rutherford O M 1999 Unilateral lower limb injury: its long-term effects on quadriceps, hamstring and plantarflexor muscle strength. Archives of Physical and Medical Rehabilitation 80: 717–720

Hortobágyi T, Katch F I 1990 Eccentric and concentric torque–velocity relationships during arm flexion and extension. European Journal of Applied Physiology 60: 395–401

Hortobágyi T, Zheng D, Weidner M et al 1995 The influence of aging on muscle strength and muscle fiber characteristics with special reference to eccentric strength. Journal of Gerontology 50: B399–B406

Huang Q-M, Thorstensson A 2000 Trunk muscle strength in eccentric and concentric lateral flexion. European Journal of Applied Physiology 83: 573–577

Kandel E R, Schwartz J H, Jessell T M 1991 Principles of neural science, 3rd edn. Elsevier, New York

Katz R T, Rymer Z 1989 Spastic hypertonia: mechanisms and measurement. Archives of Physical Medicine and Rehabilitation 70: 144–155

Kaufman R K R, An K-N, Litchy W J, Morrey B F, Chao E Y 1991 Dynamic joint forces during knee isokinetic exercise. American Journal of Sports Medicine 19: 305–316

Knutsson E 1987 Analysis of spastic paresis. In: International Congress of the World Confederation for Physical Therapy, Sydney

Knutsson E, Martensson A 1980 Dynamic motor capacity in spastic paresis and its relation to prime mover dysfunction, spastic restraint and antagonist coactivation. Scandinavian Journal of Rehabilitation Medicine 12: 93–106

Kramer J F, McDermid J 1989 Isokinetic measures during concentric–eccentric cycles of knee extensors. Australian Journal of Physiotherapy 35: 9–14

Laidlaw D, Yue G H, Alexander A L et al 1994 Non-homogenous and task-dependent activation of first dorsal interosseus muscle. Society of Neurosciences Abstracts 20: 384

Lance J W 1980 Symposium synopsis. In: Feldman R G, Young R R, Koella W P (eds) Spasticity: disordered motor control. Year Book Publishers, Chicago, pp 485–494

Levine D, Klein A, Morrissey M 1991 Reliability of isokinetic concentric closed kinematic chain testing of the hip and knee extensors. Isokinetics and Exercise Science 1: 146–152

Madsen O R, Bliddal H, Egsmose C, Sylvest J 1995 Isometric and isokinetic quadriceps strength in gonarthrosis: inter-relations between quadriceps strength, walking ability, radiology, subchondral bone density and pain. Clinical Rheumatology 14: 308–314

McMahon T A 1984 Muscles, reflexes and locomotion. Princeton University Press, Princeton, New Jersey

Nardone A, Romano C, Schieppati M 1989 Selective recruitment of high-threshold human motor units during voluntary isotonic lengthening of active muscles. Journal of Physiology (London) 409: 451–471

Nisell R, Ericson M 1992 Patellar forces during isokinetic extension. Clinical Biomechanics 7: 104–108

Nisell R, Ericson M, Nemeth G 1989 Tibiofemoral joint forces during isokinetic knee extension. American Journal of Sports Medicine 17: 49–54

Perrine J J, Edgerton V R 1978 Muscle force–velocity and power–velocity relationships under isokinetic loading. Medicine and Science in Sports and Exercise 10: 159–166

Ralston H J, Pollissar M J, Inman V T, Close J R, Feinstein B 1949 Dynamic features of human isolated voluntary muscle in isometric and free contractions. Journal of Applied Physiology 1: 526–533

Rizzardo M, Bay G, Wessel J 1988 Eccentric and concentric torque and power of the knee extensors in females. Canadian Journal of Sports Science 13: 166–169

Sapega A A 1990 Muscle performance evaluation in orthopedic practice. Journal of Bone and Joint Surgery 72A: 1562–1574

Shelbourne K D, Nitz P 1990 Accelerated rehabilitation after anterior cruciate ligament reconstruction. American Journal of Sports Medicine 18: 292–299

Shirado O, Ito K, Kaneda K, Strax T E 1995 Concentric and eccentric strength of trunk muscles: influence of test postures on strength and characteristics of patients with chronic low-back pain. Archives of Physical Medicine and Rehabilitation 76: 604–611

Shklar A, Dvir Z 1995 Isokinetic strength relationships in shoulder muscles. Clinical Biomechanics 10: 369–373

Smith A J 1975 Estimates of muscle and joint forces at the knee and ankle during jumping activities. Journal of Human Movement Studies 1: 78–86

Smith S, Mayer T G, Gatchel R J, Becker T J 1985 Quantification of lumbar function. Part I: isometric and multispeed isokinetic trunk strength measures in the sagittal and axial planes in normal subjects. Spine 10: 757–764

Stauber W T 1989 Eccentric action of muscles: physiology, injury and adaptation. Exercise and Sports Science Review 19: 157–185

Tax A, Denier G, Gielen C C, Kleyne M 1990 Differences in central control of m. biceps brachii in movement tasks and force tasks. Experimental Brain Research 79: 138–142

Taylor N A, Cotter J D, Stanley S N, Marshall R N 1991 Functional torque–velocity and power–velocity characteristics of elite athletes. European Journal of Applied Physiology 62: 116–121

Tesch P A, Dudley G A, Duvoisin M R, Hather B R, Harris R T 1990 Force and EMG signal patterns during repeated bouts of concentric or eccentric muscle actions. Acta Physiologica Scandinavica 138: 263–271

Thilmann A F, Fellows S J, Garms E 1991 The mechanism of spastic muscle hypertonus: variations in reflex gain over the time course of spasticity. Brain 145: 233–244

Timm K E 1988 Isokinetic lifting simulation: a normative data study. Journal of Orthopaedic and Sports Physical Therapy 9: 155–166

Thomas D O, White M J, Sagar G, Davies C T 1987 Electrically evoked isokinetic plantar flexor torque in males. Journal of Applied Physiology 63: 1499–1503

Trudelle-Jackson E, Meske N, Highenboten C, Jackson A 1989 Eccentric/concentric torque deficits in the quadriceps muscle. Journal of Orthopaedic and Sports Physical Therapy 11: 142–145

Wessel J, Ford D, van Drietsum D 1992 Measurement of torque of trunk flexors at different velocities. Scandinavian Journal of Rehabilitation Medicine 24: 175–180

Westing S H, Seger J Y, Thorstensson A 1990 Effects of electrical stimulation on eccentric and concentric torque–velocity relationships during knee extension in man. Acta Physiologica Scandinavica 140: 17–22

Wilkie D R 1950 The relationship between force and velocity in human muscle. Journal of Physiology 110: 249–280

Zelig G 1992 Measurement of spasticity in paraplegic patients after washout and during treatment with baclofen. Unpublished thesis, Tel-Aviv University, Tel Aviv

2

Hardware, test parameters, and issues in testing

PART 1
HARDWARE

Angular motion (AM) isokinetic dynamometers are based on the principle that the lever-arm moves at a preset angular velocity (PAV) however great the turning force, or moment, applied by the user. This principle is qualified however by the fact that in order to achieve the PAV an acceleration phase (and equally a deceleration phase at motion termination) must take place. Therefore a condition of isovelocity through the entirety of the tested range of motion (ROM) is clearly impossible (see below). However, once the PAV is reached, an increased muscular moment does not cause a concomitant increase in the angular velocity. Rather, the counter-resistance is increased so that the AM of the lever-arm remains within narrow margins about the PAV. The width of these margins is one of the performance characteristics of each system. It must be stressed that the moment generated by the muscle need not be maximal. On the contrary, using the advanced options available in some systems, users may induce perfectly smooth isokinetic motion without taxing the muscles to their utmost contractile capacity.

Each of the systems on the market has its own individual features, but all have the same basic feature, namely a rotating lever-arm which moves in a single plane. This does not necessarily mean that the motion of the joint(s) must be confined to a single anatomical plane. For instance, diagonal movements at the shoulder may be tested using isokinetic dynamometers. The general layout of a typical AM isokinetic dynamometer is illustrated in Figures 2.1 and 2.2.

The basic elements of the system are as follows:

1. *The force acceptance attachment* is the interface between the subject and the system. It consists of a metallic attachment on the lever-arm, with or without foam padding, which connects to the lever-arm via the 'load cell'. The location of the unit along the lever-arm is individually adjusted.

2. *The load cell* converts the force signal into an electric signal. The load cell may be part of the above attachment or may be located directly on the axis.

3. *The lever-arm* provides the base for the force acceptance attachment and moves radially about a fixed axis.

4. *The head assembly* (Fig. 2.1) houses the motor responsible for the motion of the lever-arm. Its orientation may normally be adjusted for:

   a. tilt, for movement in planes other than the vertical, e.g. rotations of the humerus or subtalar motions
   b. swivelling for applications such as testing of shoulder elevators.

The head may be moved up or down using an electric motor, for the purpose of alignment. Concerning the arrangement of the head assembly and the seat, there are two design approaches. One (e.g. the Cybex Norm) has a fixed head assembly positioned between two seats, which requires the subject to change seats if bilateral testing of joint/muscle systems such as the knee or shoulder is carried out. The other consists of an adjustable mechanism in which the head assembly is manually moved around the subject. The latter approach, exemplified by the KinCom 125E+ dynamometer, is also more convenient for the subjects, besides requiring less space. However, both designs must ensure the stability of the head assembly since this is a crucial factor in the reliability of the system (Herzog 1988).

Electric servomotors stand behind, literally speaking, isokinetic dynamometers. These motors move the lever-arm and may do so in either concentric or eccentric modes. In the former, the motor resists a pushing force, whereas in the latter the motor and body segment pull in opposite directions. In some systems the moment which the motor can generate in order to overcome eccentric muscle moment has deliberately been limited, with no appreciable corresponding gain in the maximal angular velocity which may be set. Other designs are characterized by high angular velocities but relatively low active (motor) moment. Consequently neither design can claim to offer genuine eccentric measurement for all joints.

5. *The seat, or plinth* serves to position the subject. The seat must have a stable frame, and

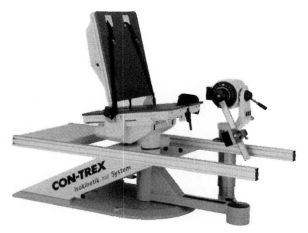

Figure 2.1 The Con-Trex isokinetic dynamometer: front view, with permission.

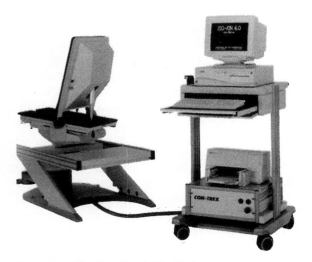

Figure 2.2 The Con-Trex isokinetic dynamometer: rear view, with permission.

independent vertical and horizontal (forward/backward) alignment options.

6. *The control unit* consists of a personal computer and its associated peripheral equipment. The mode of operation and various other parameters (see below) are fed into the computer using the keyboard. The same computer is also responsible for the real-time data processing.

7. *Specific attachments* are required for the various applications of the isokinetic dynamometer.

PART 2
CONTROL AND PERFORMANCE PARAMETERS

Isokinetic dynamometers are measurement devices, providing clinicians with information about the dynamic, i.e. moving, mechanical performance of muscle groups. It is assumed that the joint spanned by the muscles moves at a constant angular velocity, i.e. its motion is isokinetic. As mentioned above, it is really the lever-arm that moves isokinematically and only within a limited sector of the prescribed ROM. It is also possible, using these dynamometers, to measure multi-joint motion. In this case, the term 'isokinetic' bears no relevance to the actual motion that is being monitored. Moreover, biological joints do not possess a fixed axis of rotation, a situation that further impedes the derivation of an exact value for the angular motion. The extent of the error made in assuming a constant joint angular velocity depends on the joint tested, subject position etc. Isokinetic dynamometers are also useful for recording static (isometric) performance although this is not their main objective.

In isokinetic dynamometry, the basic measurement record consists of a sequence of numbers which represent the size of the force (moment in certain systems) exerted by the moving distal body segment against the force sensor. In all advanced isokinetic systems, this record is displayed in a graphical form on the computer display.

'Muscle performance' is the collective name for a set of parameters derived from the basic record. These are the 'output' parameters.

Because of the physiological and biomechanical properties of skeletal muscle, discussed in Chapter 1, the magnitudes of the output (or 'performance') parameters depend, among other variables, on a set of control (input) parameters. These variables, notably the angular velocity, determine the general framework of the test (see Table 2.1). The following sections define and describe the input and output parameters of strength testing, and of fatigue and endurance testing. All parameters are given in SI (metric) units.

CONTROL PARAMETERS OF STRENGTH TESTING

Strength testing is normally understood to consist of a minimal number of maximal effort contractions. This number may vary with different testing protocols. The objective is to produce a representative moment–angular position (MAP) curve, from which various performance parameters are derived. The control, or input, parameters which must be specified in advance, fall into two groups: the joint-dependent and joint-independent parameters.

JOINT-DEPENDENT INPUT

The joint-dependent parameters (Table 2.1) vary according to which joint is being tested. These are discussed individually in Chapters 6–10. However,

Table 2.1　Control (input) and performance (output) parameters in isokinetic testing

Control	Performance
Joint-dependent	Moment
Range of motion (ROM)	Peak
Angular velocity(ies)	Angle-based
Subject/patient positioning	Angle of peak moment
Stabilization	Average
Alignment of the axes	Contractional work
of the dynamometer	Contractional power
and the joint	Contractional impulse
Contraction mode	
Joint-independent	
Damp setting	
Isometric preactivation	
Feedback	

general descriptions of range of motion and angular velocity are given here.

Range of motion

The range of motion (ROM) which is expressed in degrees is the most basic parameter relating to isokinetic testing. It describes the allowable angular displacement of the *lever-arm* which should not be confused with the motion taking place in the *biological joint*.

The isokinetic range of motion

In specifying the ROM the examiner determines the points of motion initiation and termination. However, this arc is not equal to the angular sector in which the lever-arm moves at a constant velocity (the PAV) – the isokinetic sector (IS). The IS is always smaller than the total test ROM (as mentioned above) since at the beginning and at the end of the test ROM the angular velocity of both the lever-arm and the moving segment is, by definition, 0°/s. In order for the lever-arm to reach the PAV, it has to be accelerated. This means that a certain angular distance and a period of time elapse until the lever-arm's velocity is equal to the PAV. The same rule applies during deceleration.

Since it normally takes a longer period of time to reach a higher velocity, an inverse relationship exists between the test velocity and the IS: an increase in the preset velocity implies a smaller IS. A few studies looked into the extent to which motion was non-isokinetic. Osternig et al (1983) tested the Orthtron dynamometer at velocities ranging between 50 and 400°/s. It was found that whereas at the lower velocity the IS amounted to 92% of the total ROM, this figure was reduced to 16% upon reaching the highest velocity, respectively. This means that at the higher velocity spectrum, use of this dynamometer results in substantially ballistic rather than isokinetic motions. In a later study Iossifidou & Baltzopoulos (1996) compared ISs derived from Biodex and KinCom dynamometers. Unfortunately the measurement was performed relative to a static resistance – the weight of the lever-arm and the ROM were not

Table 2.2 Percentage of the isokinetic sector period relative to the total range of motion (From Iossifidou & Baltzopoulos 1996)

PAV (°/s)	Biodex		KinCom	
	±5%	±10%	±5%	±10%
30	63.5	76.5	40.3	66.7
60	24.0	49.4	38.5	56.4
90	22.5	39.0	16.3	47.1
120	22.5	27.5	17.2	33.3
150	14.6	20.9	19.2	43.6
210			14.0	36.8
250			21.0	28.1

The values ±5% and ±10% are the limits for the fluctuation of the actual angular velocity relative to the preset angular velocity (PAV).

specified. However Table 2.2 outlines the results of the measurements which clearly indicate that at 30°/s there was already a considerable *non-IS*. This sector increased up to about 70–80% which once again emphasizes that most of the ROM was spent on either accelerating or decelerating the lever-arm.

Moreover, it should be realized that these findings were derived using *static* resistance. However, the resistance under actual test conditions is highly *dynamic* as its magnitude is dictated by the muscle's variable length–tension, moment–angular velocity as well as by the level of recruitment. Thus studies of the type undertaken by Farrell & Richards (1986) or Iossifidou & Baltzopoulos (1996) do not fully portray the true proportional part taken up by the transients. Furthermore, it stands to reason that the IS may under realistic dynamic conditions be even smaller than what had been indicated under quasi-static calibration. At any rate the main lesson from these studies is that high velocities may be less appropriate for criterion testing – namely determination of strength status in the context of rehabilitation phase – or rating of impairment.

Size of the ROM

There is evidence that the size of the ROM has a direct effect on isokinetic performance, specifically relating to knee extensors in concentric contractions. In a study by Narici et al (1991) the effect on the peak moment (PM) of the ROM and isometric preactivation (IPA, see below) was explored. Maximal contractions of the quadriceps were performed at 180, 240 and 300°/s. The experimental conditions consisted of a ROM of 90° without IPA (condition A), 90° with IPA equal to 25% of maximal voluntary contraction (condition B) and ROM of 120° with same IPA as in B (condition C). It was revealed that condition C resulted in significantly higher PM (up to 22% at the highest velocity) compared to condition A. Condition B resulted also in higher PM compared to condition A but the differences were not equally striking. The improvement in PM was attributed to the longer *time* available for tension development as well as a greater *neural activation*. Thus although a larger ROM seems to be responsible for higher moment output, the mediating factor – time – may be responsible for this enlargement.

Angular velocity

The second input parameter is the test angular velocity (ω), measured in degrees per second (°/s). In some papers another unit, the radian per second (rad/s) has been used. As 1 rad is equal to approximately 57.3°, one can hardly see the benefit of abandoning the common and convenient units. In the case of linear motion the unit of measurement is centimeter per second (cm/s) or inch per second (in/s).

It should be restated that the test angular velocity is that of the lever-arm, not that of the distal segment. Moreover, the preset velocity does not bear any simple relationship to muscle linear contraction velocity, as indicated by Hinson et al (1979), and this relationship itself would be different for each muscle because of differing anatomical configurations.

As indicated by Iossifidou & Baltzopoulos (1996) the PAV is not absolutely constant even within the IS. Indeed, in their study it was indicated that as far as the KinCom dynamometer was concerned the difference between the actual velocity and the PAV was between −34.8 and +7.5%. As this study was based on quasi-static calibration it may underestimate the full scope of the errors

incurred. Moreover, it is possible that this measurement gap is not limited to these dynamometers and therefore acts as a general error in isokinetic dynamometry reflecting technological limits.

The ROM–angular velocity–contraction time paradigm

Regardless of the muscle-joint system, the commonly employed isokinetic test velocities typically consist of multiples of 30°/s: 60, 90, 120, 180°/s, etc. This practice has no biological, let alone, functional justification. Its roots may be traced historically to the prototype isokinetic dynamometer, the hydraulic Cybex, which was capable of measuring isometric and concentric contractions. This dynamometer was designed principally for testing knee musculature and hence the use of 90° as a 'standard' ROM was a natural choice. Bearing in mind that at the time of its development the idea of incorporating a computer as a controller and processor of this dynamometer was still very primordial, and the solution for varying the lever-arm velocity had to be mechanical and limited to a discrete number of velocities. It can therefore be assumed that by allowing some six optional equi-spaced velocities (30, 60, 90, 120, 150 and 180°/s) the designers succeeded in both using existing valve technology (velocity controller) and accommodating contraction speeds that could be described from slow to fast. However, as the typical ROM was 90°, the hidden factor was in fact lever-arm movement time. Hence, assuming ideal isokinetic conditions, and converting velocity into its precursors (time and distance) a test performed at 30°/s over a ROM of 90° should take 3 s using the formula:

$$\frac{ROM}{\text{'constant' velocity}} = \text{'time'} = \frac{90}{3} = 3\,s$$

This can be considered a 'slow' test. On the other hand covering the same ROM at the highest velocity of 180°/s would require 0.5 s – a 'fast' test.

Since the hydraulic technology was in use well into the mid-1980s, the practice of multiples of 30°/s became so well entrenched and reported in scientific publications, that little thought was given to its actual meaning. This situation is even more perplexing given the digital capacity to achieve test velocities that may be more relevant in nature. However, time as the truly other independent factor in the equation almost lost any specific value in spite of the abovementioned study by Narici et al which underlined its singular significance. Moreover, time is rarely displayed on any dynamometer's 'Results' screen. Whether this is an outcome of the reluctance of manufacturers to reveal that the ISs are really limited or due to tacit understanding that the time factor is not what users are after cannot be answered with any degree of certainty.

An attempt to find out whether time is indeed the common denominator entails the use of different ROM–velocity combinations that would result in exactly the same lever-arm movement time. Moreover, such a protocol should be applied to different ROM sectors within the allowable joint ROM. For instance if a ROM–velocity of 90°–90°/s is to be compared with a 30°–30°/s (which should ostensibly result in the same movement time, see below) then the location of the short ROM sector (30°) within the long one (90°) is definitely material. Obviously achieving such combinations while ensuring exactly the same movement time is quite impossible. It should also be borne in mind that *lever-arm movement time* is just an estimate of the *contractile period of the muscle* so that the introduction of an IPA will affect any functional relationship.

An alternative approach to this problem, although admittedly much less accurate, has recently been taken by Dvir et al (2002). Shoulder concentric and eccentric flexion strength was tested in a group of normal subjects using two distinct ROMs: 80° (long, LROM) and 16° (short, SROM) with the latter located in the middle of the former (Fig. 2.3). To each ROM a set of three angular velocities was adjusted as follows: for the LROM the velocities were 40, 80 and 160°/s whereas for the SROM they were 8, 16 and 32°/s. The adjustment was based on the equivalence of the so-called nominal movement times (NMT) of the lever-arm defined as ROM/angular velocity. Thus the experimental conditions consisted of the following NMTs: 80/40 = 16/8 (NMT = 2 s),

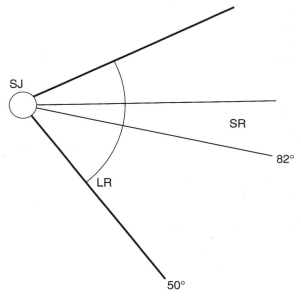

Figure 2.3 Short (16°) range of motion (SR) vs long (80°) range of motion (LR) shoulder flexion testing. Note that long range of motion (LR) start position was 50° of flexion. SJ, shoulder joint. (After Dvir et al 2002.)

80/80 = 16/16 (NMT = 1 s) and 80/160 = 16/32 (NMT = 0.5 s). No attempt was made to actually compare the NMTs since the particular dynamometer (a KinCom125E+) was not equipped with an auxiliary system for measuring the real NMT. Rather, the purpose of this experiment was to render a crude first approximation for the role of time in the outcome measure: peak moment.

The findings of this study are depicted in Figure 2.4. First it should be realized that locating different velocities and ROMs on the same coordinate system (moment–NMT as illustrated in Fig. 2.4) was possible due to the use of the NMT as the independent variable and common denominator. Second, it is recognized that the NMT units are approximations rather than an exact expression for the actual movement time of the lever-arm. With these qualifications in mind, the findings reveal three prominent features:

1. The moment–NMT curves relating to both LROM and SROM resemble the well-known sigmoidal shape of the $M–\omega$ (moment–angular velocity) curve and are approximated by third

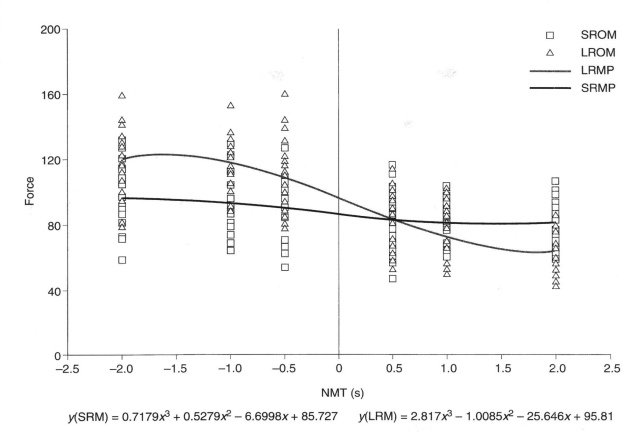

$$y(SRM) = 0.7179x^3 + 0.5279x^2 - 6.6998x + 85.727 \qquad y(LRM) = 2.817x^3 - 1.0085x^2 - 25.646x + 95.81$$

Figure 2.4   The approximate moment–angular velocity (M–ω) curves of the shoulder flexors obtained according to the protocol by Dvir et al (2002). The numbers on the X axis refer to the nominal movement times (NMT). Positive and negative X axes relate to the concentric and eccentric branches of the M–ω curve whereas the Y axis depicts the moment of the flexors. The units on this axis are in fact expression in N and should be multiplied by 0.4 for the moment value. The equations at the bottom of the graphs represent polynomial approximations of the short range of motion (SROM, left) and long range of motion (LROM, right). LRMP, polynomial fitting for long range of motion; SRMP, polynomial fitting for short range of motion.

order polynomials. Interestingly, this third order polynomial was also adjusted to M–ω curves in a previous study (Tis et al 1993).

2. For both ROMs the eccentric strength values were higher than their concentric counterparts although this was more conspicuous for the LROM protocol.

3. If the isometric strength is calculated from the polynomial equations (by setting 'x' to zero) then its values are 85 Nm and 95 Nm according to SROM and LROM protocols, respectively. Note: the SROM did not coincide with a particularly optimal sector of the total flexion strength curve.

Thus it could be argued if the SROM was located nearer to the initial part of the motion, an even better agreement between the derived SROM and LROM isometric strengths could be achieved. At any rate, put together these features add significantly to the validity of using NMT as a common basis for analyzing isokinetic strength values. Moreover, using the NMT concept may allow the scaling of previously collected data which consisted of concentric and eccentric tests in order to establish a unified model.

Equally, if indeed testing using a short ROM provides comparable data to long or full ROM testing, it opens a serious new avenue in the practice of isokinetics. Short ROM testing has at least three distinct advantages over common techniques:

1. By limiting the ROM, muscle strength may be tested effectively outside painful arcs or away from joint movement zones that may jeopardize various anatomical structures due to excess stress or strain.

2. Limited ROM reduces appreciably the effect of machine–joint misalignment since the larger the arc of movement, the lesser is the coincidence between the instantaneous axis of rotation and the motor axis.

3. In certain instances (e.g. trunk testing) long ROMs introduce significant gravitational effects such as may be found in trunk flexion and extension that span a ROM of, for example, 70°.

By limiting trunk motion to a SROM which is centered around the upright position, the values obtained may effectively reflect the net muscle strength without the need for gravitational correction. Studies along these lines indeed indicated that trunk extension strength scores were well within previously reported scores derived from much longer ROMs (Dvir & Keating 2001a,b, 2003).

JOINT-INDEPENDENT CONTROL PARAMETERS

Damp setting

The damp setting controls the acceleration and deceleration of the lever-arm and segment combination. The angular sectors occupied by the acceleration and deceleration phases, the so-called 'transients', are directly proportional to the angular velocity providing the damp setting is used (see below).

The effect of damping is demonstrated by the two MAP curves depicted in Figure 2.5. These curves are based on two consecutive concentric contractions of the quadriceps under conditions identical except for damp settings. A and B refer to undamped and maximally damped contractions. It is evident that the conspicuous spike which occurs at the beginning of the contraction in Figure 2.5A (undamped) is significantly attenuated in Figure 2.5B (maximally damped).

This spike has been termed the 'impact artifact' (Winter et al 1981), the 'torque overshoot' (Sapega et al 1982) or the 'impact torque' (Sale et al 1987). The term used in this book is 'moment overshoot' or simply 'overshoot'. This phenomenon results from the interaction between the lever-arm and the mechanism responsible for arresting its accelerated motion. It is regarded as an obstacle particularly in high velocity testing where, as explained previously, the sector of isokinetic motion is significantly reduced (Osternig 1986). Moreover, it does not reflect muscle performance at the preset velocity as it occurs long before isokinetic conditions are reached.

Some modern isokinetic dynamometers overcome the overshoot phenomenon using 'ramping', which allows acceleration of the segment to the

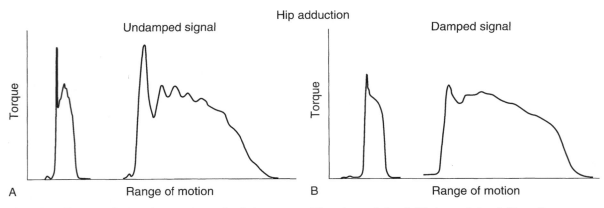

Figure 2.5   Damp settings and moment overshoot phenomena: (A) undamped signal; (B) damped signal. (From Sapega et al 1982.)

preset velocity (Farrell & Richards 1986). The role of this computer-controlled acceleration is to provide an 'absorber' for the excess force. The resulting movement is hence an overshoot-free, smooth transition from 0°/s to the preset velocity.

It should be emphasized that though the overshoot is an artifact from the point of view of isokinetic testing, physiologically it is very meaningful. First, it has been shown that the factors affecting overshoot are different from those affecting common performance parameters under isokinetic conditions (Sale et al 1987). The magnitude of the overshoot reflects the capacity to recruit the neuromuscular apparatus and generate a moment. In this respect it is reminiscent of the isometric rate of force development. The peak moment however reflects another facet of strength, that of generating moment under loading. Thus the two are very significant. In addition, one should bear in mind that the magnitude of the overshoot is also a function of the damping technology used in a particular dynamometer and hence should not be compared among different makes.

Variation of the damp setting

The effect on the peak and average moment (see below) of knee extensors, of varying the damp setting has been examined (Rathfon et al 1991). The authors used three damp settings, low, medium and high, which corresponded to a long, medium and short delay in reaching the PAV, which in this study consisted of 90°/s. Both concentric and eccentric modes were tested. The findings indicated that the choice of the damp setting did not appear to have a clinically significant effect on either the peak or average moments. This conclusion can reasonably be extended to lower velocities but its validity for higher velocities is unknown at present.

Isometric preactivation

Isometric preactivation (IPA) refers to static tension which is generated in the tested muscle(s) before motion of the lever-arm and segment ('preloading'). The use of IPA was first reported by Gransberg & Knutsson (1983) who indicated that it had a restraining effect on the initial moment oscillations. Later studies failed to reach a clear answer concerning its effect, probably because of different protocols. Table 2.3 outlines the basic experimental designs and the findings.

As evident from Table 2.3 there are three approaches to setting the IPA: absolute force, absolute moment and relative %MVIC (maximal voluntary isometric contraction) values. The latter approach conforms to the practice of normalizing muscle performance, and should be preferred. The inclusion of IPA has an obvious positive effect on the average moment but whether or not this also affects the peak moment is a controversial issue.

Table 2.3 Isometric preactivation (IPA): control parameters and effects*

Source	Velocity (°/s)	IPA	Effect
Gransberg & Knutsson (1983)	30, 120, 240	5, 140 Nm	Increase in initial moment, damping of oscillations
Piette et al (1986)	30, 180	50, 100%MVIC	Increase in initial moment
Gravel et al (1988)	30	0 100%MVIC	Decrease in mid-ROM moment
Jensen et al (1991)[†]	90	50 N, 75%MVIC	Increase in average moment, shift in peak moment angle
Narici et al (1991)	180, 240, 300	25%MVIC	Damping of oscillations, shift of angle-based moment, marginal increase in moment
Kramer et al (1991)[†]	45, 135	20, 50, 100 N	Increase in average moment, increase in mid-ROM eccentric moment, initial proportional increase in moment

* Except for Gravel et al (1988) all studies refer to knee extension.
[†] Contractions performed concentrically and eccentrically.
  MVIC, maximal voluntary isometric contraction.

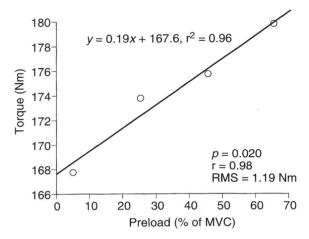

Figure 2.6 Group mean moment (torque) for each preload condition regressed against preload. MVC, maximal voluntary contraction; RMS, root mean square. (From de Morton & Keating 2002.)

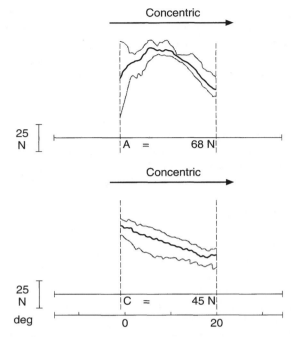

Figure 2.7 Different shapes of the moment–angular position (MAP) curve during ankle eversion strength testing. Top trace, IPA = 50 N; bottom trace IPA = MVC (maximal voluntary contraction).

Worth mentioning is a recent well-conducted study (de Morton & Keating 2002) which looked not only into the effect of the IPA on the moment output but also on the variability of the measurements. Subjects performed maximal knee extensions subject to IPAs of 5, 25, 45 and 65% of the maximal voluntary contraction (MVC). A strong and significant relationship was indicated between the IPA and the moment (Fig. 2.6). There was also a strong inverse relationship between the magnitude of the moment and the variability.

Another effect of the IPA relates to the situation when its magnitude is close to the MVC. In such a case the shape of the MAP concentric curve may change quite dramatically from resembling an inverted U to one which is similar to a hyperbola (Fig. 2.7). The reason for this phenomenon lies in the fact that concentric strength is smaller than the isometric strength at a given point in the range of motion. If the test ROM starts at a point which is not far from the optimal (e.g. 45–60° flexion in the knee), movement towards extension will result in a moment which is lower than the isometric. Moreover, as the knee comes closer to full extension the dynamic moment becomes smaller, hence the hyperbolic character of the MAP curve.

With respect to eccentric contractions, Kramer et al (1991) highlight the point that IPA eccentric knee flexion (quadriceps activity) demands a higher initial contractile moment since, at the usual initial horizontal position, gravity adds about 9 Nm. A relevant comparison of the differential effect of IPA on concentric and eccentric contractions would be possible through, for instance, setting of equivalent demands using different IPAs. In addition it would naturally be erroneous to compare muscle performances which are not based on the same IPA.

Lower isometric bias and upper moment limit

Another form of demand on isokinetically contracting muscle(s) is the imposition of a lower isometric bias (LIB). The LIB is by definition the minimal magnitude of moment that has to be maintained in order to ensure a smooth progression of isokinetic motion. It thus serves as a complement to IPA.

In addition to the latter, an upper moment limit (UML) may be incorporated for the purpose of ensuring the safety of potentially vulnerable structures. The use of LIB together with UML may be beneficial in non-maximal efforts (e.g. post anterior cruciate ligament reconstruction) or for the purpose of fine motor performance analysis.

Feedback

Similar to the performance of a large range of other motor-sensory modalities, the performance of an isokinetic task is also influenced by provision of feedback to the subject. Termed also 'knowledge of results' (KR) the purpose of the feedback is three-fold: maintenance/elevation of the performer's motivation, reinforcement of good performance and provision of error–correction information (Annett 1969). Feedback may be described in terms of form, amount, delay (Peacock et al 1981) and content (see Box 2.1).

In one of the first uses of an isokinetic system for analyzing the effect of feedback, it was revealed that isometric quadriceps performance was significantly improved (by about 10%) by combined visual and auditory feedback but not by either of them separately (Peacock et al 1981).

Isokinetic performance with and without visual feedback was examined in a study by Figoni & Morris (1984). The performance criteria were strength (peak moment) and fatigue of knee flexors and extensors, at slow and fast test velocities of 15 and 300°/s, respectively. The major finding was an improvement of performance at the slow but not at the high velocity, which amounted to about 12% in strength and 24–30% more fatigue (strength decrement) in both muscle groups. The selectivity of the effect was explained by the much longer period of time available for processing the feedback information in the slow test. Also, since the visual feedback consisted of the moment trace

and not its numerical value, it was more regular in the slow velocity as opposed to more oscillatory in the fast velocity test. The increase in fatigue was related to higher initial strength values. The general extent of improvement in isokinetic performance and its dependence on the test angular velocity was later confirmed in studies by Hald & Bottjen (1987) and Baltzopoulos et al (1991).

The effect of three types of visual information, as sources of error–correction, on maximal knee extension effort as indicated by PM has been the focus of a study by Hobbel & Rose (1993). The three feedback cues related to distinct presentation of the test results, graded by the degree of precision. The tests consisted of two angular velocities: 120 and 240°/s. A no-feedback pre-test was followed by two practice sessions during which the three feedback modules were provided to three experimental groups respectively while one group served as control (no feedback). A post-test without feedback was administered one day following the test. It was indicated that although no within-practice variations took place, comparison of pre-test to post-test changes in mean PM revealed that the groups receiving feedback improved significantly compared to the control (no feedback). This improvement included the slower as well as the faster performances. Therefore the conclusion that the use of visual feedback may be limited to strength testing at low angular velocities, at least in terms of retention over short periods of time, depends in part on the informational quality of the feedback.

Auditory feedback in the form of verbal encouragement, is far more difficult to standardize, which is probably the reason for a lack of information concerning it. It has however been found by Wilk et al (1991) that aggressive verbal commands and encouragement resulted in earlier occurrence of fatigue. It was their recommendation that if encouragement was given, it should be consistent and moderate in intensity.

PERFORMANCE PARAMETERS OF STRENGTH TESTING

A typical moment–angular position (MAP) curve is depicted in Figure 2.8. Though it is the force, expressed in newtons (N), which is the most basic

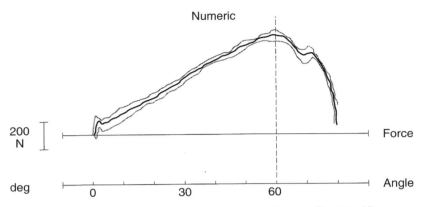

Figure 2.8 Peak moment (force) of an isokinetic strength curve. The dotted line shows the highest point and maximum force value on the moment–angular position (MAP) curve (623 N). Multiplication of this force value by the length of the lever-arm gives the peak moment.

mechanical parameter, all isokinetic findings relate to its rotational effect, namely the moment (see below). The latter serves in turn as the basis from which all other performance parameters are derived. In recent years a scattered number of studies preferred to expand the MAP curve by adding a 'third' dimension: the angular velocity. The surfaces generated by these moment–angle velocity functions have been used by Signorile & Applegate (2000) to examine the isokinetic knee extension performance of competitive runners. The authors claimed that it was possible to distinguish among the four different runner groups using discriminant function analysis of the generated surfaces. Eccentric contractions were not included in this presentation. It is doubtful however if this particular form of presentation adds substantially to the interpretation of isokinetic findings, particularly in the clinical environment. It should be realized that besides rendering an already complicated picture more complex, the error (see Chapter 3) is increased. Therefore it would be more constructive, when indicated, to assess velocity-based variations on a velocity-by-velocity basis rather than try to include all data in one representation, however compact that may seem to be.

SHAPE OF THE MAP CURVE

This is one of the most interesting and controversial issues associated with isokinetic measurements.

The advent of active dynamometers, capable of measuring eccentric performance led to the production of even more complex curves. These led to correspondingly higher expectations that the shape of the MAP curves could furnish information that went beyond the performance parameters. To what extent have these expectations been fulfilled?

Problems of interpretation

There are a number of difficulties that must first be addressed. First, it would be of prime importance to know the extent to which simple visual analysis can reveal the same idiosyncrasies to different observers. Although human perception lacks the mathematical probing power of the computer, it is capable of good pattern recognition. It was suggested in a few studies that the shape of the curve could be instrumental in identifying various knee pathologies (Blackburn et al 1982, Hoke et al 1983, Grace et al 1984, Grace 1985). However, none of these studies attempted to investigate this using an interobserver analysis.

Second, it would indeed be necessary to use processing techniques that so far have not been applied in this field. An original attempt has been reported by Afzali et al (1992) who found a mathematical expression which described quadriceps MAP curves. As pointed out by Mayhew (1992) the study suffered some weaknesses, notably a lack of reproducibility. From another point of view a major drawback was that the curves analyzed were derived from normal subjects or from the uninvolved side of patients with knee problems. Thus the curves could be described as 'simple' or 'regular' with the characteristic inverted U shape. However most problematic of all seemed to be the use of averaged MAP curves rather than original curves as the database. Hence the applicability of the findings, which did not deal with outstanding curves, is questionable.

There is a third difficulty concerning the issue of the MAP curve shape: reiterating Mayhew's criticism, unless 'reproducibility of shape' can be confirmed, the question is pointless. In fact, when performing an isokinetic test, examiners are looking for a 'representative' or 'the same' curve but this convergence is not always achieved, and is estimated using visual inspection only. The real obstacle is, however, consistency from one session to another. Whereas parameters like peak moment or contractional work may manifest acceptable reproducibility, this may not necessarily be the case with respect to shape.

Specificity in MAP curves

On the positive side it should be recognized that not all isokinetic curves have the same typical inverted U shape. Consequently there is a certain degree of specificity associated with these curves. A typical example is the difference between the quadriceps and hamstring concentric MAP curves, obtained upon testing the muscles in the sitting position. Whereas the quadriceps curve starts and normally ends at near zero moment, the hamstring is characterized by a monotonously increasing curve which peaks near or at the end of the ROM.

Another example is the phenomenon of 'break' or 'dip' in the curve, which has been associated with pain in the knee joint (Nordgren et al 1983, Dvir et al 1991b) (see detailed discussion in Chapter 6). These breaks disappeared following surgical intervention (Nordgren et al 1983), a finding which correlated well with the alleviation of pain in the joint. On the other hand the reproducibility of this phenomenon in terms of both magnitude and location has not been confirmed.

Paradoxically it does not mean that this is an invalid criterion as the source of pain (e.g. tissue stretching) may vary its responsivity even within the same testing session. Nevertheless the shape may vary quite considerably and thus few inferences may be drawn from it.

Clearly these issues must be investigated before the incorporation of shape analysis into clinical decision making can be considered.

CALCULATION OF THE MOMENT

In systems based on a resistance pad and load sensor assembly, whose position on the lever-arm is adjustable, the moment (M) is obtained using the following formula:

$$M = \text{lever-arm length} \times \text{force}$$

where the term lever-arm length refers to the distance between the axis of rotation of the lever-arm and the location of the load sensor. In some systems the load sensor is located differently but the calculation is the same.

As long as the PAV is relatively low, the error incurred by assuming that the recorded moment is equal to the joint moment, is also small. However, as shown in studies by Iossifidou & Baltzopoulos (1998a,b) certain parameters, particularly the peak moment, are exposed in relatively high PAV.

Moment and torque

The practice of using the term 'torque' rather than moment must be traced to the early days of isokinetic testing. Though torque, like moment, is associated with a force which acts at a distance from an axis, the mechanical connotation of the two is different. When a torque acts on a body it exerts torsional stresses and may in addition impart axial rotation (winding). When a moment acts on a body it exerts bending stresses and may in addition impart rotation. The difference is therefore in the axes about which the force acts. In this respect, major joint motions along the common anatomical planes are interpretable in terms of *moment* (flexor moment, abductor moment, etc.) whereas those relating to internal and external rotations would more correctly be described in terms of *torque*. One of the purposes of proper alignment of the joint axis with that of the dynamometer head is to minimize the effect of torque in tests of muscle performance taking place along the major planes (Oberg et al 1987). The opposite is also true when the purpose of the test is measurement of axial rotations. As a greater proportion of isokinetic testing is devoted to moment-related measurements, the term 'moment' is used in this book (e.g. peak or average moment). This will apply for both major planes and axial rotations (though in the latter, the term torque would have been even more appropriate).

Unit of measurement

The unit of measurement of moment is the newton-meter (Nm). Some sources prefer a different notation, N.m which might be misleading. Furthermore, the unit Nm should be reserved for moment (see below) whereas the joule, which may also be expressed as newton-meters, should specifically relate to work. Providing gravity is accounted for, the value of the moment at any point on the curve (Fig. 2.8) represents the strength of the tested muscles at that point.

Peak moment

The maximal value of the MAP curve is termed the peak moment (PM). In this book the terms peak moment and maximal strength are synonymous. The peak moment does not involve specifying its location. For instance, based on the MAP curve depicted in Figure 2.8, the strength of the muscle is 199 Nm (based on a lever arm of 32 cm and a peak force of 623 N).

The identification of the peak moment is not always straightforward. This is particularly apparent in two instances:

1. Eccentric contractions sometimes involve oscillations of varying amplitude in the moment–angular position curve. In pain-free tests, repeated trials and averaging normally serve to smooth out the curve, yet in certain instances the difficulty persists.

2. If the sampling rate of the data processing unit is fixed at 100 Hz (100 readings per second,

the isokinetic industry standard) curves based on very high test velocities appear as dotted rather than solid lines. In this case the accuracy of determining the peak moment may be compromised. Higher sampling rates solve this problem.

Angle-based moment

This is an alternative method of presentation, relating to the value of the moment at a predetermined angular position. It has been used in several studies. Since time and angular position are directly related to each other, except during the transient acceleration periods, the angle-based moment (ABM) is also a time-based value and it may be used for comparing moment generation capacity. Its reproducibility as a performance parameter of the knee extensors has been examined by Kramer et al (1991). Findings revealed that the reproducibility of ABM at 15° of knee flexion was consistently smaller than the corresponding value at 50° of knee flexion at two velocities and three different IPAs. This difference probably derives from the fact that the MAP curve had not settled by 15° of knee flexion. The ABM is less commonly used than the PM and the two are almost never coincident. On the other hand, the ABM allows a more standardized method of comparison, as it relates to the same muscle length. Hence the angle-based form of strength was indicated for multiple velocity measurements (Perrine & Edgerton 1978). It was also used in a recent study of an optimal isokinetic test protocol (Kues et al 1992). However, the decision concerning the specific angle to which reference should be made is basically arbitrary, and on retesting one has to assume absolute reproducibility of the alignment. Such an assumption is not realistic particularly with respect to joint systems such as the shoulder.

The potential benefit of using angle-based versus moment-based strength was studied in a group of patients suffering from chronic insufficiency of the anterior cruciate ligament (Kannus et al 1991). It was indicated that the angle-based method offered little additional information on thigh muscle performance compared with that obtained by the moment-based method. In view of this, and the points already mentioned the use of peak moment is strongly indicated.

Angle of peak moment

The angle at which the peak moment occurs (60° in Fig. 2.8) is called the angle of peak moment (APM). The APM is known to vary as a function of the test velocity (Rothstein et al 1987). A higher test velocity results in a delay in reaching the peak moment and hence a greater APM. In addition, the APM varies widely among subjects, particularly in the case of the shoulder (Ivey et al 1985). Therefore its value as a basis for clinical judgment, at least as far as the shoulder is concerned, is very questionable.

Average moment

Very often strength is expressed in terms of the average moment (AM), also expressed as newton-meters, rather than the peak moment. Clearly the average moment is measured over the IS. The use of average moment as an alternative strength parameter demonstrates the controversy over the definition of the theoretical construct 'strength': should strength be represented by a single moment value, i.e. the peak moment, or by the totality of all moment values which produce a single contraction? Since at present there is no unequivocal definition of strength (Rothstein et al 1987) average moment is no less a legitimate descriptor of strength than peak moment.

Some insight concerning this issue is provided by a recent study of the strength of trunk flexors (Wessel et al 1992). The peak concentric moment of the flexors bore a *positive* relationship to the test angular velocity, contrary to the well established moment–angular velocity (MAV) relationship. However, when the average concentric moment was considered the same trend was not apparent, although the expected relationship was only very weakly inverse. Furthermore, compared to their eccentric peak moment the average moment of the trunk flexors increased significantly less with the increase in velocity (30, 60 and 90°/s). The authors suggested that the relatively high mass of the trunk was responsible for the unevenness of

the moment curve and thus created an artifact which was the cause of this effect. It followed that the average moment was less affected than the peak moment. Since similar problems could potentially be encountered during testing of muscles operating on other heavy segments (e.g. hip region muscles), the use of average rather than peak moment is strongly recommended.

It is however suggested that a possible way to examine the appropriateness of peak or average moment parameters would be to determine the coefficient of variation (CV) associated with each, based on a fixed number of contractions. Since a smaller coefficient of variation indicates a more consistent measure, it could help resolve this issue.

Calculation of the average moment

The average moment is obtained from summing the moment values at each sampling point in the relevant isokinetic range of movement (IROM) and dividing the result by the number of points (Fig. 2.9). Consider a test performed at an angular velocity of 90°/s, along a ROM of 90°, with a sampling rate of 100 Hz. In theory, this test will last 1 s and hence if the required average moment is based on the full ROM, the database would consist of 100 moment values. The average moment ($M_{average}$) is therefore:

$$M_{average} = \frac{M_1 + M_2 + \cdots + M_{100}}{100}$$

where $M_1, M_2, ..., M_{100}$ denote the moment values at each sampling point.

If the number of moment values is n, the average moment value is given by:

$$M_{average} = \frac{M_1 + M_2 + \cdots + M_n}{n}$$

or more concisely:

$$M_{average} = \frac{1}{n} \sum_{x=1}^{x=n} M_x$$

To eliminate the transients (moment overshoot, initial oscillations) as already mentioned, the average moment is normally based on a sector of,

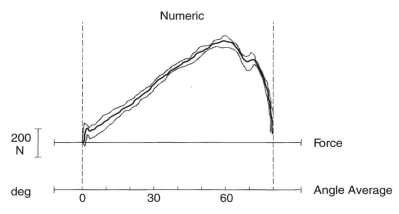

Figure 2.9 Average moment (force) of an isokinetic strength curve identical to the one depicted in Figure 2.8. Note the approximately 40% difference between the numerical values of the peak force and the average force (384 N).

rather than the full ROM. There are no rules concerning the extent of this sector; for instance in knee testing where the common test ROM is 90° the accepted practice is to ignore the first and last 10°. Obviously with a smaller ROM or high test velocities this practice becomes problematic and use of the peak moment is indicated. Also, limiting the average moment to a smaller sector, as described here means that it approximates to the peak moment.

Relationship of peak and average moments

The relationship between average and peak moments has been reported in a few studies (Morrissey 1987, Kramer & MacDermid 1989, Dvir et al 1989, Bandy & Lovelack-Chandler 1991). It was indicated that the two parameters were strongly correlated, in concentric and eccentric contractions alike, with correlation coefficients (Pearson's r) generally greater than 0.9. Since the peak moment represents, by definition, the greatest moment value, and the average moment is a linear combination incorporating the peak moment, the very high correlation coefficients are not surprising.

Kramer & MacDermid (1989) reported an interesting relationship between the test angular velocity (45, 90, 135 and 180°/s) and the peak-to-average moment ratio (PM:AM) in concentric and eccentric contractions. For concentric contractions there was an inverse relationship, for eccentric contractions it was direct. Specifically the ratio varied from 1.3 to 1.21, at 45 and 180°/s respectively, in concentric mode, and in eccentric mode the variation was from 1.3 to 1.36. Although not discussed by the authors, it seems from the findings that the concentric peak moments declined more rapidly than the corresponding average moments whereas this was not the case in eccentric contractions. In other words, the shape of the moment–angular velocity curve was different for peak moment and average moment. Consequently, although correlation coefficients of between 0.94 and 0.96 were found in both modes of contraction for a given velocity, this degree of correspondence may not hold for comparisons at different velocities. This leads to the conclusion that average and peak moments cannot be used interchangeably because of their different magnitudes, and their probably different relationships to angular velocity.

In this study the relationship between concentric and eccentric PM and AM was explored for both maximal conditions and efforts. The findings indicated that in maximal as well as submaximal conditions there was a very strong correlation between these parameters with Pearson's r for the trunk extensors ranging between 0.922 and 0.995. The respective scores for the knee extensors were lower: 0.628–0.992. The low end of the distribution in the case of the knee related to the production of 50% of the maximal effort which probably indicates an attempt to control the muscular tension in a way which was not compatible with maximal output. Taking into account the phenomenon of initial transients in both contraction modes and oscillations in eccentric contractions the application of AM in bilateral comparison was advised.

Strength normalization

Both the peak and average moments are commonly quoted in Nm units. In quite a number of papers, the preferred unit is Nm/kilogram of bodyweight (Nm/kgbw) or ft-lb/lb, i.e. the absolute strength values are 'normalized' according to the subject's weight.

The relationship between strength and body mass has been the focus of a number of studies but a conclusive decision regarding the validity of expressing strength as a normalized unit is still elusive. For instance, Jaric et al (2002) tested six muscle groups in normal subjects with the purpose of exploring the use of either an allometric scaling or by ratio standards. According to both methods the relationship is of the form $S = km^b$ where S, k, m and b are the muscular strength, a constant, body mass and the exponential constant, respectively. However, whereas allometric scaling implies that strength increases at a slower rate than body mass – namely S per kilogram$^{2/3}$ – ratio standards assume that S increases proportionally to bodyweight. Isokinetic measurements of the elbow, knee and hip flexors and extensors have indicated that while b was very close to 1 for elbow flexors and extensors and knee flexors, it was substantially greater and lesser than 1 for knee extensors and hip flexors and for the hip extensors, respectively. Thus in the absence of clear-cut indications the current approach seems to be against the practice of normalization (see, for instance, Delitto et al 1991, Newton et al 1993). Users are therefore advised to quote the average or peak moment in Nm (or ft-lb).

Contractional work

A parameter which is closely associated with average moment is the contractional work (CW),

whose unit of measurement is the joule (J). It is a measure of the work done, or energy expended, by the muscle(s) under test. It is equal to the area under the MAP curve or alternatively to the average moment times the angular displacement (A) (Fig. 2.5). In mathematical form, where work is represented by W:

$$W = M_{average} \times A$$

A normally refers to the angular displacement in the truly isokinetic sector of the MAP curve, as with the calculation of the average moment, described earlier.

Since contractional work is derived from the average moment through multiplication by a constant (the angular sector) their correlation coefficient is r = 1.0. Like average moment, contractional work eliminates the intricacies of the MAP curve.

Contractional power

Contractional power (CP), which is measured in watts, is an important performance parameter which relates to the average time rate of work namely:

$$Power = \frac{Work\ done}{Time\ taken}$$

or, if T is the total time for the movement through the angular sector (A):

$$P = \frac{W}{T}$$

This can be expressed:

$$P = \frac{M_{average} \times A}{T}$$

Hence:

$$P = M_{average} \times \omega$$

where ω is the test angular velocity.

The importance of this parameter derives from the fact that it reflects aspects other than strength although it bears a close relationship to the latter (Rothstein et al 1983, Bandy & Lovelack-Chandler

1991). For instance, although the concentric peak moment is inversely related to the test velocities (moment–angular velocity relationship), contractional power may be positively related to the latter as has been indicated with respect to the ankle plantarflexors (Gerdle & Fugl-Meyer 1985). This phenomenon results from the non-linear (decelerated) decay in the moment–velocity curve. Although it is theoretically valid to relate to an instantaneous P (the power based on a small angular sector), it probably has no value for the purpose of interpreting test findings based on normal or patient populations.

The relationship between CP and velocity has been the object of a study by Iossifidou & Baltzopoulos (2000). Peak power was calculated based on the product of:

1. preselected angular velocity and PM without considering the velocity at PM
2. actual velocity and respective moment values
3. instantaneous velocity at the point of PM
4. actual constant velocity and the PM during this period.

Quadriceps served as the model muscle and tests were carried out at 30, 90, 180 and 300°/s. Significant differences were found among the methods. Analysis has shown that only method 4 (highest moment during constant angular velocity period) provided a valid measure of power.

Contractional impulse

The performance parameter contractional impulse (CI) is the product of the moment multiplied by the time for which it acts, i.e. where I is the value of the impulse namely:

$$I = M_{average} \times T$$

Impulse is measured in Nms. Studies of athletes and patients have shown that impulse has a special significance. Sale (1991) analyzed the performance of sprinters versus cross-country skiers, using knee extension performance. The contractional impulse at 180°/s was the best discriminator between the two groups, while the peak moment at 30°/s revealed no differences. In another study in patients suffering from patellofemoral pain syndrome, the contractional impulse was highly correlated with the subjective pain ratings whereas the average moment was not (Dvir et al 1991a). Both studies have suggested the wider application of this parameter.

Suggested convention for specification of parameters

Used correctly, all of the above parameters must be applied relative to test angular velocity and mode of contraction. Since it is the concentric strength that is most commonly referred to, the latter should be used as a default. The following is suggested as a convenient way of quoting isokinetic parameters: parameter, angular velocity, contraction mode (only if eccentric). Examples are PM-120, AM-30 or CI-60E (PM, peak moment; AM, average moment; CI, contractional impulse).

Table 2.4 outlines the performance parameters of strength testing, their acronyms, measurement metric units, conversion factors and mechanical relationships.

FATIGUE AND ENDURANCE TESTING

Isokinetic testing of fatigue and endurance (F & E) is much more complex than the testing of strength. The complexity derives from the various criteria used and the serious void in terms of test standardization. Furthermore, fatigue is often confused with endurance where the former is used to describe elements of the latter.

In principle, isokinetic fatigue and endurance testing involves the repetitive exertion of maximal effort of one (agonist) or two (agonist and antagonist) muscle groups. These efforts are performed, by definition, at a PAV. Some protocols use a predetermined number of repetitions (Thorstensson & Karlsson 1976, Gleeson & Mercer 1992, Manou et al 2002) as the outcome criterion whereas others are based on a predetermined period of time during which subjects are instructed to perform as many repetitions as possible (Emery et al 1994, Felicetti et al 1994). Another approach has relied on examination of the shape of the fatigue curve using repeated contractions to exhaustion (Patton et al 1978),

Table 2.4 Performance and related parameters: units, conversion formulae and mechanical relationships

Parameter	Abbreviation	Symbol	Unit	Conversion	Relation to other parameters
Force		F	newton (N)	1 N = 0.2248 lb 　　 = 0.102 kgf	$F = M/r$ (r = lever length)
Moment		M	newton-meter (Nm)	1 Nm = 0.738 ft-lb 　　 = 0.102 kg m 1 ft-lb = 1.356 Nm 1 kg m = 9.81 Nm	$M = rF$
Peak	PM	M_{peak}	Nm		$M = rF_{peak}$
Average	AM	$M_{average}$	Nm		
Angle-based moment	ABM		Nm		
Angle of peak moment	APM		degree (°)	1° = 0.0174 rad	
			radian (rad)	1 rad = 57.3°	
Contractional work	CW	W	joule (J)	1 J = 1 Nm 　 = 0.737 ft-lb	$W = M_{average}A$ (A = angular displacement)
				1 ft-lb = 1.356 J	$W = \int_0^a M\,da$
Angular velocity		ω	degree per second (°/s)	1°/s = 0.0174 rad/s	$v = r\omega$ (v = linear velocity)
			radian per second (rad/s)	1 rad/s = 57.3°/s	
Contractional power	CP	P	watt (W)	1 W = 1 J/s 　 = 0.00134 hp	$P = W/T$ (T = contraction time) $P = M_{average}\omega$ $T = M_{average}T$
Contractional impulse	CI	I	newton-meter-second (Nms)		$I = M_{average}T$ $I = \int_0^t M\,dt$

while using a predetermined reduction (quoted as a percentage relative to the initial output) was the method of Schwendner et al (1995). Once the various *within-contraction* parameters (e.g. ROM, velocity, IPA, etc.) are considered, the likelihood of arriving at comparable results is very low indeed.

During the performance of repeated exertions mechanical output parameters such as the PM, work or power will exhibit two phases: initially (the number of contractions depending on the test conditions), the output will decrease relatively steeply, a phenomenon known as *fatigue*. Thereafter, a steady state level of output will be established. This phase is known as *endurance* (Gerdle et al 1998). Determination of the transition from one phase to another is an important index which is known to be subjective and to vary between groups. An illustration of the transition is given in Figure 2.10.

CONTROL PARAMETERS IN F & E TESTING

Number of repetitions

It follows from the dichotomy of fatigue and endurance that the number of repetitions may determine the quality of the phenomenon being measured. Obviously, where this number is maximal, the endurance phase is not attained without first passing through the fatigue phase. Thus for example the isokinetic 'endurance' test of the elbow flexors and extensors in a study by Motzkin et al (1991) probably related to fatigue.

There is no rule governing the number of repetitions required in a fully fledged fatigue and endurance test although some guidelines have been formulated. In various reports this number ranged between 10 (Barnes 1981) and 150 (Elert & Gerdle 1989, Gerdle et al 1989). However, the majority of cases used the middle sector: between

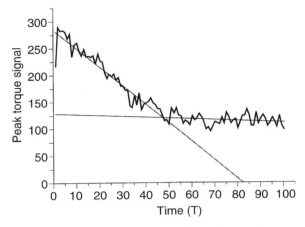

Figure 2.10 Fatigue–endurance shift based on peak moment scores (lines are fitted statistically). (From Gerdle et al 1998.)

40 and 100 repetitions. It should also be mentioned that fatigue and endurance may be explored in terms of submaximal effort, a factor that can greatly confound the interpretation of the findings. On the other hand, if the objective of the test is the assessment of repeated motions in a work environment, using submaximal rather than maximal effort is the logical choice.

Contraction time

This parameter refers to the ratio between the time actually spent in contractional activity and the total testing time (Mathiassen 1989). Contraction time (CT) which is expressed as a percentage reflects therefore the relationship between the activity and pause time.

PERFORMANCE PARAMETERS IN F & E TESTING

Reductions in peak moment (PM), contractional work (CW) and contractional power (CP)

Reduction in peak moment (PM) is probably the most commonly used performance measure. It is based on the percentage ratio of the last and first contractions. There are some variations. Thorstensson & Karlsson (1976), for instance,

compared the average peak moment of the first five contractions with that of the last five, whereas Gray & Chandler (1989) selected the three highest peak moment values from the five initial and five final contractions.

Reductions in contractional work and contractional power are used as performance measures in a way comparable to peak moment (Elert & Gerdle 1989, Gerdle et al 1989). Mathiassen (1989) used a variant of contractional work reduction in fatigue and endurance analysis of the quadriceps. Instead of dividing the final by the initial work output, the initial work output was replaced by a contractional work value based on a strength test.

Time to 50% of peak moment

This performance parameter refers to the period of time in which a subject can maintain a repetitive peak moment level of 50% or above the peak moment obtained at the initial contraction (Motzkin et al 1991). It is therefore a time-based rather than repetitions-based indicator. One disadvantage associated with this parameter is the inability to predict the exact number of contractions. Moreover, whether or not a single contraction with a peak moment value of 50% that of the initial peak moment should be sufficient to terminate the test is as yet unresolved.

A fatigue and endurance protocol which utilized a number of parameters has recently been described by Manou et al (2002). In this study 12 male subjects performed 40 maximal knee flexion/extension repetitions along a ROM of 100° at an angular velocity of 120°/s. Testing took place on two different occasions and test-retest correlations relate to the following parameters:

- *Total work* (TW): the amount of work (in joules) exerted during the full test. This parameter was also divided by bodyweight for normalizing (in J/kgbw)
- *Endurance ratio*: defined as $(TW_{1-20}/TW_{21-40}) \times 100$ where the subscripted numbers refer to the TW performed between repetitions numbered 1–20 and 21–40
- *50% fatigue work*: the amount of work performed when 50% of the maximal work was reached

Table 2.5 Mean (SD) scores and correlation coefficients of knee flexion/extension fatigue and endurance tests (From Manou et al 2002)

Parameter	Flexors			Extensors		
	Test	Retest	r	Test	Retest	r
TW (J)	3737(597)	3765(689)	0.96	6381(824)	6436(836)	0.92
TW/bodyweight	43.4(9.2)	48.6(9.3)	0.97	82.2(11.3)	82.7(9.6)	0.92
ER (%)	54.1(8.9)	53.9(8.0)	0.90	53.1(4.0)	54.7(3.8)	0.91
50% FW (J)	3029(695)	2903(830)	0.96	5041(659)	5091(846)	0.89
50% FT (s)	26.5(4.6)	23.9(4.4)	0.84	25.0(3.4)	25.5(4.4)	0.88
50% FR (N)	27.4(4.3)	25.3(5.3)	0.90	26.5(1.9)	27.2(3.6)	0.82

ER, endurance ratio; FR, fatigue repetitions; FT, fatigue time; FW, fatigue work; TW, total work.

- *50% fatigue time*: the period of time required to reach 50% of the maximal work
- *50% fatigue repetitions*: the number of repetitions performed before 50% of the maximal work was reached.

Table 2.5 summarizes the main findings and the Pearson's r correlation coefficients. As may be judged by both the pictorial and numerical representations this protocol yields stable fatigue and endurance parameters.

PART 3
ISSUES IN ISOKINETIC MEASUREMENT AND REHABILITATION

THE MEASUREMENT SCALE AND ISOKINETIC RATIOS

The classification of isokinetic measurements as consisting of interval and not ratio scales has been advocated in a review article by Rothstein et al (1987). It was stated that:

... isokinetic torque measurements must be considered to be interval scaled; that is, the zero level on the torque curve does not represent a true absence of muscularly generated torque. The torque curve actually represents the resistive torque generated by the machine to keep a limb segment from accelerating. The torque generated by the muscle to move the limb segment up to the machine speed is not registered. Ratios, or percentages, thus cannot be formed from interval-scaled data.

Although from the strictly mathematical viewpoint this remark is correct, in practice zero moment levels (which in this case are equivalent to grade 3 in manual muscle testing) are never compared. Therefore, the question whether, for instance, a muscle which generates a PM of 80 Nm is twice as strong as another muscle which generates 40 Nm must be answered affirmatively. The relevance of these ratios is discussed in the chapters on the isokinetics of the trunk (extension/flexion), the knee (extension/flexion) and the shoulder (internal/external rotation).

INDICATIONS AND CONTRAINDICATIONS FOR ISOKINETIC PROCEDURES
Indications

These have been finely elaborated by Timm (1992), regarding the special case of the trunk. They may be generalized, with the appropriate limitations, to other joint systems, and include:

1. *Trunk deconditioning syndrome* (Mayer & Gatchel 1987) or general muscle weakness. With respect to the trunk, the syndrome refers to a general decline in muscle and cardiovascular performance which results from chronic low back dysfunction without a definite spinal pathology. General muscle weakness in other joint systems may result from long periods of significantly reduced activity such as those following cast immobilization. However, there is a definite pathology associated with the immobilization and

the status of the injured tissues must carefully be considered (see contraindications).

2. *Testing and correction of muscle imbalance* which is often closely related to muscle weakness, may be reduced through the use of isokinetics. However, the precise extent of the imbalance must be assessed and confirmed. For instance, one views with alarm the common practice of determining the balance between trunk flexor and extensor performance without regard to the gravitational effect. Imbalance may be revealed between various muscle groups, like the glenohumeral rotators, and its rectification, as a therapeutic means, has been indicated (Glousman et al 1988).

3. *Provision of additional data* when the patient's available information cannot be satisfactorily interpreted, or where symptoms do not diminish using other therapeutic approaches. In this instance also, attention must be paid to any existing contraindications.

4. *An alternative source of information* may be provided by isokinetic testing when reporting the results of new forms of treatment (Sapega 1990).

Contraindications

The use of preset moment and force levels, an option which is available in modern systems, has drastically reduced the risk associated with isokinetic exertions. These levels work two ways: they

---

Box 2.2   Contraindications spectrum (based on Davies 1992)

1. Severely limited ROM ..... limited ROM
2. Severe pain .... pain
3. Severe effusion .... effusion or synovitis
4. Acute sprain .... chronic third degree sprain
5. Acute strain .... subacute strain of the musculotendinous unit
6. Soft tissue healing constraints
7. Unstable bone fracture or joint

---

ensure the generation of muscular tension greater than a certain threshold yet protect the involved structures from a potentially damaging stress. Moreover, as previously stated, an isokinetic motion pattern can be produced even without maximal contraction. Consequently the 'relative' versus 'absolute' classification of contraindications, as suggested by Davies (1992), may be modified to consist of a spectrum (Box 2.2). The clinical status appearing on the left hand side of Box 2.2 signifies the 'no testing permitted zone' whereas that on the right shows those clinical situations in which the decision to test is left to the clinician, while exercising maximal caution.

In addition, isokinetic testing of maximal muscle performance is *absolutely contraindicated in patients suffering from heart disease.*

REFERENCES

Afzali L, Kuwabara F, Zachazewski J, Browne P, Robinson B 1992 A new method for the determination of the characteristic shape of an isokinetic quadriceps femoris muscle torque curve. Physical Therapy 72: 585–595

Annett J A 1969 Feedback and human behavior. Penguin Books, Middlesex, UK

Baltzopoulos V, Williams J G, Brodie D E 1991 Sources of error in isokinetic dynamometry: effects of visual feedback on maximum torque measurements. Journal of Orthopaedic and Sports Physical Therapy 13: 138–142

Bandy W D, Lovelack-Chandler V 1991 Relationship of peak torque to peak work and peak power of the quadriceps and hamstring muscles in a normal sample using an accommodating resistance measurement device. Isokinetics and Exercise Science 1: 87–91

Barnes W S 1981 Isokinetic fatigue curves at different contractile velocities. Archives of Physical Medicine and Rehabilitation 62: 66–69

Blackburn T, Eiland W, Bandy W 1982 An introduction to the plica. Journal of Orthopaedic and Sports Physical Therapy 3: 171–177

Davies G J 1992 Isokinetic testing. In: Davies G J (ed) A compendium of isokinetics in clinical usage. S & S Publishers, Onalaska, Wisconsin, p 37

Delitto A, Rose S J, Crandell C C, Strube M J 1991 Reliability of isokinetic measurements of trunk muscle performance. Spine 16: 800–803

de Morton N A, Keating J L 2002 The effect of preload on variability in dynamometric measurements of knee extension. European Journal of Applied Physiology 86: 355–362

Dvir Z, Keating J 2001a The reproducibility of isokinetic trunk extension: a study using very short range of motion. Clinical Biomechanics 16: 627–630

Dvir Z, Keating J 2001b Identification of feigned isokinetic trunk extension effort: an efficiency study of the DEC. Spine 26: 1046–1051

Dvir Z, Keating J 2003 Trunk extension strength and validation of trunk extension effort in chronic low-back dysfunction patients. Spine, in press

Dvir Z, Eger G, Halperin N, Shklar A 1989 Thigh muscles activity and anterior cruciate ligament insufficiency. Clinical Biomechanics 4: 87–91

Dvir Z, Halperin N, Shklar A, Robinson D 1991a Quadriceps function and patellofemoral pain syndrome. Part I: pain provocation during concentric and eccentric isokinetic activity. Isokinetics and Exercise Science 1: 26–30

Dvir Z, Halperin N, Robinson D, Shklar A 1991b Quadriceps function with patellofemoral pain syndrome. Part II: the break phenomenon during eccentric activity. Isokinetics and Exercise Science 1: 31–35

Dvir Z, Steinfeld-Cohen Y, Peretz C 2002 The identification of feigned isokinetic shoulder flexion weakness in normal subjects. American Journal of Physical Medicine and Rehabilitation 81: 178–183

Elert J, Gerdle B 1989 The relationship between contraction and relaxation during fatiguing isokinetic shoulder flexions. An electromyographic study. European Journal of Applied Physiology 59: 303–309

Emery M, Sitler I, Ryan J 1994 Mode of action and angular velocity fatigue response of the hamstrings and quadriceps. Isokinetics and Exercise Science 4: 91–95

Farrell M, Richards J E 1986 Analysis of the reliability and validity of the kinetic communicator exercise device. Medicine and Science in Sports and Exercise 18: 44–49

Felicetti G, Zelaschi F, Di Patrizi S 1994 Endurance tests during isokinetic contraction: reliability of functional parameters. Isokinetics and Exercise Science 4: 76–80

Figoni S F, Morris A F 1984 Effects of knowledge of results on reciprocal isokinetic strength and fatigue. Journal of Orthopaedic and Sports Physical Therapy 6: 190–197

Gerdle B, Fugl-Meyer A R 1985 Mechanical output and iEMG of isokinetic plantarflexion in 40–64 year old subjects. Acta Physiologica Scandinavica 124: 210–211

Gerdle B, Elert J, Hendriksson-Larsen K 1989 Muscular fatigue during repeated isokinetic shoulder forward flexions in young females. European Journal of Applied Physiology 59: 666–673

Gerdle B, Karlsson S, Crenshaw A G, Fridén J, Lennart N 1998 Characteristics of the shift from fatigue phase to the endurance level (breakpoint) of peak torque during repeated dynamic maximal knee extensions are correlated to muscle morphology. Isokinetics and Exercise Science 7: 49–60

Gleeson N P, Mercer T H 1992 Reproducibility of isokinetic leg strength and endurance characteristics of adult men and women. European Journal of Applied Physiology and Occupational Physiology 65: 221–228

Glousman R, Jobe F, Tibone J et al 1988 Dynamic electromyographic analysis of the throwing shoulder with glenohumeral instability. Journal of Bone and Joint Surgery 70A: 220–226

Grace T G 1985 Muscle imbalance and extremity injury: a perplexing relationship. Sports Medicine 2: 77–82

Grace T G, Sweetser E, Nelson M, Skipper B J 1984 Isokinetic muscle imbalance and knee joint injuries. Journal of Bone and Joint Surgery 66A: 734–740

Gransberg L, Knutsson E 1983 Determination of dynamic muscle strength in man with acceleration controlled isokinetic movements. Acta Physiologica Scandinavica 119: 317–320

Gravel D, Richards C L, Filion M 1988 Influence of contractile tension development on dynamic strength measurements of the plantarflexors in man. Journal of Biomechanics 21: 89–96

Gray J C, Chandler J M 1989 Percent decline in peak torque production during repeated concentric and eccentric contractions of the quadriceps femoris muscle. Journal of Orthopaedic and Sports Physical Therapy 10: 309–313

Hald R D, Bottjen E J 1987 Effect of visual feedback on maximal and submaximal isokinetic test measurements of normal quadriceps and hamstrings. Journal of Orthopaedic and Sports Physical Therapy 9: 86–93

Herzog W 1988 The relation between the resultant moments at a joint and the moments measured by an isokinetic dynamometer. Journal of Biomechanics 21: 5–12

Hinson M N, Smith S C, Funk S 1979 Isokinetics: a clarification. Research Quarterly 50: 30–35

Hobbel S L, Rose D J 1993 The relative effectiveness of three forms of visual knowledge of results on peak torque output. Journal of Orthopaedic and Sports Physical Therapy 18: 601–608

Hoke B, Howell D, Stack M 1983 The relationship between isokinetic testing and dynamic patellofemoral compression. Journal of Orthopaedic and Sports Physical Therapy 4: 150–153

Iossifidou A N, Baltzopoulos V 1996 Angular velocity in eccentric isokinetic dynamometer. Isokinetics and Exercise Science 6: 65–70

Iossifidou A N, Baltzopoulos V 1998a Relationship between peak moment, power and work corrected for the influence of inertial effects. Isokinetics and Exercise Science 7: 79–86

Iossifidou A N, Baltzopoulos V 1998b Inertial effects on moment curves and angle of peak moment during isokinetic knee extension. Isokinetics and Exercise Science 7: 87–93

Iossifidou A N, Baltzopoulos V 2000 Peak power assessment in isokinetic dynamometry. European Journal of Applied Physiology 82: 158–160

Ivey F M, Calhoun J H, Rusche K, Bierschenk J 1985 Isokinetic testing of shoulder strength: normal values. Archives of Physical Medicine and Rehabilitation 66: 384–386

Jaric S, Radosavljevic-Jaric S, Johansson H 2002 Muscle force and muscle torque in humans require different methods when adjusting for differences in body size. Journal of Applied Physiology 87: 304–307

Jensen R C, Warren B, Laursen C, Morrissey M C 1991 Static pre-load effect on knee extensor isokinetic concentric and eccentric performance. Medicine and Science in Sports and Exercise 23: 10–14

Kannus P, Jarvinen M, Lehto M 1991 Maximal peak torque as a predictor of angle-specific torques of hamstring and quadriceps muscles in man. European Journal of Applied Physiology 63: 112–118

Kramer J F, MacDermid J 1989 Isokinetic measures during concentric–eccentric cycles of the knee extensors. Physiotherapy Canada 35: 9–14

Kramer J F, Vaz M D, Hakansson D 1991 Effect of activation force on knee extensor torques. Medicine and Science in Sports and Exercise 23: 231–237

Kues J M, Rothstein J M, Lamb R L 1992 Obtaining reliable measurements of knee extensor torque produced during maximal voluntary contractions: an experimental investigation. Physical Therapy 72: 492–504

Manou P, Arseniou V, Kellis S 2002 Test–retest reliability of an isokinetic muscle endurance test. Isokinetics and Exercise Science, in press.

Mathiassen S E 1989 Influence of angular velocity and movement frequency on development of fatigue in repeated isokinetic knee extensions. European Journal of Applied Physiology 59: 80–88

Mayer T G, Gatchel R 1987 A prospective two-year study of functional restoration in industrial low back injury. Journal of the American Medical Association 258: 1763–1767

Mayhew T P 1992 Commentary. Physical Therapy 72: 593–594

Morrissey M C 1987 The relationship between peak torque and work of the quadriceps and hamstring after meniscectomy. Journal of Orthopaedic and Sports Physical Therapy 8: 405–408

Motzkin N, Cahalan T D, Morrey B F, An K-N, Chao E Y S 1991 Isometric and isokinetic endurance testing of the forearm complex. American Journal of Sports Medicine 19: 107–111

Narici M V, Sirtori M D, Mastore P, Mognoni P 1991 The effect of range of motion and isometric preactivation on isokinetic torques. European Journal of Applied Physiology 62: 216–220

Newton M, Thow M, Somerville D, Henderson I, Waddell G 1993 Trunk strength testing with isomachines part II: experimental evaluation of the Cybex II back resting system in normal subjects and patients with chronic low back pain. Spine 18: 812–824

Nordgren B, Nordesjo L, Rauschning W 1983 Isokinetic knee extension strength and pain before and after advanced osteotomy of the tibial tuberosity. Archives of Orthopaedic and Traumatic Surgery 192: 95–101

Oberg B, Bergman T, Tropp H 1987 Testing of isokinetic muscle strength in the ankle. Medicine and Science in Sports and Exercise 19: 318–322

Osternig L R 1986 Isokinetic dynamometry: implications for muscle testing and rehabilitation. Exercise and Sports Science Reviews 14: 45–80

Osternig L R, Sawhill J A, Bares B T, Hamill J 1983 Function of limb speed on torque pattern of antagonistic muscles. Biomechanics VIII-A. Human Kinetics, Champaign, Illinois

Patton R W, Hinson M M, Arnold B R, Lessard B 1978 Fatigue curves of isokinetic contractions. Archives of Physical Medicine and Rehabilitation 59: 507–509

Peacock B, Westers S, Walsh S, Nicholson K 1981 Feedback and maximum voluntary contraction. Ergonomics 24: 223–228

Perrine J, Edgerton V R 1978 Muscle force–velocity and power–velocity relationships under isokinetic loading. Medicine and Science in Sports 10: 159–166

Piette V, Richards C, Milton F 1986 Use of static preloading in estimation of dynamic strength with the KinCom dynamometer. In: Proceedings of the North American Congress on Biomechanics, Montreal, pp 261–262

Rathfon J A, Matthews K M, Yang A N, Levangie P K, Morrissey M C 1991 Effects of different acceleration and deceleration rates on isokinetic performance of the knee extensors. Journal of Orthopaedic and Sports Physical Therapy 14: 161–168

Rothstein J M, Delitto A, Sinacore D R, Rose S J 1983 Electromyographic, peak torque and power relationships during isokinetic movements. Physical Therapy 63: 926–933

Rothstein J M, Lamb R L, Mayhew T P 1987 Clinical uses of isokinetic measurements: critical issues. Physical Therapy 67: 1840–1844

Sale D G 1991 Testing strength and power. In: MacDougall J D, Wenger H A, Green H J (eds) Physiological testing of the high performance athlete, 2nd edn. Human Kinetics, Champaign, Illinois

Sale D G, MacDougall J D, Alway S E, Sutton J R 1987 Voluntary strength and muscle characteristics in untrained men and women and male bodybuilders. Journal of Applied Physiology 62: 1786–1793

Sapega A A 1990 Muscle performance evaluation in orthopaedic practice. Journal of Bone and Joint Surgery 72A: 1562–1574

Sapega A A, Nicholas J A, Sokolow D, Saraniti A 1982 The nature of torque 'overshoot' in Cybex isokinetic dynamometry. Medicine and Science in Sports and Exercise 14: 368–375

Schwendner K I, Mikeski A E, Wigglesworth J K, Burr D B 1995 Recovery of dynamic muscle function following isokinetic fatigue testing. International Journal of Sports Medicine 16: 185–189

Signorile J F, Applegate B 2000 Three-dimensional mapping. In: Brown L E (ed) Isokinetics in human performance. Human Kinetics, Champaign, Illinois

Thorstensson A, Karlsson J 1976 Fatiguability and fibre composition of human skeletal muscle. Acta Physiologica Scandinavica 98: 318–322

Timm K E 1992 Lumbar spine testing and rehabilitation. In: Davies G J (ed) A compendium of isokinetics in clinical usage. S & S Publishers, Onalaska, Wisconsin, pp 497–532

Tis L L, Perrin D H, Weltman A, Ball D W, Gieck J H 1993 Effect of preload and range of motion on isokinetic average and peak torque of the knee extensor and flexor musculature. Medicine and Science in Sports and Exercise 25: 1038–1043

Wessel J, Ford D, Van Driesum D 1992 Measurement of torque of trunk flexors at different velocities. Scandinavian Journal of Rehabilitation Medicine 24: 175–180

Wilk K E, Arrigo C A, Andrews J R 1991 Standardized isokinetic testing protocol for the throwing shoulder: the throwers' series. Isokinetics and Exercise Science 1: 63–71

Winter D A, Wells R P, Orr G W 1981 Errors in the use of isokinetic dynamometers. European Journal of Applied Physiology 46: 397–408

Reproducibility of isokinetic measurements

INTRODUCTION

Since the publication of the first edition of this book the number of studies and in-depth analyses relating to various aspects of reproducibility of isokinetic findings has risen quite profoundly. This development and the pivotal importance of reproducibility for the correct interpretation of isokinetic data has led to the dedication of a full chapter to this subject. Due to some misconceptions regarding the use of reproducibility assessment techniques, this chapter introduces a number of basic tools along with more advanced techniques as well as their application in the field of isokinetics.

Although a high degree of reproducibility is essential to all kinds of human-related measurements, meeting this demand satisfactorily takes up significantly harder proportions where subject (patient) *performance* is at stake. Unlike tests which do not require active participation of the subject (e.g. ECG), what singles out performance measurements is the complex part played by the subject or patient. This element introduces inherent as well as interactive sources of measurement variations. In this respect, measurements derived from isokinetic dynamometry incorporate all sources of such variations extending from purely (and seemingly simple) technical factors such as axis alignment to complex neurobehavioral elements like motivation. The cumulative effect of the vast number of factors involved in strength testing, particularly upon using isokinetic dynamometry, ensures that no two tests, believed to be the product of identical conditions (e.g. two consecutive exertions of maximal knee extension) will, strictly speaking, yield exactly the same findings. Although it may be argued that detection of differences depends on the precision of the system, it has to be realized that variations in strength output as measured by any instrument possess a random component and are an inherent and a normal expression of human motor behavior. Reproducibility analysis is meant to assess these variations and quantitatively define their range.

Thus, in trying to define the most important role reproducibility has in the context of clinical isokinetic measurements, the impression emerging from hundreds of papers which have applied this technology relates to two issues:

1. *How representative is a strength score?* The mere testing of strength relating to a given muscle and patient (subject) group does not ensure that the results are of any *clinical* significance unless on repeated tests, sufficiently similar results are produced under the same circumstances (e.g. test protocol and environment). In other words, if the variations observed upon repeated tests are judged *clinically* to be too wide, such scores may not be acceptable. The emphasis on clinical is not a vain one; whether a particular methodology and its associated findings are clinically acceptable is a clinically based and not a statistically based decision. Needless to say, a positive decision regarding reproducibility does not render the findings clinically valid.

2. *How to divide observed changes* into those that reflect a true change from those that could be attributed to normal variations – namely the so-called measurement error – is equally important from the clinical point of view. Since reproducibility analysis is based on statistical concepts, in its very essence it is intimately connected with the theory of probability. In other words, the margin of *normal variations* or *measurement error* must eventually be defined with respect to the applied level of confidence. Wider margins require, by definition, that larger variations take place in order to indicate a genuine change and vice versa.

In view of the apparent diversity of opinions concerning the interpretation of the concept of reproducibility, this chapter opens with a description of the relevant measurement scale, types of error and definition and types of reproducibility. These will be followed by a systematic description of various reproducibility indices and their application in analyzing isokinetic data. A summary and recommendations for a standard format conclude this chapter.

THE ISOKINETIC MEASUREMENT SCALE, TYPES OF ERROR AND REPRODUCIBILITY

Measurement scale

While isokinetic test results are expressed in discrete units – newton-meters (Nm), ft-lb, joules (J) – it should be emphasized that this is a result of the conversion of the analog force signal to a digital format rather than the nature of the measurement. The force or moment that is being measured is a continuous variable and whereas no question arises as to its upper limit (the maximum recorded capacity for the particular muscle group), the meaning of zero moment (strength) requires elaboration as it is this factor that ultimately determines whether isokinetic findings are to be interpreted in terms of interval or ratio scale. To explore this problem, it is convenient to use terms taken from the method of manual muscle testing (MMT). Strictly speaking zero strength signifies that the relevant muscle is not capable of developing any contractility, a state equivalent to grade 0 in MMT. Furthermore, it is not until muscles reach grade 3 that they are, by definition, capable of moving the distal segment against gravity. Thus, although developing enough tension to counteract the force of gravity, a muscle that is graded 3 on MMT may not be able to move the dynamometer's lever-arm. Therefore a record of 0 Nm does not necessarily mean that the tested muscle is not contracting and therefore as pointed out by Rothstein et al (1987) a true zero is an elusive entity as far as isokinetic measurements are concerned.

This deficiency can however be rectified by subtracting or adding the gravitational moment which in principle is the missing term. Consider for instance extension of the knee from 90° of flexion (leg hanging freely) to full extension when performed at the standard sitting position. Initially, the gravitational moment is zero and hence as soon as the tension which is developed by the quadriceps is greater than the minimal possible isometric preactivation bias (IPB), motion ensues. The gravitational demand rises with movement towards extension and reaches its maximum when the leg is in the horizontal position. The true moment developed by the muscle is then the combined recorded and gravitational moments. If the previous is 160 Nm and the latter is 10 Nm, quadriceps strength is 170 Nm. Admittedly, the gravitational correction procedures may not operate very satisfactorily, particularly with respect to trunk strength (Bygott et al 2001a,b), yet they seem to go some way for other segments. It should also be borne in mind that other than in the case of testing of trunk muscles in the upright and hip abductors in the side-lying position, the size of the gravitational effect relative to maximal isokinetic strength is quite low: between 5 and 10% (Dvir 1997). Furthermore, for some muscles (e.g. those operating in grip) and positions (testing all major hip muscles in standing using a very short range of motion) this effect is quite negligible. Consequently, despite the above reservations, isokinetic measurements may justifiably be considered in terms of a ratio, rather than an interval, scale (Atkinson & Nevill 1998). This means that from the statistical point of view test findings may be processed using any of the available procedures. It also allows the application of 'ratios of agreement', a novel and promising technique for expressing and interpreting variations in strength (Atkinson & Nevill 1998).

Reproducibility, also known by terms such as reliability and repeatability, relates to the consistency of measurements where consistency may relate to repeated events that are measured within seconds, days or weeks (see below). It is by no means an absolute concept in that it reflects the 'amount of *measurement error* ... deemed acceptable for the effective [and] practical use of the measurement tool' (Atkinson & Nevill 1998). The term *error* deserves special attention as its statistical connotation is not equivalent to the commonly perceived meaning of this word. In measurement theory error refers to all sources of variability within a set of data that cannot be explained by the independent variable (Portney & Watkins 2000). A measurement (rather than, for example, simple counting) relating to any physical or behavioral variable incorporates two components: the *true* score (T) and an *error* score (E). The relationship between the measure (X), T and E is expressed by the following formula:

$$X = T \pm E \qquad \text{(Equation 1)}$$

Since a perfect measurement would require an infinite precision which is an unattainable goal, the *true* value of the measurand is never known. As a result all measuring instruments have a limited precision and therefore provide only *estimates* of the measurand. It should be emphasized that the *operational* precision of the measurement device derives from technological, commercial and practical constraints. For instance, isokinetic muscle strength could be measured in units of ± 0.1 Nm but given the absolute magnitude of most muscle groups and the inherent error, such precision may not add significantly to interpretation of the findings.

Types of error

Irrespective of the measurant, all measurements involve *random* errors and some also include *systematic* errors. Random errors reflect unpredictable fluctuations in the scores. However providing a sufficiently large number of measurements is performed, these fluctuations are distributed around the mean score of the measurements in such a way that they cancel each other out. This leaves the mean as the best estimate of the true score.

Random error

Sources of random error abound in isokinetic testing. Consider for example some of the errors introduced in measurement of hip flexion strength. This test is best performed at the functional position of standing but for that to be effected the tested limb must be clear of the support platform if zero flexion (upright) position is to be included in the range of motion. Assuming this is the case some test-to-test variations in pelvic lateral tilt are inevitable introducing a source of error due to resulting length changes in the contracting muscles. Moreover, stabilization for testing in the upright position requires that the trunk, pelvis, thigh and shank are firmly controlled otherwise contributions from other muscle groups are likely to take place. Unavoidable and unpredictable changes of slackness in the stabilizing belts introduce error.

Random variations are also typical with respect to the location of the flexion axis of the hip joint and their effect on the alignment error. Although the greater trochanter serves invariably for the purpose of marking the axis, identifying this anatomical landmark is very problematic with obese subjects. Assuming a dynamometer lever-arm of 30 cm, fluctuations of at least ±1 cm are very likely, and these alone would introduce an error of 3%. If hip muscles are to be tested in other positions (e.g. sitting, side-lying, prone or supine) other, probably more severe difficulties may arise.

The most typical indicator for random error is the variance, s^2, which reflects the difference between the mean ('true' value) and the individual measurements. Similar to Equation 1, the total variance of a set of scores consists of the variances of the true and error scores respectively:

$$s_X^2 = s_T^2 + s_E^2 \qquad \text{(Equation 2)}$$

where s_X^2 is the total variance. The ratio of the true variance to the total variance:

$$r_X = \frac{s_T^2}{s_X^2}$$

is known as the *reliability coefficient* and since all terms in the equation must be positive the extreme values of r_X are 0 and 1. Strictly speaking, the reliability coefficient is not a practical index in the present context (human performance measures) since a gold standard (the true score) is unknown. On the other hand it delineates in relative terms how much of the variance in a set of measurements is due to variations in the true (error) scores. Thus if r_X is equal to 0.9 this means that 90% of the variance in the total score reflects variance in the true score, in other words the measured scores are a good representation of the true score.

Systematic error

Alongside the random error, systematic error is another source for the observed non-similarity in test findings. A systematic error signifies a unidirectional change in scores (larger or smaller) than a parallel set of scores obtained typically from another instrument or another test occasion. Consider for instance the strength scores obtained from six subjects performing maximal shoulder flexion during two test sessions (Table 3.1).

In view of the similar standard deviations within each testing session it is reasonable to assume that a general shift of scores has taken place, probably due to familiarization with the system. Situations where a systematic increase is apparent do not constitute a special *reproducibility* problem. The difficulty is in deciding which of the two (or more) 'true' scores is a genuine representation of the measured quantity, i.e. *validity* of the test findings is being challenged.

Reproducibility

One of the most confusing elements in reproducibility analysis is the simultaneous use of the term for describing the so-called 'internal consistency' and 'stability' of measurements (Baumgartner 1989). *Internal consistency* or repeatability normally refers to variability between repeated trials within the same day (typically

Table 3.1 Hypothetical test-retest scores of isokinetic shoulder flexion strength

Subject	Test	Retest	Difference
1	56	65	9
2	48	53	5
3	41	47	6
4	53	63	10
5	61	70	9
6	43	50	7
Mean	50.3	58.0	7.7
SD	7.4	9.3	

within the same testing session), for instance the variations in average moment scores based on four consecutive intermittent concentric and eccentric contractions. This type of reproducibility will invariably lead to a lesser variance among the individual scores and should be compared with *stability* which relates to day-to-day variability. The value of monitoring the internal consistency within a test cannot be overlooked, particularly in the context of pain provocation or the patient's understanding of the task. However since rehabilitation periods are measured in weeks rather than in days, the more challenging and possibly meaningful type of reproducibility is stability.

In addition to the consistency–stability classification another dichotomy deserves special attention. Reproducibility indices have been divided into *relative* and *absolute* (Baumgartner 1989):

- *Relative reproducibility* is 'the degree to which individuals maintain their position in a sample with repeated measurements' (Atkinson & Nevill 1998) and is normally associated with the use of correlation coefficients such as r and ICC.
- *Absolute reproducibility* is the degree to which repeated measurements vary for individuals. The indices used in this case are expressed using the units of the actual measurement (e.g. the standard error of measurement, SEM) or as a proportion of the measured values (e.g. the coefficient of variation, CV).

Although widely used in the isokinetic literature, it is now being recognized that the value of relative indices for describing reproducibility is rather limited and may even be misleading. On the other hand, since the publication of Bland & Altman's paper (1986), an ever-increasing number of studies have used absolute indices. One of the main objectives of this chapter is therefore a comparative assessment of relative and absolute indices.

Reproducibility indices

This assessment is ultimately concerned with the question: how relevant is a given reproducibility index? Viewed from another perspective, does the fact that a specific index is found to be statistically significant for a given set of data also mean that it is also clinically meaningful? In their excellent review of reliability Atkinson & Nevill (1998) try to answer these questions by introducing several concepts, the most important of which is *analytical goal* or the 'acceptance of a certain degree of measurement error'. Analytical goals move from focusing the analysis on statistical techniques and levels of significance to establishing well-defined criteria which provide clinicians with a more appropriate answer to the question: how far do consecutive sets of measurements need to differ in order to be considered as really different? In the following sections it will be demonstrated that some of the commonly employed reproducibility indices fail to address this critical question and therefore studies that relied on them to prove that a certain protocol led to reproducible findings can no longer serve as a guide.

TESTS AND INDICES EMPLOYED IN ANALYZING REPRODUCIBILITY
The t-test and ANOVA

In the past, one of the most commonly used techniques in assessing the stability of findings was the t-test. In principle, the test is intended to indicate whether a difference exists between the mean scores of the test and the retest. In other words if the resulting t value is significant, the only conclusion that may be permitted concerns the existence of a systematic error (bias). It should be borne in mind that the t score derives from a ratio whose numerator represents the difference between the means and the denominator – their variance. Thus if the variance, which stands for the random error, is relatively large (which it invariably is) the ratio would indicate non-significant differences and therefore lead to a conclusion that the test protocol yields reproducible results. Such a conclusion may often be unwarranted. To demonstrate this situation consider the data in Table 3.2 which is based on a hypothetical isokinetic study of trunk extension strength conducted with 10 subjects. The data refer to two retesting occasions.

For the combination test-retest$_1$ the t score for paired samples (0.53) implies good stability.

Table 3.2	Hypothetical trunk extension scores		
Subject	Test	Retest$_1$	Retest$_2$
1	189	135	191
2	176	137	180
3	171	139	172
4	157	148	159
5	155	151	156
6	149	162	151
7	143	169	145
8	130	172	133
9	126	182	127
10	121	193	122
Mean	151.7	158.8	155.5
SD	22.5	20.0	23.9
$r_{test-retest_1}$	−0.965	$r_{test-retest_2}$	0.998

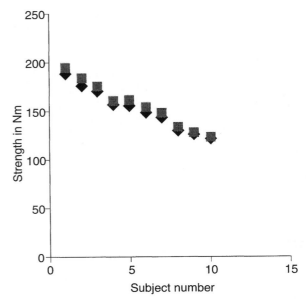

Figure 3.2   Association of strength scores: test-retest$_2$.

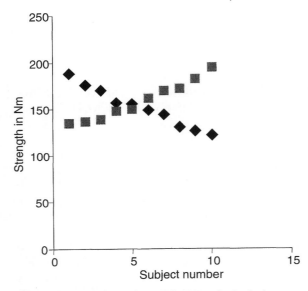

Figure 3.1   Association of strength scores: test-retest$_1$.

However examination of the results (Fig. 3.1) reveals a large variance between the tests and a reverse trend in the scores as evidenced by an almost perfect negative correlation. This strongly suggests very low reproducibility.

On the other hand, consider now the combination of test-retest$_2$ in which a strong positive correlation exists between the findings. In this case the value of t (2.27) indicates a significant difference (at 0.05 level) which ostensibly denotes poor reproducibility. However, inspection of the numerical values and Figure 3.2 reveals that for all subjects,

the strength scores in the retest were larger than the corresponding values in the test indicating a systematic error (bias). The average value of the bias was relatively small: 1.9 Nm (about 1.2% of the average strength) so that together with the almost perfect correlation (r = 0.998) this protocol yields in fact excellent reproducibility.

These two examples serve also to highlight the significance of the term 'analytical goal'. Neither the individual t scores nor their corresponding level of significance facilitate interpretation of the data. For that matter the t scores for the combination test-retest$_2$ could be any number greater than 2.26 (if $a = 0.05$ is the required level of significance) or 3.25 ($a = 0.01$) and still a wrong implication would have been drawn. Moreover, the actual score would not permit scaling of the difference between the test and retest$_2$ scores. Clearly, the same logic is applicable to the combination test-retest$_1$. It may therefore be concluded that as a tool for analyzing reproducibility, the t-test is quite inferior (particularly in comparison to modern techniques) and its use for this specific objective should consequently be especially limited.

More complex study designs may call for the application of analysis of variance (ANOVA) as the preferred statistical tool. Commonly employed for the detection of bias (systematic error) ANOVA is impaired, as much as the t-test, by its vulnerability to large random variations. One reason for performing ANOVA is the ability to use its component variances to calculate the intraclass correlation coefficients (ICC). However, relative reproducibility indices, such as the ICC, and the parameters derived from the ANOVA cannot function as independent analytical goals.

Correlational indices

Though different correlation coefficients have been described in the isokinetic literature the two most widely used are Pearson's r (heretofore r) and the ICC. The latter was described in a classical paper by Shrout & Fleiss (1979) and has since been reported in almost every paper dealing with reproducibility of dynamometric findings. Both are classified as indices of relative reproducibility which is concerned with the question: to what extent will individual measurements within a group maintain their position over repeated measurements? (Myrer et al 1996).

Pearson's r

Pearson's r is a bivariate index, i.e. it measures the covariation of two sets of measurements derived from two independent variables. Thus, strictly speaking, r is *not* supposed to be applied to two separate sets of measurements derived from the *same* variable. However there are two major problems with using r in reproducibility analysis. First, this index measures the *strength of relation* between two sets of measurements, not their *agreement*. The term 'strength of relation' means that the independent sets vary in the same way, namely individual measurements retain their relative position in both sets. This does not necessarily mean that they repeat each other (i.e. demonstrate stability). Consider for example five original measurements: 10, 20, 30, 40, 50 (set I). If on retesting (set II) the values are: 13, 23, 33, 43 and 53 the test-retest r will be the same compared to yet another set (III) of assigned values: 18, 36, 54, 72, 90 which clearly is much different from set II. In both cases r = 1.00 as indicated by a single line which passes through all

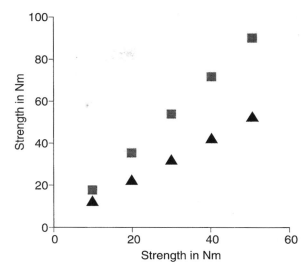

Figure 3.3 Test-retest correlations: triangles, sets I–II; squares, sets I–III.

points relating set I to set II and set III respectively (Fig. 3.3). Furthermore inspecting these lines reveals that in comparison to set III, set II demonstrated a much better agreement with the original set (I) as the difference between the respective sets (II vs I) was uniform: 3 Nm. This fact is not borne out by r. This is a significant drawback where systematic errors induced by fatigue or experience-based improvement ('learning') effects are analyzed using Pearson's r.

The second weakness of r is its dependence on the range of measurements within the sets, the larger the range the higher the correlation. Consider for instance the test-retest results obtained from knee flexion strength measurement of two hypothetical groups (Table 3.3). The difference between Group I and Group II is only one subject (10).

As evident from Figures 3.4 and 3.5 the replacement of subject 10 in Group I whose scores were similar to his peers with a subject who had particularly low scores shifted r from what can be described as a moderate to a very strong association. This drastic variation results directly from the way r is calculated, i.e. its reliance on the variance of the scores. Furthermore as mentioned by Bland & Altman (1986) highly correlated sets of findings can conceal considerable disagreement so that exclusive reliance on r may lead to gross

Table 3.3   Hypothetical knee flexion scores

Subject	Group I		Group II	
	Test I	Retest I	Test II	Retest II
1	121	124	121	124
2	129	128	129	128
3	119	125	119	125
4	130	136	130	136
5	125	127	125	127
6	118	121	118	121
7	122	132	122	132
8	117	128	117	128
9	125	130	125	130
10	126	127	104	105

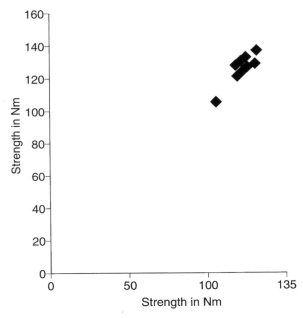

Figure 3.5   Group II: r = 0.89.

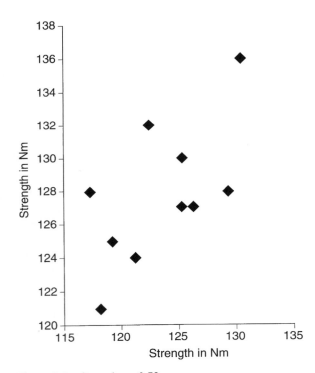

Figure 3.4   Group I: r = 0.58.

misinterpretation of the reproducibility of find-ings. To highlight the serious drawbacks asso-ciated with the use of a relative reproducibility index like r, a comparison to the consequences drawn from the application of absolute indices to the same database is essential. However, it is safe to state that previous isokinetic reproducibility studies that consisted of heterogenous popula-tions and expressed the outcome in terms of Pearson's r must be viewed with great caution.

Ostensibly the use of heterogenous samples renders the results more generalizable. However, this may lead to misinterpretation of the results. On the other hand homogenous samples, particu-larly those relating to groups with a special pathol-ogy, are invariably more difficult to comprise and their results will, by definition, apply only to the selected groups. Thus a fine line passes between these two ends. How heterogenous a sample is is not an easy question to answer. Nevertheless in the context of isokinetic dynamometry and subject/patient characteristics, mixing of genders, age decades, physique and activity levels could intro-duce extreme scores and result in irrelevantly high r values. Needless to say, the incorporation of find-ings derived from different protocols into one data set would be strictly inadvisable.

Intraclass correlation coefficients

Intraclass correlation coefficients (ICC) are derived from analysis of variance (ANOVA) with repeated measures and would be interpretable only if F is significant. Similar to Pearson's r the ICC can assume any value between 0 and 1. This index is supposed to reflect not only the strength of association but the actual *agreement* between scores and unlike r it can assess the correlation among a number of factors (e.g. raters). The ICC main strength is in providing information about the ability of a given test or measure to differentiate among subjects or patients (Stratford & Goldsmith 1997). Thus in assessing the comparative differentiating strength of a test a higher ICC score indicates a better discriminatory power.

As outlined by Shrout & Fleiss (1979) there are six ways to calculate the ICCs. However not all of these are commonly used in analyzing reproducibility of isokinetic data. The six types are based on three *models* and two *forms* (Portney & Watkins 2000):

- In Model 1 each subject is measured by a *different* set of k raters and hence it is rarely, if at all, applicable in studying reproducibility of human performance data.
- In Model 2 each subject is measured by the same raters who are selected at random.
- In Model 3 each subject is measured by the same raters who are intentionally selected – no generalization beyond this group of raters is allowed.

In Model 3, for instance, such a situation may occur when two highly trained clinicians, out of a group of clinicians working at the same site, conduct a reproducibility study of a specific isokinetic protocol. Obviously the findings obtained cannot be extended to any clinician. However this element is often of minor relevance as it is assumed that only those skilled in performing isokinetic tests are the only ones who actually do them.

The two forms relate to either a single score or a mean score as the unit of interest. Thus when prescribing ICC(2,1) it is understood that all subjects were tested by same raters and that the score quoted represented a single unit of measurement. As a general rule, ICCs that are based on the mean value of k scores – namely (1,k), (2,k), (3,k) – are higher than their counterparts which are based on a single score: (1,1), (2,1), (3,1). This is a direct

outcome of the way the ICC is calculated. Moreover, the size of the ICC obtained from the same data set follows the order Model 3 > Model 2 > Model 1. This again reflects the fact that as the extent of randomness in selecting the raters is limited a higher agreement between them should be indicated (Walmsley & Amell 1996). Therefore, when quoting ICC it is imperative that the model is explicitly specified as the clinical significance of, say ICC = 0.86, which is based on model (2,1) is materially different from that which applies to model (3,k). Furthermore, citing the confidence intervals for a given ICC has been advocated (Stratford 1997). Consequently, depending on the specific confidence intervals the discriminating power of a test or measure could be less than the ostensibly acceptable cutoffs (e.g. 0.75). Because most isokinetic tests are performed by the same clinician reproducibility of measurements often relates to the intrarater set-up and therefore the most common method for assessing this type of reproducibility is based on ANOVA with repeated measures incorporating a single measurement, namely model (3,1).

The great popularity of ICC in human performance testing literature must however be qualified by the fact that ICC are prone to the same limitations which apply to Pearson's r, i.e. they are affected by the sample heterogeneity. In other words a high ICC is not mutually exclusive with unacceptable measurement error for some analytical goals (Bland & Altman 1990, Atkinson & Nevill 1998). As correctly pointed out by Bland & Altman '... we want a method of assessing agreement which is not dependent on the particular subjects we choose to investigate'. Another qualifier concerns the absolute value of the ICC as a measure of reproducibility. It has been suggested, in however muted terminology, that an ICC of 0.90 or greater was essential for ensuring reasonable validity (Portney & Watkins 2000). On the other hand ICC < 0.75 indicates poor reproducibility. Apart from the fact that the validity of applying these cutoffs was never tested in the context of isokinetic assessments, the strong effect the sample variance has on the size of the ICC renders them much less relevant. Thus although the ICC provides some useful information the mere reliance on this index to prove that the data are stable is unjustified.

SUMMARY OF TESTS AND INDICES

To sum up this section, none of the three indices mentioned so far – t-test, r and ICC – provide a number which can be singularly applied for interpretation of isokinetic tests. The t score relates to the question of whether a difference exists between two sets of measurements. On its own it is quite meaningless and even when leading to a conclusion, namely no difference or significant difference, this conclusion, as outlined by the above examples, may be erroneous. Both r and ICC provide *numerical scores* which strongly depend on the variance of the test findings. Thus, unless the range of raw scores and their variances are outlined, their clinical significance is limited. Especially noteworthy, neither r nor ICC can be interpreted in terms of percentage, a conceptual extension adopted by many users when trying to explain the meaning of a given score, for example ICC (3,1) = 0.9. Often incorrect notions such as the test-retest scores are identical 90% of the time are heard. In other words, as a guide to interpreting the stability of the data and hence to deciding whether a true change has taken place, none of the above indices is suitable. Recognition of these serious drawbacks provided the impetus for searching for alternative and clinically interpretable indices. These indices are the main issue of the next section.

Absolute indices

Absolute indices indicate the extent to which a score varies on repeated measurement (Myrer et al 1996). They differ from their *relative* counterparts by not being variance dependent. Consequently the relative rank of an individual subject within a group is irrelevant. These indices which are expressed in units that are readily interpretable allow extrapolation to new individuals as well as comparison between different measurement tools (Atkinson & Nevill 1998) and hence the significant increase in their application in reproducibility analysis. In the following, each of the four main indices – standard error of measurement,

coefficient of variation, method error and limits of agreement – is described.

The standard error of measurement (SEM)

An often used statistic for assessing reproducibility is the SEM. It is derived from the test-retest correlation, Pearson's r or ICC, and the SD of the individual measurements and is expressed by the following formula:

$$SEM = SD\sqrt{1 - r_{xx}} \quad \text{or} \quad SEM = SD\sqrt{1 - ICC}$$

Thus in case of a *perfect agreement* (zero bias; r, ICC = 1) the SEM is zero and any change is a true one. One of the significant features of the SEM is that it is expressed in the same units as the base measurements namely Nm (or ft-lb) for strength. Therefore it provides a satisfactory tool for comparing different test protocols or measurement systems given the same study samples.

It should be noted that since the SD is integral to its formula, the SEM is still affected by the extent to which the sample is homogenous. In other words, if the data are homoscedastic (i.e. the error is unaffected by the absolute magnitude of the measurand) the SEM will be valid across the range of measurements irrespective of their magnitude. On the other hand if a positive relationship exists between the absolute magnitude of the variable and the associated error, a situation defined by the term heteroscedasticity, the SEM will not be applicable to all data points. That heteroscedasticity is often characteristic of isokinetic strength scores has been indicated by a number of studies and highlighted extensively in an excellent meta-analytic paper by Keating & Matyas (1998). Using data reported in the following papers they were able to reconstruct the SEM versus the magnitude of isokinetic strength scores.

In a study by Frontera et al (1993) flexion and extension strength in the knee and elbow were measured twice over 7–10 days at two different test velocities: 60 and 240°/s (knee) and 60 and 180°/s (elbow). Of the between-session variability in measurements, 88% was attributable to changes in strength (mean scores) reflecting variations in muscle group and velocity. The same analysis was carried out with respect to the elbow muscles although the relationship was not equally strong. Upon combination of the knee and elbow scores the correlation was, as expected, even higher than for knee musculature alone. Two other studies referring to measurements of knee flexors and extensors were analyzed. Molczyk et al (1991) measured the isometric and concentric strength at 60, 180 and 300°/s whereas Thompson et al (1993) used the same velocities without the isometric conditions. The results reflect the same trends both in absolute as well as relative (line slope term). The variability–magnitude relationship was also explored with respect to muscles operating predominantly on the ankle joint. Karnofel et al (1989) applied test velocities of 30 and 120°/s whereas Wennerberg (1991) used a slightly different paradigm of 60 and 120°/s. The derived relationships indicate a very strong relationship. Nevill & Atkinson (1997) have measured human performance in terms of parameters derived from the Åstrand rhyming, grip strength, vertical jump and isokinetic leg and trunk strength tests. They were able to show quite unequivocally that all of the 13 parameters were heteroscedastic. It is unfortunate that no studies were available for studying this relationship in eccentric performance. This would have been an important addition in terms of studying the nature of error associated with a contraction mode that is possibly controlled by different neural mechanisms compared to its concentric counterpart.

Although a detailed discussion of the reasons for the heteroscedastic nature of isokinetic exertions is beyond the scope of this book it should be emphasized that the motion pattern associated with moving the dynamometer lever-arm using maximal muscle force may not be compared with static situations or instances when the kinematic profile is self-selected. Yet, the fact that variability does increase with magnitude bears evidence to the possible effect of the peripheral noise in the neuromotor circuitry. As proposed by Schmidt et al (1979) this factor is random both within and across contractions as well as muscle groups. It may also be related to the way the neuronal information arriving at the motor pool in the cord is being translated

into the activation of a given number of motor units which ultimately take part in deciding the level of force produced by the muscle.

The main lesson derived from the above collection of studies relates to the interpretation of the SEM in different subject or patient groups. In particular, since the error is positively correlated with score magnitude, the application of SEMs obtained from low scoring subjects to high scoring subjects would be erroneous. For the latter group higher SEMs are indicated leading inevitably to the result that small but significant differences are more difficult to confirm in stronger subjects. On the other hand, using high scores-based SEMs for weaker subjects reflects extra (probably unwarranted) caution. Thus if under a given set of test parameters a difference of 30 Nm in knee extension strength proved to be an indicator of a real change at 95% confidence level in strong normal subjects, any change equal or exceeding this cutoff would automatically be considered significant in relatively weak subjects. Consequently, within the context of isokinetic test data, valid use of an absolute error index like the SEM requires that it is incorporated within a regression equation that allows the user to adjust the expected error to the particular subject group (Keating & Matyas 1998). Alternatively, this situation calls for a relative (rather than an absolute) index to be used as detailed below.

In addition to its strong relationship with test conditions, the SEM has some links with subject factors relating to gender and health status. In the abovementioned study by Frontera et al (1993) it was revealed that men had systematically larger error variance than females and that this variance was highly compatible with the gender-based strength differences. On the other hand the significance of health status is not unequivocal. Grabiner et al (1990) tested trunk extension and flexion strength in normal versus subjects with low back disorder (LBD). In four out of six test conditions, impairment resulted in a higher variance although in all tests LBD subjects scored considerably less than their normal counterparts, particularly in extension. The same trend, although statistically insignificant, was pointed out by Durand et al (1991) who compared knee extension and flexion strength in subjects with meniscal injury versus normal controls. In contrast to these findings Estlander et al (1992) indicated that subjects with LBD performing an isokinetic lifting task had a lower unpredictable error. Similarly, in a test-retest study of patients with spastic hemiparesis which compared the involved with the uninvolved side (Tripp & Harris 1991) impairment was generally associated with smaller variance.

Before looking at the next variability index it is worth noting that any decision regarding the nature of strength change (genuine or not) must incorporate explicit reference to the degree of certainty with which it was made. Thus if it is the SEM that serves as the criterion for decision making, quoting the confidence level and intervals is essential. Contrary to some sources, the SEM covers about 68% of the variability and not 95%. Therefore, in order to differentiate between a real change and one which may be attributable to error, at a level of confidence of 95%, the correct index is $1.96\sqrt{2}$SEM (Eliasziw et al 1994).

The coefficient of variation (CV)

The CV has been in fairly common use in isokinetic measurements, so much so that in at least one dynamometer it was incorporated into the result report. The CV is calculated based on an ensemble of measurements and is defined by the formula:

$$CV = \frac{SD}{Mean} * 100$$

For example the following scores were recorded during four consecutive eccentric contractions of the shoulder external rotators at 60°/s: 51, 54, 56 and 55 Nm. The mean score is 54 Nm and the SD 2.16. Therefore the CV for this particular test is:

$$\frac{2.16}{54} * 100 = 4\%$$

Because the mean and SD are given in the same units, the CV is dimensionless and therefore allows comparison of the reproducibility of different methods. In applying this index to isokinetic test data the element of heteroscedasticity is of a positive value as it is assumed that the CV is particularly suitable in cases where the error increases with the magnitude of the measurement. Consider for example an ensemble of test scores obtained from a plantarflexion strength test using two protocols, A and B, which incorporate different warm-up procedures both consisting of various paradigms of submaximal and maximal contractions prior to the criterion test. For A the scores are 101, 94, 87 and 98 for the first, second, third and fourth repetition whereas for B they are 102, 109, 115 and 118, respectively. The CVs are 6.37% (for A) and 6.36% (for B) indicating excellent compatibility in terms of the internal consistency in spite of a considerable difference in the mean ensemble score (95 in A vs 111 in B). Interestingly as a derivate of the mean and SD, the CV (much like the SEM) pays no respect to the conspicuous variation in trend demonstrated in these protocols: whereas the findings in protocol A showed no definite pattern, those from protocol B demonstrate a clear rise in values as a function of repetition number. As a further example, both of these protocols should be compared to protocol C involving stretching only in which the results 61, 79, 88 and 96 lead to a much inferior CV of 18.6%.

Similar to the SEM, application of the CV assumes the findings exhibit normal distribution. Thus a CV of 7% means that 68% of the differences between tests are within 7% of the mean of the data. In order to cover 95% of the cases, it has been suggested that the SD should be multiplied by 1.96. However, such a mathematical operation is still short of being applicable to all subjects as pointed out by Quan & Shih (1996). As an analytical goal the CV has in the past been utilized to indicate whether muscular efforts were performed at maximal or submaximal levels. Specifically it was suggested that if the CV of an ensemble of repeated contractions (isometric or isokinetic) exceeded 10% there was a real likelihood that they reflected submaximal effort. It is now well established that this analytical goal in particular or the use of CV for this particular application is generally without merit (see Chapter 5).

Method error (ME)

This index is a measure of the discrepancy between two sets of repeated scores (Portney & Watkins

2000) and is calculated using the following formula:

$$ME = \frac{S_d}{\sqrt{2}}$$

where S_d is the SD of the difference in scores between the test and retest. In order to be appropriately interpreted the ME is divided by the mean differences and converted to percentage using the CV. In this case the CV_{ME} is:

$$CV_{ME} = \frac{2ME}{(X_{test} + X_{retest})}$$

A variant of this index has also been used by Holmbäck et al (1999) to establish the reproducibility of ankle dorsiflexion strength. In this paper the formula was of the form:

$$CV = \frac{ME}{Xc} * 100$$

where Xc is the mean for all observations. It appears that in this particular case the authors have treated X_{test} and X_{retest} as equal in magnitude and hence the use of a global rather than test-based mean.

The limits of agreement (LOA)

As mentioned before, the various correlation coefficients which have been the mainstay of reproducibility analysis, are greatly influenced by the range of the measurements and describe the association rather than the agreement between the measured variables. In a similar fashion, the matched pairs t-test or repeated measures ANOVA would be affected by the variance within subjects returning a 'no difference' answer in the face of an unacceptable extent of random variation (Nevill & Atkinson 1997). Cognizant of these limitations, Bland & Altman (1986) suggested a different approach, termed the limits of agreement (LOA) which is strongly linked to the standard deviation of the *differences* between two sets of measurements, derived from *two* different methods. Thus the original intention was to explore whether two methods of measurement could be used interchangeably (Bland & Altman 1990). This paradigm was later extended to include

Table 3.4 Hypothetical shoulder internal rotation strength (peak moment) scores

Subject	Test 1	Test 2	Mean	Difference	Absolute difference
1	30	26	28	4	4
2	32	34	33	−2	2
3	41	46	43.5	−5	5
4	62	62	62	0	0
5	27	30	28.5	−3	3
6	42	51	46.5	−9	9
7	43	53	48	−10	10
8	66	66	66	0	0
9	46	57	51.5	−11	11
10	39	43	41	−4	4
11	42	44	43	−2	2
12	56	48	52	8	8
13	60	59	59.5	1	1
14	41	42	41.5	−1	1
15	48	47	47.5	1	1
16	48	43	45.5	5	5
17	43	48	45.5	−5	5
18	50	52	51	−2	2
19	39	40	39.5	−1	1
20	51	56	53.5	−5	5
Mean	45.3			−2.05	
SD				4.605	

assessment of differences recorded using the same method on two different occasions.

In using the LOA for assessing the reproducibility, the findings of the second session are subtracted from the respective scores of the first session and presented against their mean score. For instance, if a subject scores 84 Nm on test and 94 Nm on retest, the individual 'bias' is −10 Nm (84 − 94) and the mean score is 89 Nm. The mean of the individual 'biases' is considered the global bias. Obviously a positive bias indicates that the retest scores were on average lower than the test scores and vice versa. The SD of the differences (individual 'biases') is then calculated and multiplied by 1.96 to yield the 95% limits within which the two tests (or testing systems) 'agree'.

To illustrate the way in which LOA is applied to reproducibility analysis of isokinetic findings consider the statistics in Table 3.4 derived from hypothetical test-retest data ($n = 30$) of shoulder concentric internal rotation strength. The graphical presentation is called a Bland–Altman plot and depicts the relationship between the error and the mean score (Fig. 3.6).

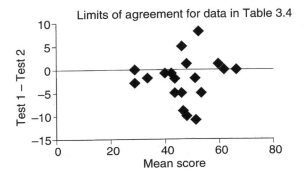

Figure 3.6   Bland–Altman plot for data in Table 3.4.

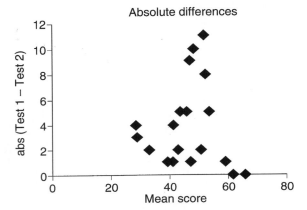

Figure 3.7   Limits of agreement: absolute differences versus mean scores.

The calculated bias for the data is −2.05 and the SD is 4.605. The negative *bias* indicates that the scores were higher in test 2 compared to test 1. The LOA is formulated in terms of bias ± error where error is equal to 1.96 SD. In this case the 95% LOA is therefore equal to −2.05 ± 9.03 Nm. Assuming the data behave homoscedastically (see below), i.e. the error does *not* change with magnitude of mean score, a group-based improvement in internal rotation strength would, at 95% level of confidence, require at least 7 Nm. Notably, although Pearson's r in this case is 0.89, a comparable criterion regarding the magnitude of variation necessary for a significant change will by no means be provided by this index.

Figure 3.7 is an alternative presentation for the Bland–Altman plot relating to the absolute difference between the test and retest scores. Visual inspection does not reveal a heteroscedastic character and indeed a correlational analysis between the error and the measurements returned a very low value, r = −0.05. This means that the LOA of −2.05 ± 9.03 Nm will be valid throughout the spectrum of strengths. If on the other hand a positive relationship exists between the error and the magnitude of the measurant, a different approach should be adopted.

Indeed in most other studies a clear tendency for heteroscedasticity was observed, notably in a comprehensive study of various performance parameters where isokinetic strength behaved in such manner (Nevill & Atkinson 1997). In this study, heteroscedasticity was judged to take place even when the correlation between the absolute difference and the mean score was as low as 0.3. Furthermore only four out of the 12 correlation coefficients relating to isokinetic tests reached an acceptable level of significance (Table 3.5 refers to the raw (absolute) data). Nevertheless, an alternative approach was taken which is based on the natural log transformed (nlt) values of the original scores. Providing the differences between the nlts are normally distributed, the analysis is valid.

Suppose K_1 and K_2 are such scores deriving from two consecutive tests. The difference between the nlt of these scores:

$$D = \log_e(K_1) - \log_e(K_2) = \log_e\left(\frac{K_1}{K_2}\right)$$

In other words D is equal to the ratio between K_1 and K_2. By taking antilog the resulting 'LOA' the result constitutes a ratio which relates to the bias which is multiplied by another ratio that spans the LOA. It should be emphasized that the bias is no longer the arithmetic mean of the differences but a dimensionless geometric mean obtained by dividing the two measurement methods. Thus instead of a LOA which derives from differences, this approach yields a LOA that is based on ratios and should preferably be termed RLOA. In practical terms this manipulation means that in order to indicate a genuine change the second test score must differ from the first not by a given absolute difference but by a given percentage. Table 3.6

Table 3.5 Findings of reproducibility analysis of several strength tests: absolute limits of agreement

Strength variable	Velocity	n	Test	Retest	Difference (SD)	Absolute limits (95%)*	R
Grip (right)	Isometric	12	39.9	40.5	−0.6 (3.0)	−0.6 ± 6.0	0.33
Grip (left)	Isometric	12	36.6	37.2	−0.6 (1.09)	−0.6 ± 2.1	0.24
Extension[K]	60°/s	10	217.3	225.0	−7.7 (21.3)	−7.7 ± 41.8	0.44
	180°/s	10	162.0	162.2	−0.2 (8.4)#	−0.2 ± 15.8	0.32
	300°/s	10	126.1	126.2	−0.1 (9.2)	−0.1 ± 18.0	0.40
Flexion[K]	60°/s	10	128.0	129.2	−1.2 (16.3)	−1.2 ± 32.0	0.31
	180°/s	10	105.5	101.6	3.9 (8.5)	3.9 ± 16.7	0.45
	300°/s	10	89.6	86.5	3.1 (7.0)	3.1 ± 13.6	0.69
Extension[T]	60°/s	31	147.6	165.4	−17.7 (35.8)	−17.7 ± 70.2	0.37
	90°/s	23	164.6	176.8	−12.2 (45.0)	−12.2 ± 88.1	0.34
	120°/s	31	153.2	159.5	−6.4 (47.3)	−6.4 ± 92.7	0.51
Flexion[T]	60°/s	31	179.6	198.8	−19.2 (48.1)	−19.2 ± 94.3	0.60
	90°/s	23	197.5	206.3	−8.8 (52.7)	−8.8 ± 103.3	0.31
	120°/s	31	190.8	202.0	−11.2 (49.7)	−11.2 ± 97.4	0.56

* in Nm; [K] knee; [T] trunk; # differences not normally distributed. All numbers rounded to first decimal.
From Nevill & Atkinson 1997.

Table 3.6 Findings of reproducibility analysis of several strength tests: ratio-based limits of agreement

Strength variable	Velocity	n	Test	Retest	Difference (SD)	Ratio limits (95%)*	R
Grip (right)	Isometric	12	3.665	3.673	−0.0082 (0.073)	0.99(* /)1.15	0.01
Grip (left)	Isometric	12	3.567	3.582	−0.0156 (0.031)	0.98(* /)1.06	−0.18
Extension[K]	60°/s	10	5.349	5.387	−0.0383 (0.088)	0.96(* /)1.19	0.16
	180°/s	10	5.063	5.069	−0.006 (0.047)	0.99(* /)1.10	0.03
	300°/s	10	4.806	4.814	0.0072 (0.069)	0.99(* /)1.14	0.01
Flexion[K]	60°/s	10	4.811	4.912	−0.0118 (0.129)	0.99(* /)1.29	−0.20
	180°/s	10	4.631	4.598	0.0337 (0.076)	1.03(* /)1.16	0.34
	300°/s	10	4.472	4.435	0.0370 (0.071)#	1.04(* /)1.15	0.35
Extension[T]	60°/s	31	4.918	5.048	−0.1298 (0.220)	0.88(* /)1.54	−0.16
	90°/s	23	5.038	5.125	−0.0869 (0.245)	0.92(* /)1.62	−0.03
	120°/s	31	4.957	5.007	−0.0501 (0.273)	0.95(* /)1.71	0.23
Flexion[T]	60°/s	31	5.129	5.218	−0.0895 (0.234)	0.91(* /)1.58	0.21
	90°/s	23	5.222	5.284	−0.0617 (0.247)	0.94(* /)1.62	−0.03
	120°/s	31	5.176	5.251	−0.0751 (0.233)	0.93(* /)1.58	−0.02

* in %; [K] knee; [T] trunk; # differences not normally distributed.
From Nevill & Atkinson 1997.

outlines the RLOA for the absolute LOA scores in Table 3.5.

To illustrate the use of absolute LOA versus ratio-based LOA consider one of the tests outlined in Tables 3.5 and 3.6. The sample of 31 college students, females and males (no number specified) were twice tested for trunk flexion strength at 60°/s. At test 1 the mean score was 179.6 Nm and in the following session the mean score was 198.8 Nm, i.e. a practice-based improvement took place. The differences between the testing sessions were normally distributed using the Anderson-Darling test for normality. The calculated bias was −19.2 Nm with an SD of 48.1 Nm. The 95% LOA in this case was therefore −19.2 ± 94.3 Nm, namely between −113.5 Nm (−19.2 − 94.3) and 75.1 Nm (−19.2 + 94.3). Notably the test-retest correlation was 0.6 and significant. To illustrate the meaning of these limits suppose that under these testing conditions a relatively weak subject scored 132 Nm on Test I. At a 95% level of confidence, this subject would be likely to score, on retest, between as low as $132 - 113.5 = 18.5$ Nm and as high as $132 + 75.1 = 207.1$ Nm. On the other hand, consider a strong subject with an initial score of 244 Nm. The LOA for this subject will be 130.5 and 319.5 Nm. As guides for reproducibility, both of these margins are totally unacceptable.

As an alternative consider now the RLOA. In Table 3.6 the mean scores are expressed as their nlts. The mean nlt for the mean scores of Test I and Test II are 5.129 ($\log_e$ 179.6) and 5.218 respectively and the difference $5.129 - 5.218 = -0.089$. The SD of the nlt values is 0.234. The RLOA is now expressed as:

$$-0.0895 \pm (0.234 * 1.96)$$

To find the actual numerical values, the antilog of the bias is first calculated: antilog(-0.0895) = 0.914. The nlt of the limits are $-0.0895 - 0.234 * 1.96 = 0.548$ and $-0.0895 + 0.234 * 1.96 = 0.369$, respectively. The agreement ratio $0.548/0.369 = 1.485$ is to be multiplied or divided by the bias, i.e. the RLOA is now expressed as $0.914*/1.485$ or between 0.62 and 1.353. Multiplied by the absolute individual score these values set the 95% LOA.

For instance, consider the abovementioned subject with a 132 Nm of trunk flexor strength. In this case the 'bias' is $132 * 0.914 = 120.6$ Nm. The 95% RLOA is spanned between $120.6/1.485 = 81.2$ Nm and $120.6 * 1.485 = 179.1$ Nm. This is a considerable narrowing of the absolute LOA interval of $18.5 - 207.1$ Nm. In a similar fashion, consider the RLOA for the stronger subject (244 Nm). In this case the 'bias' is $244 * 0.914 = 223$ Nm and the 95% RLOA is between 150.2 Nm ($223/1.485$) and 331 Nm ($223 * 1.485$). In this case the interval does not contract to the same extent but is still a little smaller than the corresponding absolute LOA. In assessing the significance of the latter results it should be realized that in this study the findings derived from a mixed sample of women and men, low n, no gravitational corrections and poorly outlined protocols. Furthermore, some of the results were in sharp variance with expected physiological results.

It should also be mentioned that with respect to the *bias* (assuming equal error) a smaller value results in a more equally balanced LOA around the score. For RLOA the same applies as the bias approaches unity (1.0). Furthermore, for RLOA the error term signifies the percentage deviation from the bias and therefore provides an instant idea about the extent of deviation required for indicating a significant change. A comparable facility is not afforded by the LOA as the error is not related to the magnitude of the individual score. Thus an ideal reproducibility would in terms of RLOA be expressed by the form $1.0*/(1.0)$, namely on retest, any deviation from the original score will be considered significant. By analogy the parallel expression in terms of LOA will be 0.0 ± 0.0. Notably, for the particular purpose of assessing reproducibility of isokinetic data none of the relative indices – t-test, Pearson's r or the various forms of the ICC – is as informative and clinically revealing.

In assessing the suitability of any of the above indices to analyzing the reproducibility of test data, Bland & Altman (1990) suggest that 'The magnitude of the difference which is acceptable is not a statistical decision but a clinical one. We should ask whether the agreement is good enough for a particular purpose, not whether it conforms to some absolute, arbitrary criterion.' Quite paradoxically, in some respects this conclusion is unfortunate as it does little to help practitioners draw a line between what may be considered an acceptable change or alternatively what should be regarded as falling within the margins of measurement error. Thus some of the quantitative flavor of reproducibility analysis is still lost to what, for the want of a better term, should be good clinical judgment.

Doubtless, the more robust the protocol, the less error is expected. Furthermore, elements such as practice-based improvement ('learning') would play a progressively lesser role when multiple isokinetic tests are undertaken (e.g. in the course of rehabilitation or strength conditioning). In such cases the error margin would be expected to decrease irrespective of individual performance. These all lead to an acute need for basic research which will encompass all of the above statistical methods in a systematic manner that would allow the formulation of more realistic goals. Such research may also indicate that inasmuch as isokinetic findings are concerned, no generalization from one muscle group to another is permitted. Finally one should be aware that judging variations in human performance parameters depends on the level of significance employed. A more lenient approach (e.g. at 95% level of confidence) may enable a decision that cannot be accepted at 99% level of confidence. This does *not* mean that the former is wrong to the same extent that it does not vindicate the application of the latter.

In the following section a number of studies will be discussed. These will serve to put the ideas presented so far in their correct perspective. In the first papers, Ottenbacher & Tomchek (1994) examine the way in which 'random error, systematic or proportional variation (bias) affect the results of statistical procedures used to analyze data from method comparison studies'. Although derived from another performance measurement, this study serves as a proper general platform for reiterating some of the misconceptions inherent in the use of relative indices. In the other studies, by Madsen (1996a,b), Holmbäck et al (1999) and Mandalidis et al (2001) reproducibility analyses of isokinetic data obtained from various muscle groups are

presented. Collectively they portray what may possibly constitute a format for future studies. By the same token, previous reproducibility research that consisted of particularly mixed populations or relied exclusively on the t-test or Pearson's r should be regarded with particular reservation.

REPRODUCIBILITY ANALYSIS: APPLICATION OF MODERN CONCEPTS

In an often-quoted study Ottenbacher and Tomchek (1994) used an artificial set of 40 reference values relating to range of shoulder flexion. Table 3.7 presents a section of the full table which explains the data structure.

Random variation was obtained by mathematically generating another set of 40 values under the constraints that it had a similar mean and SD. A third set was formed by alternately adding and subtracting 5° to each of the reference scores (variable bias). A fourth set consisted of adding an absolute value of 5° (constant bias) whereas in the fifth set 10% of the reference score was added, for example 150° became 165° (proportional bias). The statistical analysis was based on using the following indices: Pearson's r, ICC (2,1) and ICC

Table 3.7 Reference range of motion (ROM) values and test data representing different types of measurement variation: the first five and the last five values

	Reference ROM values	Random variation	Alternate variation	Constant variation	Proportional variation
First 5 values	20	11.55	25	25	22
	30	16.40	25	35	33
	40	29.58	45	45	44
	50	31.53	45	55	55
	55	36.49	60	60	60
Last 5 values	170	155.67	165	175	187
	172	161.29	177	177	189.2
	175	162.02	170	180	192.5
	180	163.47	185	185	198
	185	182.25	180	190	203.5
Number	40	40	40	40	40
Minimum	20	11.55	25	25	22
Maximum	185	182.25	185	190	203.5
Mean	104.5	102.8	104.57	109.57	115.03
SD	42.4	42.19	42.43	42.39	46.64

From Ottenbacher & Tomchek 1994.

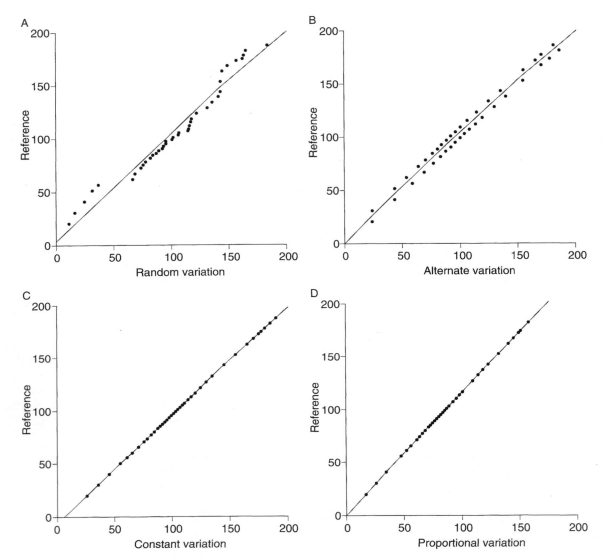

Figure 3.8   Graphs displaying random (A), alternate (B), constant (C) and proportional (D) variations constructed using ordinary least square regression. (From Ottenbacher & Tomchek 1994.)

(3,1), least square regression (in terms of the slope, intercept and standard error), t-test and LOA. The main question related to the differential sensitivity of each of the indices to the different types of measurement variation.

Figures 3.8A–D and 3.9A–D display the values for different statistical parameters and limits of agreement presentation, respectively. Table 3.8 outlines the associated sensitivities.

Clearly none of the relative parameters was capable of adequately detecting the nature of the variations although the ICCs performed slightly better with respect to the random and proportional forms. In a large number of analytical studies, comparable numerical results (of r and ICC) would have been interpreted as indicating excellent reproducibility, a particularly misleading consequence as far as the proportional perturbation is concerned.

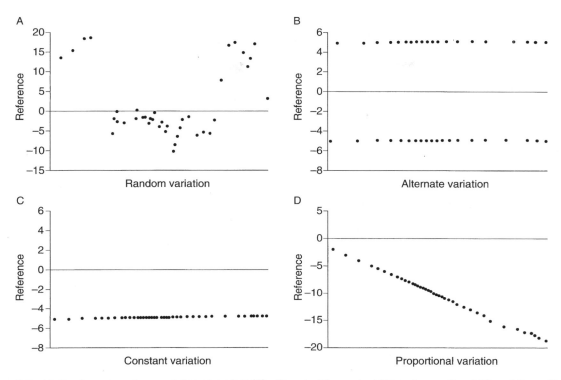

Figure 3.9 Limits of agreement presentation of random (A), alternate (B), constant (C) and proportional (D) variations. (From Ottenbacher & Tomchek 1994.)

Table 3.8 Statistical parameters, their values and sensitivities to different types of measurement variation

Parameter	Ideal	Random	Alternate	Constant	Proportional
Correlation (r)	1.00	0.98 –	0.99 –	1.00 –	1.00 –
Bias	0.00	1.77 ±	0.00 –	5.00 +	−10.46 +
LSR – slope	1.00	0.98 –	0.99 –	1.00 –	0.90 +
LSR – intercept	0.00	3.45 ±	0.83 ±	5.00 +	0.00 –
Standard error	0.00	0.03 –	0.02 –	0.00 –	0.00 –
t-test	Undefined	1.29 –	0.00 –	−201.0 +	−15.6 +
ICC (2,1)	1.00	0.94 ±	0.98 –	0.98 –	0.93 ±
ICC (3,1)	1.00	0.94 ±	0.98 –	1.00 –	1.00 –
Limits of agreement		+	+	+	+

(+) sensitive to variation; (−) not sensitive to variation; (±) minimally sensitive to variation. ICC, intraclass correlation coefficients; LSR, least square regression. Modified from Ottenbacher & Tomchek 1994.

Table 3.9 Coefficients of variation of knee extensor strength measurements in 24 healthy women measured in three sessions with median intervals of 2–30 days

Parameter	Isometric[a]	30°/s[a]	240°/s[a]	30°/s[b]	240°/s[b]	30°/s[c]	240°/s[c]
Intrasession 1							
CV_p	4.3	7.7	3.2	4.8	3.7	4.9	6.0
CV_m	1.2	3.0	0.9	3.2	1.9	2.5	3.1
CV_r	0.0–9.7	0.5–13.4	0.0–4.5	0.9–8.5	0.4–8.3	1.0–10.0	0.1–12.2
Short term 1 and 2							
CV_p	8.4	7.8	5.2	5.5	6.2	6.4	9.2
CV_m	4.4	5.9	3.2	3.5	4.5	3.5	7.1
CV_r	1.2–17.7	0.6–16.5	0.9–9.0	0.2–13.5	0.4–12.1	0.0–14.1	0.5–16.1
Long term 1 and 2							
CV_p	6.0	6.9	7.6	5.2	10.2	6.0	12.7
CV_m	4.4	3.4	13.7	4.2	4.6	4.5	11.9
CV_r	0.8–10.6	0.0–13.4	1.4–42.8	0.8–10.1	1.0–21.5	0.0–12.8	0.5–23.1

[a] strength; [b] work; [c] power; CV_p, CV pooled; CV_m, median of individual CVs; CV_r, 80% central range of individual CVs.
From Madsen 1996a.

On the other hand, the LOA was effective in every instance although the authors did not proceed with expressing the limits in the form of bias $\pm$ error. However it clearly emerges from the figures that in the case of random, alternate and constant variations the error was, as expected, homoscedastic whereas the proportional variation was by definition heteroscedastic.

In a series of papers, a Danish physician, OR Madsen, has studied the reproducibility of several muscle systems, applying the CV of the test-retest differences as the predominant index. In one study, within-session consistency, short and long term reproducibility of knee and elbow muscle extension isokinetic performance variables and isometric strength were assessed in a group of 24 healthy women aged 18–52. In addition to reproducibility the other objectives were to explore the effect of warming up and practice-based improvement ('learning'). This necessitated an intricate experimental design consisting of four testing sessions (Madsen 1996a) which incorporated intrasession, short term and long term test-retest paradigms. For assessing the reproducibility of the repeated measurements, the CV_{ME} was used and expressed as a percentage, namely $100 * CV_{ME}$ (termed CV_p% in the original paper). Intra- and intersession CV_ps were determined using the highest values of each strength variable. The CV for each of the above performance variables in each individual subject was calculated similarly: $CV_i\% = 100(0.5d_i^2)^{1/2}/x_i$ where d_i is the difference between two repeated measurements in the same subject and x_i is the mean. The median score of CV_i% (50%) as well as the 10th and 90th percentiles (80% central range) of the CV_is were calculated.

No positive effect for either practice or warming up took place. CV-based findings are presented in Tables 3.9 and 3.10 including the medians and 80% central ranges of CV_is and CV_ps.

Intrasession CV_is tended to be lower than their short and long term counterparts. Substantial between-subject variation in CV_is was apparent. Relatively high CV_ps characterized all muscle groups ranging (accounting for all recorded variables) from 5.2 to 21.6% and 9.4 to 14.8% for knee and elbow extensors respectively. In this study the critical differences were based on the 10–90th medians as recommended in another study (Costong et al 1985). This means that if the individual (subject/patient) difference between repeated measure is less than the 90th median, the change may be due to expected individual variations. For instance, if for a given subject and under the test input parameters outlined in this study, knee extension strength was 66 Nm at 240°/s then a

Table 3.10 Coefficients of variation of elbow extensor strength measurements in 24 healthy women measured in three sessions with median intervals of 2–30 days

Parameter	Isometric[a]	30°/s[a]	240°/s[a]	30°/s[b]	240°/s[b]	30°/s[c]	240°/s[c]
Intrasession 1							
CV_p	7.6	7.6	4.5	4.6	6.4	6.5	8.0
CV_m	3.7	4.4	2.7	2.4	3.2	6.1	5.3
CV_r	0.0–13.2	0.0–11.7	0.0–9.5	0.0–9.9	0.0–15.4	0.0–10.6	0.4–15.7
Short term 1 and 2							
CV_p	11.3	12.5	8.3	10.8	9.8	13.0	9.4
CV_m	7.8	6.6	2.8	7.1	6.1	11.2	6.5
CV_r	3.4–19.7	0.8–24.9	0.0–14.2	1.1–18.6	0.0–19.1	0.0–22.6	1.4–17.3
Long term 1 and 2							
CV_p	10.1	10.6	9.4	11.2	13.2	14.0	14.8
CV_m	5.7	6.3	7.4	4.5	8.4	6.7	10.8
CV_r	2.3–16.2	0.0–20.2	0.0–13.5	0.0–22.2	1.2–23.9	0.0–27.0	2.2–26.8

[a] strength; [b] work; [c] power; CV_p, CV pooled; CV_m, median of individual CVs; CV_r, 80% central range of individual CVs.
From Madsen 1996a.

minimum of 94 Nm would be required to indicate a real improvement ($CV_{i90\%}$ is 42.8%). As the corresponding figure for the strength at 30°/s is 13.4% and to the extent that low velocity strengths are indicative, this test condition is to be preferred as it is associated with a significantly smaller error. Another point worth mentioning with respect to this study is the nature of the error observed. It seems that the non-symmetrical spread of the 10 and 90th tails around the median is indicative of heteroscedasticity. For instance the median elbow extension strength (CV_{im}) at 30°/s was 6.3% whereas the central 80% (CV_{ir}) was delimited by the 10 and 90th tails at 0.0 and 20.2%, respectively. More recent analysis in this case would have indicated the possible application of RLOA. Attention is drawn to the fact that unlike the critical difference approach which applies to a *reference group* the median-based analysis looks at *individual* performance.

In a similar study, trunk extensor and flexor strength was measured in a group of 24 healthy women who were tested using a range of motion (ROM) of 65° and angular velocities of 30, 120 and 180°/s. The main purpose was to assess the extent of intrasession, short term and long term reproducibility (Madsen 1996b). A secondary objective was the exploration of possible effect of practice. In

this study the same indices were applied: CV_i and CV_p. In addition the critical difference ($CD_{0.05} = z_{0.05} * \sqrt{2} * CV_p$, where $z_{0.05} = 1.96$ is the standard deviate for $p = 0.05$) was calculated. Table 3.11 relates to the strength, work and power parameters as the acceleration time and energy parameters were associated with such extremely large CV_ps that they were rendered irrelevant. Table 3.12 relates to variations in the CV_ps, CV_{im}s, CV_{ir}s and $CD_{0.05}$.

The results revealed no practice effect, in line with the previous study. In terms of the CVs, the intrasession variations were smaller than their short and long term counterparts. Furthermore, a correlational analysis failed to discover any significant association between intrasession and long term CVs. Table 3.12 also reveals that the CDs of the three parameters were roughly within the same range, a tribute to the fact that they are to a great extent linearly dependent as evidenced by the relatively high correlations among them. However, the absolute values of the CDs were particularly large, ranging from 19.7% for total work during flexion at 30°/s to 77.6% for extension power at 180°/s. With respect to strength, the range was 24.9–55.7%. This means that based on these values any change in performance will have to be considered as non-consequential unless it is

Table 3.11 Coefficients of variation and critical differences (in %) of trunk extensor strength measurements in 24 healthy women

Parameter	Isometric[a]	30°/s[a]	180°/s[a]	30°/s[b]	180°/s[b]	30°/s[c]	180°/s[c]
Intrasession (S1)*							
CV_p	4.3	6.2	15.4	5.5	20.0	10.6	21.0
CV_m	2.0	4.3	12.3	3.3	11.2	6.9	13.4
CV_r	0.4–7.7	0.2–9.7	0.8–28.6	0.3–9.1	1.0–42.9	0.6–21.3	1.3–46.1
Short term (S1 vs S2)							
CV_p	9.7	10.0	17.2	9.5	24.9	12.2	22.6
CV_m	6.9	8.0	11.3	7.2	10.4	7.3	17.3
CV_r	0.9–20.9	1.2–17.8	1.6–32.6	0.7–18.2	1.3–43.7	1.7–25.2	2.4–56.0
Long term (S1 vs S3)							
CV_p	12.5	10.9	22.2	8.9	30.2	11.9	29.0
CV_m	10.4	6.2	13.7	5.4	17.0	9.7	21.1
CV_r	1.4–26.5	0.0–18.1	1.4–42.8	0.6–16.8	4.8–62.5	0.0–22.9	3.5–55.9
Long term (S2 vs S3)							
CV_p	24.9	11.1	20.1	10.0	24.4	12.6	28.0
CV_m	6.9	7.7	8.8	7.8	16.7	6.8	11.7
CV_r	0.7–24.2	2.5–19.5	0.6–42.1	1.5–18.8	0.5–58.2	0.0–23.9	1.3–68.8
CD	68.9	30.5	55.7	27.7	67.6	34.9	77.6

* session; [a] strength; [b] work; [c] power; CV_p, CV pooled; CV_m, median of individual CVs; CV_r, 80% central range of individual CVs; CD, critical differences for long term reproducibility: session 2 vs session 3.
From Madsen 1996b with permission of Lippincott Williams & Wilkins.

Table 3.12 Coefficients of variation (in %) of trunk flexor strength measurements in 24 healthy women

Parameter	Isometric[a]	30°/s[a]	180°/s[a]	30°/s[b]	180°/s[b]	30°/s[c]	180°/s[c]
Intrasession (S1)*							
CV_p	4.9	4.0	6.1	3.0	7.5	4.9	11.0
CV_m	2.9	1.6	5.0	2.2	7.1	3.6	8.5
CV_r	0.0–8.1	0.0–7.0	1.3–9.9	0.4–5.7	0.0–11.9	0.0–9.2	0.8–14.3
Short term (S1 vs S2)							
CV_p	10.8	10.4	10.5	7.4	10.1	9.8	13.1
CV_m	7.1	3.4	10.1	3.6	8.3	6.1	8.6
CV_r	0.8–14.9	0.0–22.6	1.4–19.2	0.0–14.0	0.4–21.7	0.0–19.2	0.0–30.2
Long term (S1 vs S3)							
CV_p	9.6	10.5	12.3	8.3	12.5	9.8	14.3
CV_m	5.4	6.4	6.1	5.7	7.5	6.2	12.2
CV_r	0.9–13.8	0.5–19.3	0.7–26.9	1.2–16.9	1.2–27.0	1.6–17.6	1.7–28.4
Long term (S2 vs S3)							
CV_p	9.8	9.0	12.3	7.1	10.5	9.0	14.4
CV_m	6.9	3.0	4.9	5.3	4.5	7.3	8.8
CV_r	2.2–18.5	0.5–17.1	1.2–18.5	0.6–14.2	0.5–19.4	1.6–15.9	3.2–27.8
CD	27.1	24.9	34.1	19.7	29.4	24.9	39.9

* session; [a] strength; [b] work; [c] power; CV_p, CV pooled; CV_m, median of individual CVs; CV_r, 80% central range of individual CVs; CD, critical differences for long term reproducibility: session 2 vs session 3.
From Madsen 1996b with permission of Lippincott Williams & Wilkins.

at least 25% higher or lower than the base value. These critical differences are actually smaller than those reported by Nevill & Atkinson (1997) which were based on RLOA and therefore should have been smaller. The CDs in the latter study which included testing of trunk flexion and extension at 30, 60 and 120°/s ranged from 0.88*/(1.54) to 0.95*/(1.71), a general percentage change of more than 50%. Interestingly the LOA-based CDs were even higher. Coefficient of variations of this magnitude and their associated CDs impose a significant limitation on the use and interpretation of isokinetic trunk testing in subjects and patients alike and indicate an acute need for improved protocols.

In a study of ankle doriflexion Holmbäck et al (1999) analyzed findings based on a test-retest paradigm (a week apart) using a set of indices which included the ICC (2,1), Pearson's r, SEM, t-test and and the CV of the method error (ME). Of the three variables that were analyzed only strength (PT) will be reported since 'work' is closely related to PT and 'torque * time' is a rarely used parameter besides being relatively impractical as it necessitates scanning of each moment curve and partitioning into segments. Thirty healthy subjects, 15 women and 15 men, were tested using a ROM of 45° and angular velocities of 30, 60, 90, 120 and 150°/s. In analyzing the results, the authors concluded that in view of no discernible differences between the men and women pooling of the findings was permissible. As outlined before, mixing of groups will increase correlational coefficients and therefore attention is called to the numerical values of ICC and r.

Table 3.13 depicts the results from which it emerges that the ICC and r were generally high and very similar. Although higher ICCs allow detection of smaller differences, the results offer no guide regarding the absolute discrepancy between test and retest scores necessary to indicate change. On the other hand the absolute indices provide cutoff values which at a given level of significance may demonstrate such change. The results show the SEM and ME are in close agreement, an expected outcome in view of the relatively large n and sufficiently small mean. Moreover, these indices do not seem to exhibit a clear velocity dependence, supporting previous analysis (Keating & Matyas 1998). On the other hand, the CV did increase steadily with the rise in velocity. What are the relations between SEM and ME on one hand and the CV on the other?

In order to indicate change the SEM (ME) has to be multiplied by 1.96 ($z_{0.05}$) and hence the CD for this index is around 4 Nm which for the pooled group and strength at 30°/s will be roughly

Table 3.13 Reproducibility indices of ankle dorsiflexion strength at five angular velocities

Index	30°/s	60°/s	90°/s	120°/s	150°/s
ICC	0.91	0.93	0.90	0.78	0.80
R	0.91	0.93	0.88	0.79	0.82
SEM (Nm)	2.01	1.69	1.71	2.16	2.15
ME (Nm)	2.03	1.71	2.00	2.35	2.25
CV (%)	6.40	6.60	9.20	12.60	13.50

CV, coefficient of variation; ICC, intraclass correlation coefficients; ME, method error; R, Pearson's r; SEM, standard error of measurement.
From Holmbäck et al 1999.

equivalent to 12%. For the CV the corresponding CD is slightly higher: 18% (2.77 * 6.04). These figures are quite low and better than those quoted by Nevill & Atkinson (1997) for the LOA of knee flexion and extension. It should also be emphasized that inspection of difference versus mean presentation (Figs 3.6 and 3.7) does reveal a heteroscedastic trend and it is possible that using the RLOA would have resulted in even narrower limits of agreement.

In a recently published series of papers Mandalidis et al (2001) have examined several aspects of shoulder muscle performance. In one study, the reproducibility of shoulder elevation strength (peak and average) was analyzed with respect to the inclusion or exclusion of transient moment oscillations (TMO), sectors that occur typically at the initiation and termination of movement and roughly correspond to the non-isokinetic sectors of the curve (Mandalidis et al 2001, see also Chapter 9). The test-retest period was 6–7 days. No practice-based changes were indicated. The reproducibility indices appear in Table 3.14.

Using the ICC (3,1) formula the correlations between test and retest ranged from 0.86 to 0.95 (for both sides) which would indicate excellent agreement. For the TMO-free data, the 95% SEM ranged from 9.2 to 12.7 Nm. The 95% LOA exhibited a small bias ⩽1 Nm and an error component of 9.4 and 12.6 Nm, closely resembling the SEM for the TMO-free data. The non-free TMO was characterized by higher SEMs and LOAs although the ICCs were very similar to the TMO-free data. These scores will be interpreted slightly differently for the average and peak moment. Judged against

Table 3.14 Reproducibility indices of shoulder elevation strength based on data with and without filtering of transient moment oscillation (TMO)

Index	Average moment				Peak moment			
	TMO data*		TMO-free data**		TMO data		TMO-free data	
	60°/s	120°/s	60°/s	120°/s	60°/s	120°/s	60°/s	120°/s
D: Strength	51.1	56.0	63.3	58.8	69.7	69.1	68.9	63.1
D: ICC (3,1)	0.91	0.92	0.91	0.92	0.92	0.87	0.93	0.92
D: 95% SEM[a]	10.3	9.4	10.6	9.9	10.1	14.4	9.7	10.8
D: ±95% LOA[a]	0.4 ± 10.3	−1.3 ± 9.2	0.9 ± 10.7	−0.6 ± 9.7	0.9 ± 10.6	−1.8 ± 14.7	1.7 ± 9.8	−0.4 ± 10.6
ND: Strength	62.5	54.9	64.3	57.9	71.1	68.4	70.0	62.7
ND: ICC (3,1)	0.95	0.91	0.95	0.88	0.94	0.86	0.94	0.92
ND: 95%SEM	8.9	10.1	9.2	12.7	10.9	14.9	10.3	10.6
ND: ±95% LOA	−1.2 ± 8.9	−0.9 ± 10.5	−1.0 ± 9.4	−0.3 ± 12.6	−1.7 ± 11.6	−1.9 ± 15.9	−1.4 ± 10.6	−0.3 ± 11.3

D, dominant; ND, non-dominant; ICC, intraclass correlation coefficients; [a]standard error of measurement (SEM) and limits of agreement (LOA) in Nm; * without filtering of transient moment oscillations; ** with filtering of transient moment oscillations. For the strength data, the higher score between the test and retest was quoted as the maximal intersession difference as in the great majority of cases the difference was less than 1 Nm.
From Mandalidis et al 2001.

the peak moment at 60 and 120°/s (test and retest, dominant and non-dominant pooled) the 95% SEM would be roughly equivalent to about 15%, a figure closely in agreement with Holmbäck et al (1999) but significantly at variance with Madsen (1996a) or Nevill & Atkinson (1997) who reported RLOA-based cutoffs as large as 65%.

Worth mentioning are two recent studies which allow comparison with these cutoffs. Focusing on the reproducibility of eccentric as well as concentric contractions of the knee flexors, Dauty & Rochcongar (2001) used a non-reciprocal protocol based on five concentric contractions at 180°/s and five eccentric contractions at 30 and 60°/s (each). The findings revealed a 95% SEM which was equivalent to between 16 and 24% of the peak moment. Smith et al (2001) have examined the reproducibility of shoulder rotational strength and found 95% SEMs of between 11 and 16%. These relatively low cutoffs reflect in particular the dependence of the SEM on the associated ICCs which in both studies were quite high.

In trying to explain the diversity of results one has to consider all of the factors that determine the reproducibility of data: examiner(s), examinee, protocol, system and environment. To date no acceptable testing protocols exist for any of the body muscle systems. Moreover, even if two

protocols resemble each other closely, a variation in each and every parameter which takes part in defining the protocol becomes quite automatically a source of error. Adding to these, the application of different statistical tools unfortunately helps in confounding the picture even further.

SUMMARY AND RECOMMENDATIONS

In spite of drawbacks, some firm conclusions and recommendations emerge from this chapter:

1. Strength scores derived from normal subjects as well as patients do vary upon retesting. This is a universal trait and should be interpreted as a normal phenomenon characterizing any measurement process.
2. Exploring the nature of these variations is best conducted using absolute indices of reproducibility which are not affected by factors such as extreme individual scores.
3. Moreover, absolute indices yield cutoff values which enable clinicians to decide whether the variations observed are within the boundaries of the error or indicate a true change.
4. There is also evidence that the variation of error with the magnitude of the measurement

is not unidirectional; some cases evidence homoscedasticity whereas others indicate heteroscedasticity.

5. In case the behavior is indeed heteroscedastic, the use of RLOA would be preferable, otherwise application of simple LOA or other absolute indices should suffice.

6. Taken together, in the absence of a comprehensive analysis a very rough estimate dictates that unless a 20% difference (invariably, improvement) is found on retesting, no real change is indicated. This benchmark should be varied according to emerging published research.

REFERENCES

Atkinson G, Nevill A M 1998 Statistical methods for assessing measurement error (reliability) in variables relevant to sports medicine. Sports Medicine 26: 217–238

Baumgartner T A 1989 Norm-referenced measurements: reliability. In: Safrit M J, Wood T M (eds) Measurement concepts in physical education and exercise science. Human Kinetics, Champaign, Illinois

Bland J M, Altman D G 1986 Statistical methods for assessing agreement between two methods of clinical measurement. Lancet 1: 307–310

Bland J M, Altman D G 1990 A note on the use of the intraclass correlation coefficient in the evaluation of agreement between two methods of measurement. Computations in Biology and Medicine 20: 337–340

Bygott I L, McMeeken J, Carroll S, Story I 2001 Gravity correction in trunk dynamometry: is it reliable? Isokinetics and Exercise Science 9: 1–10

Bygott I L, McMeeken J, Carroll S, Story I 2001b A preliminary analysis of the validity of gravity correction procedures applied in trunk dynamometry. Isokinetics and Exercise Science 9: 53–64

Costong G, Janson P, Bas B 1985 Short-term and long-term intra-individual variations and critical differences of haematological laboratory parameters. Journal of Clinical Chemistry and Clinical Biochemistry 23: 69–76

Dauty M, Rochcongar P 2001 Reproducibility of concentric and eccentric isokinetic strength of the knee flexors in elite volleyball players. Isokinetics and Exercise Science 9: 129–132

Durand F, Malouin C, Richards L, Bravo G 1991 Intertrial reliability of work measurements recorded during concentric isokinetic knee extension and flexion in subjects with and without meniscal tears. Physical Therapy 71: 804–812

Dvir Z 1997 Grade 4 in manual muscle testing: the problem with submaximal strength assessment. Clinical Rehabilitation 11: 36–41

Eliasziw M, Young S L, Woodbury M G et al 1994 Statistical methodology for the concurrent assessment for inter-rater and intra-rater reliability: using goniometric measurements as an example. Physical Therapy 74: 777–788

Estlander A M, Mellin G, Weckstrom A 1992 Influence of repeated measurements on isokinetic lifting strength. Clinical Biomechanics 7: 149–152

Frontera W R, Hughes V A, Dallal G E, Evans W J 1993 Reliability of isokinetic muscle strength testing in 45–78 year old men and women. Archives of Physical Medicine and Rehabilitation 74: 1181–1185

Grabiner M D, Jeziorowski J J, Diverkar A D 1990 Isokinetic measurements of trunk extension and flexion performance collected with the Biodex clinical data station. Journal of Orthopaedic and Sports Physical Therapy 11: 590–598

Holmbäck A M, Porter M M, Downham D, Lexell J 1999 Reliability of isokinetic ankle dorsiflexion strength measurements in healthy young men and women. Scandinavian Journal of Rehabilitation Medicine 31: 229–239

Karnofel K, Wilkinson K, Lentell G 1989 Reliability of isokinetic muscle testing at the ankle. Journal of Orthopaedic and Sports Physical Therapy 11: 150–154

Keating J L, Matyas T A 1998 Unpredictable error in dynamometry measurements: a quantitative analysis of the literature. Isokinetics and Exercise Science 7: 107–121

Madsen O R 1996a Torque, total work, power, acceleration energy and acceleration time assessed on a dynamometer: reliability of knee and elbow extensor and flexor strength measurements. European Journal of Applied Physiology 74: 206–210

Madsen O R 1996b Trunk extensor and flexor strength measured by the Cybex 6000 dynamometer. Assessment of short-term and long-term reproducibility of several strength variables. Spine 21: 2770–2776

Mandalidis D G, Donne B, Regan M O, O'Brien M 2001 Effect of transient moment oscillations on the reliability of isokinetic shoulder elevation in the scapular plane. Isokinetics and Exercise Science 9: 100–109

Molcyzk L, Thigpen L K, Eickhoff J, Coldgar D, Gallagher J C 1991 Reliability of testing the knee extensors and flexors in healthy adult women using a Cybex II isokinetic dynamometer. Journal of Orthopaedic and Sports Physical Therapy 14: 37–41

Myrer J W, Schulthies S, Fellingham G W 1996 Relative and absolute reliability of the KT-2000 arthrometer for uninjured knee. American Journal of Sports Medicine 24: 104–108

Nevill A M, Atkinson G 1997 Assessing agreement between measurements recorded on a ratio scale in sports medicine and sports science. British Journal of Sports Medicine 31: 314–318.

Ottenbacher K J, Tomchek S D 1994 Measurement variation in method comparison studies: an empirical examination. Archives of Physical Medicine and Rehabilitation 75: 505–512

Portney L G, Watkins M P 2000 Foundations of clinical research: applications to practice, 2nd edn. Prentice Hall Health, Upperdale Saddle River, New Jersey

Quan H, Shih W J 1996 Assessing reproducibility by the within subject coefficient of variation with random effect models. Biometrics 52: 1195–1203

Rothstein J M, Lamb R L, Mayhew T P 1987 Clinical uses of isokinetic measurements: critical issues. Physical Therapy 67: 1840–1844

Sapega A A 1990 Muscle performance evaluation in orthopaedic practice. Journal of Bone and Joint Surgery 72A: 1562–1574

Schmidt R A, Zelaznik H, Hawkins B, Frank J S, Quinn J T 1979 Motor-output variability: a theory for the accuracy of rapid motor acts. Psychological Reviews 86: 415–451

Shrout P, Fleiss J 1979 Intraclass correlations: uses in assessing rater reliability. Psychological Bulletin 66: 629–639

Smith J, Padgett D J, Kotajarvi B R, Eischen J J 2001 Isokinetic and isometric shoulder rotation strength in the protracted position: a reliability study. Isokinetics and Exercise Science 9: 119–128

Stratford P W 1997 Confidence limits for your ICC. Physical Therapy 69: 237–238

Stratford P W, Goldsmith C H 1997 Use of the standard error as a reliability index of interest: an applied example using elbow flexor strength data. Physical Therapy 77: 745–750

Thompson C R, Paulus L M, Timm K 1993 Concentric isokinetic test-retest reliability and testing interval. Isokinetics and Exercise Science 3: 44–49

Tripp E J, Harris S R 1991 Test-retest reliability of isokinetic knee extension and flexion torque measurements in persons with spastic hemiparesis. Physical Therapy 71: 390–396

Walmsley R P, Amell T K 1996 The application and interpretation of intraclass correlations in the assessment of reliability in isokinetic dynamometry. Isokinetics and Exercise Science 6: 117–124

Wennerberg D 1991 Reliability of an isokinetic dorsiflexion and plantarflexion apparatus. American Journal of Sports Medicine 19: 519–522

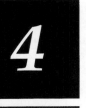

4

Application of isokinetics to muscle conditioning and rehabilitation

PART 1
INTRODUCTION

Compared with the use of isokinetics in testing, where there are relatively well-established rules and procedures, its clinical role in the conditioning of muscle performance is far less researched and understood. A number of difficulties seriously undermine and sometimes even preclude the establishment of pathology- or intervention-specific protocols. These difficulties result from a range of factors which may be divided into two groups: methodological and patient-linked on one hand, and the predominantly logistic on the other.

From the methodological viewpoint, there are complex interactions between factors ranging from the type of injury or pathology to the patient's motivation. This is reflected in a paper by Zarins et al (1985), discussing rehabilitation after the relatively straightforward meniscectomy procedure:

Thus a large amount of variability exists in rehabilitation patterns following meniscectomy. Patient-to-patient differences dictate that each recovery program be tailored to meet the individual needs.

For instance for surgical cases the following factors must be taken into account when designing the rehabilitation protocol (Zarins et al 1985, Wilk & Andrews 1992):

1. surgical approach, e.g. arthrotomy versus arthroscopy
2. amount of periarticular soft tissue dissection

3. type of tissue used (in reconstruction)
4. grafting factors
5. coexisting lesions and concomitant surgery
6. preoperative status
7. patient compliance and expectations.

Protocol problems

Muscle conditioning protocols are another critical methodological component. The difficulties in managing isokinetic testing variables effectively were described in Chapter 2. The complexity associated with rational implementation of conditioning protocols is considerably greater. Problems arise in various quarters, for instance, the impact on tissues other than muscle. During isokinetic conditioning significant loads may be exerted on structures such as the articular surfaces, capsule or ligaments. The cumulative effect of this, which is notoriously hard to determine, must be considered.

The question of submaximal versus maximal exertions has to be answered with regard to healing stage, pain and the potential of the muscles and/or other involved tissues. The issues of protocol structure, mainly the conditioning dose and which performance criteria should be optimized, have never been settled in a systematic manner. Clinicians have therefore to rely either on a very limited number of studies and/or on their own experience which may be even more restricted.

Logistic limitations

The logistic problems, though not necessarily limited to isokinetic conditioning are no less daunting. The time frame for significant improvements in muscle performance is measured in weeks rather than minutes. Moreover, within this period, subjects have to attend all sessions, typically at least three per week. Hence, even a 'minimal size' study consisting of 20 patients, who exercise at this rate for a period of 6 weeks, necessitates 360 sessions, an undertaking which can be met only by large and well-equipped centers.

This obstacle is associated with the difficulty of obtaining a large homogeneous sample for a given symptom and/or interventions. Small clinics and some medical centers rarely treat more than a handful of patients afflicted with the same pathology during a limited period. Consequently, the likelihood of generating original conditioning (rather than testing) protocols and more significantly, their objective assessment, is very low. For instance, the body of knowledge relating to the isokinetic testing of thigh muscles in chronic deficiency of, or reconstruction of, the anterior cruciate ligament (ACL) is disproportionately larger than that relating to isokinetic-based rehabilitation.

Moreover, the success rate reported by one center may not apply to others in spite of the same conditioning philosophy being used. This may, for example, be the case with the 'accelerated rehabilitation' approach for patients with reconstructed ACL (Shelbourne & Nitz 1990); surgical skills accumulated after many hundreds, perhaps thousands, of reconstructions at a particular center are bound to be reflected in the immediate postoperative status of the patient. Although this issue is common to all conditioning methods, its effects are more pronounced with isokinetic rehabilitation in view of the large range of options inherent in this technology.

Limitations of knowledge base

Finally, the studies which form the conceptual background of this chapter were based almost exclusively on young and healthy individuals, and practically all studies were based on a single muscle system, that of the thigh. It should also be noted that whereas the quadriceps and hamstring muscle groups frequently operate within the framework of a closed isokinetic chain, these muscles have usually been isokinetically conditioned in the open kinetic chain configuration. Consequently, although the results may be valid for other major muscle groups, the specific joint and dysfunction would dictate the individual approach.

Issues in therapeutic use of isokinetics

These difficulties (and probably others) contribute to a situation in which professionals, who are well known in the practice of muscle performance rehabilitation, advocate the use of specific methods without the backing of solid research and its later recognition in peer-reviewed literature. For example, in one of the few books dedicated to isokinetics, one author quoted certain protocols which allegedly were implemented in the rehabilitation of more than 1000 patients. These patients were reported to have significantly benefited from these protocols. The present author believes that since, in the present context, muscle conditioning refers to the therapeutic use of isokinetics, it must be considered with the utmost care. Consequently, one may rely only on those studies which systematically pursued relevant issues such as the principle of physiological overflow or the comparison of resistance training methods.

The purpose of this chapter is to review a number of issues which are relevant to the use of isokinetic dynamometry in the conditioning–rehabilitation context. These issues include:

- physiological interactions in the course of muscle conditioning
- specificity of muscle performance conditioning
- principles of isokinetic conditioning programs in clinical rehabilitation.

PART 2
PHYSIOLOGICAL INTERACTIONS IN MUSCLE CONDITIONING

This subject has received considerable attention and hundreds of papers have been published, representing the scientific output of the fields of exercise physiology, physical therapy, rehabilitation medicine, athletic training, kinesiology, biomechanics and motor behavior. The interactions that are commonly referred to in the scientific literature concern the relationships between biochemical correlates of muscle conditioning, morphological changes particularly in terms of fiber and whole muscle area and neural adaptations on the one hand and the major outcome criteria – strength, work and/or power – on the other.

Obviously it is beyond the scope of this book to encompass all existing knowledge even when this refers exclusively to isokinetic conditioning. Rather, the purpose of this section is to highlight a number of developments that have taken place since the publishing of the first edition.

Overloading

Muscle performance enhancement is reflected in adaptive processes, both in the muscle tissue itself and in the neural apparatus associated with motor activity. These processes can be realized by 'almost any method provided that the frequency of the exercises and the loading intensities sufficiently exceed those of normal activation of an individual muscle' (Komi 1986). This statement defines the principle of overloading. However, the 'loading intensities' vary quite dramatically from one muscle group to another and depend heavily on individual functional demand. Thus as a general guideline it has been suggested that the overloading stimulus should not be lower than 60% of the maximum since gains in strength had not been recorded using levels lower than this benchmark (Fleck & Kraemer 1987).

Isokinetic dynamometry provides an ideal platform for overloading since the level of the overloading stimulus may be determined with a precision that can hardly be matched by other methods, static or dynamic. It will also be realized that studies relating to improvement of performance in patients are generally different from those targeting normal subjects in that the latter are very often requested to exert maximal effort. In other words, whereas the stimulus for patients will be set as a percentage of the maximal allowable performance (e.g. 1 RM) the parallel stimulus for normal subjects will invariably be equal to the maximal level. Therefore a direct comparison between clinical and 'normal' conditioning protocols is, strictly speaking, not possible.

Neural activity and conditioning

Electromyographic (EMG) changes, as evidenced by recording using surface electrodes, highlight the interaction between the conditioning process and the neural adaptations. It is now well recognized that during the initial stage of conditioning, increase in muscle moment is due to neural adaptations and possibly improved force transmission from individual sarcomeres to the skeletal apparatus (Enoka 1988). These changes may take place quite rapidly although one should be aware of the intensity of loading stimuli. Thus 2 weeks were sufficient to cause sizeable improvements in knee extension (Akima et al 1999) and ankle dorsiflexion (Connelly & Vandervoort 2000) strength.

On the other hand, the size changes, which characterize the later stage of strength conditioning, are brought about mainly by the increase in size of individual muscle fibers, and probably by some proliferation of the latter (hypertrophy and hyperplasia respectively). Moreover, the conditioning process targets fast twitch (type II) compared with slow twitch (type I) fibers (Tesch 1988).

The extent to which EMG during the course of *isokinetic* muscle conditioning is different from *non-isokinetic* conditioning is not clear and may depend on subtle elements. Indeed in two important studies (see below) that explored EMG variations in the course of isokinetic conditioning, the results were almost opposite, emphasizing the serious dearth in protocol standardization including the specific modes of data handling. It should also be realized that EMG changes are but one facet of the neural adaptations and that interpreting the latter in terms of EMG variations must be made with utmost care as none of the studies reported the measurement error associated with post-training EMG variations (a design that would have involved two measurement sessions before the training regime and two after).

Concentric versus eccentric conditioning

Higbie et al (1996) compared the relative effectiveness of concentric versus eccentric conditioning of the quadriceps using normal women who trained using the protocol: 10 weeks (w) × 3 days (d) × 3 sets (s) × 10 maximal repetitions (mr). During each training session subjects were asked to exert maximal effort either in concentric (group Con) or eccentric (group Ecc) mode, both at 60°/s. The performance of a control group was measured parallel to the experimental groups at the start and end of the study. Results revealed a significant increase in neural excitation as evidenced by increases in the maximal integrated (i) EMG: 22% in concentric action for the Con group versus 16.7% in eccentric action for the Ecc group. The crossover effects did however differ as the Con conditioning induced a significant 20% increase in iEMG during the eccentric tests whereas the opposite effect amounted to about 7%. The authors suggested that these effects occurred due to increased recruitment and/or frequency of stimulation of the motor units. Moreover, previous argument relating to a lower activation level during eccentric contraction and therefore a higher recruitment potential as a result of training could not be substantiated as the Con and Ecc groups' improvements in iEMG were nearly the same.

In a similar study by Hortobágyi et al (1996) adaptations of knee extensors and flexors to concentric and eccentric conditioning was explored in men who trained at 60°/s according to the following protocol: 12 w × 3 d × (4–6) s × (8–12) mr. The dynamic EMG output was calculated based on normalization to its isometric counterpart. The proportional gains in the EMG were profoundly different from those indicated in the previous study. Eccentric training increased EMG activity about seven times more than concentric training increased EMG activity during concentric test contractions. The crossover effects were of a generally similar magnitude, approximately 10%. At variance with Higbie et al (1996) the authors reasoned that incomplete muscle activation at the initial stages of exercise represented a greater reserve for neural adaptation. Previous work indicated that the phenomenon of incomplete activation was apparent in untrained individuals who displayed depressed forces especially in eccentric exertions. Moreover, EMG analysis of repeated eccentric contractions revealed incomplete muscle activation. As potential mechanisms for increasing mechanical output such as a greater number of operating motor units or a higher discharge rate were largely ruled out, the authors claimed that the training effect resulted from 'learning to recruit more of the available type II fibers within a motoneuron pool after training'.

A later study by Hortobágyi et al (1997) examined the effect of ipsilateral knee extensor and flexor training on contralateral EMG changes using the above paradigm: 12 w × 3 d × (4–6) s × (8–12) mr. It was found that the surface EMG in the untrained quadriceps increased significantly more during eccentric (77%) compared to concentric (30%) training with no concomitant changes in the hamstring. Obviously, cross-education is a form of neural adaptation and in the absence of morphological contralateral changes, the authors suggested that this adaptation was an expression of the increase in central drive.

In a recent, as yet unpublished, study of strength and EMG correlates of short range of motion isokinetic concentric and eccentric conditioning (6 w × 3 d × 4 s × 10 mr) motor unit excitation frequency increased significantly due to training (Barak 2003). It was further indicated that this effect bore a direct relationship to the velocity of training. Increased excitation frequency up to a certain level can result in an increase in the maximal voluntary contraction (MVC). A higher frequency does not contribute to a greater muscular tension; rather it probably reduces the time required to achieve maximal tension, the so-called rate of force development (RFD). Various studies have shown that it was possible to increase significantly the excitation frequencies prior to any discernible morphological change in the muscular tissue. Simultaneous with the rise in frequency, the threshold for activation of fast twitch units may be lowered following strength training at high joint angular velocities. This reduction may result in some type II fibers firing even before type I fibers. Thus, the dual effect of higher frequency and lower threshold may be behind the changes seen during conditioning of this type. The source of this enhanced activity may reside at the spinal and/or supraspinal levels.

Reaction time

Quite on a different front, a single study which looked into the effect of isokinetic training on a specific neural function – reaction time – has revealed an interesting interaction (Wojtys et al 1996). Normal volunteers were placed into one of four groups: isokinetic, isotonic, agility, or control. Each group trained the quadriceps based on a 6 w × 3 d × 3 s × 12 mr paradigm. The agility-trained group significantly improved the spinal reflex times of the lateral and medial quadriceps in response to anterior tibial translation. The cortical response time of the agility group was also significantly improved in the gastrocnemius, medial hamstring and the lateral quadriceps. Interestingly, the cortical response time of the medial hamstring and the medial quadriceps muscles in the isokinetic group *slowed* significantly following training. Thus both isotonic and isokinetic strength training of the lower extremities does not appear to improve muscle reaction time to anterior tibial translation.

Morphological changes in muscle cross-sectional area and fibers area

The time course of neural and morphological adaptations in the context of isokinetic conditioning, using the commonly employed regimes, is not immediately obvious. Earlier studies have shown no adaptive hypertrophy within the first weeks of conditioning at slow or medium velocities (Costill et al 1979, Caiozzo et al 1981, Coyle et al 1981), but did indicate a significant increase for type II fibers at the high conditioning velocity of 300°/s (Coyle et al 1981). Komi (1986) suggested a period of 8 weeks before hypertrophy is apparent, though not with particular reference to isokinetics. However, later studies presented other views with respect to this issue.

Cote et al (1988)

In this study 23 sedentary individuals trained concentrically the quadriceps and hamstring using the following protocol: 10 w × 5 d × 3 s × 10 mr. Seven subjects then participated in the latter part of the study which consisted of 50 days without training, and then retraining according to the same protocol as before. Biopsies were performed on the vastus lateralis for histological and biochemical analyses. While the strength of the quadriceps increased by 54%, no overall increase in the fiber area was observed. However the percentage of type IIa fibers did increase significantly in number and area. Retraining after a 50-day detraining period did not result in any significant variation, either in strength or fiber area. It was concluded that although isokinetic conditioning could increase the functional capacity of skeletal muscle, it did not appear to induce hypertrophy.

Ewing et al (1990)

Isokinetic and biopsy studies of muscle performance and adaptation following conditioning were also undertaken by Ewing et al (1990) and Esselman et al (1991). In the former study subjects trained using maximal concentric quadriceps and hamstring contractions according to the following protocol: $10\,w \times 3\,s \times 3\,d \times 8–20\,mr$. Relatively modest increases in performance criteria (peak moment and contractional power) were recorded. Although there were no significant increases in the percentage of any fiber type (I, IIa or IIb) the area of type I and IIa fibers increased significantly, contrasting with the findings of Cote et al.

Esselman et al (1991)

The sophisticated protocol of Esselman et al (1991) consisted of $12\,w \times 5\,s \times 1\,d \times 20–60\,mr$ of quadriceps conditioning with a different input for the opposite lower extremity of each subject. Twenty men were randomized into four groups. Subjects in group I trained at 36°/s (low velocity) with 20 or 60 repetitions (reps), group II did 20 reps at 36°/s with one limb and 60 reps at 108°/s (medium velocity) contralaterally, and group III trained at 108°/s with 20 or 60 reps. Group IV (control) did not train. The significant increases in strength, especially in the low velocity conditioning group, following this relatively long period of conditioning, were not correlated with muscle hypertrophy, as no significant changes in type I and II fiber area were indicated. On the other hand, there was a significant increase in glycolytic and mitochondrial enzyme activity, in line with the findings of Cote et al (1988).

Whereas the low velocity group showed consistent gains up to the eighth week of conditioning, strength improvement in the medium/low velocity group leveled off after only 4 weeks. The authors suggested that these variations were consistent with neural adaptation and concluded that, in view of the absence of hypertrophy, the muscle adaptation had a smaller role in the overall strength gains.

Petersen et al (1989, 1990, 1991)

In this series of studies the cross-sectional area (CSA) of muscle (quadriceps, hamstring or both) was shown to increase significantly following different protocols of concentric conditioning, lasting 6 and 12 weeks respectively (see section on specificity of conditioning for description of the regime used).

In the first study, various hydraulic strength conditioning devices were used to overload the lower limb. In the second study, maximal knee extension was used as the overloading stimulus, whereas in the third study, conditioning was based on a combination of loading patterns for the lower limb, some of which were identical to those used in the first study. The authors used computed tomography (CT) for the calculation of thigh muscle cross-sectional area.

In all the studies significant hypertrophy was indicated, but the effect was not uniform; whereas quadriceps area increased during the first 6 weeks, a significant change in hamstring area occurred only after 12 weeks. The latter finding should be compared with a significant increase in hamstring strength, half-way into the program, which could be explained by neural adaptation.

The weekly variations in strength found in the 1990 study of Petersen et al are shown in Figure 4.1. The accelerating gain in strength shown in this study contrasts notably with the decelerating gain shown in that of Esselman et al (1991). This discrepancy, doubtless the result of the different protocols used by the investigators, serves to emphasize the complexities associated with interpretation of conditioning outcome.

Housh et al (1992)

In this study subjects trained concentrically their non-dominant knee and elbow flexors and extensors according to the protocol: $8\,w \times 3\,d \times 6\,s \times 10\,mr$. Using magnetic resonance imaging

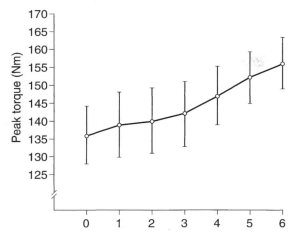

Figure 4.1 Peak concentric extension moment (mean ± SE) observed during the final training session of each week at 60°/s. (From Petersen et al 1990.)

(MRI) the cross-sectional area (CSA) of the relevant muscles and their component members in the proximal, medium and distal levels, in both the trained and untrained extremity were calculated before and after training. Significant CSA increases (8–34%) were demonstrated in the trained elbow extensors (proximal and middle levels) and flexors (all levels) but not in the contralateral muscles. For the trained knee extensors, increases were noted for the rectus femoris, vastus lateralis and intermedius (middle level). Significant differences were also noted for the semitendinosus and biceps femoris (middle level). No contralateral changes were discernible for either the extensors or flexors of the knee.

These results are in line with other studies such as those of Coyle et al (1981) or Narici et al (1989) and indicate that concentric isokinetic training without an eccentric component is a sufficient stimulus for inducing hypertrophy. This conclusion is at variance with that drawn by Cote et al (1988). Furthermore, there was a preferential increase in CSA of member muscles (i.e. rectus femoris) which could not be directly related to the level of activation. The authors suggest that in view of the specific location of those component members that increased the most, it is possible that a more sagittal orientation results in a more intense stimulus and thus a larger proportional increase. The authors argue that previous negative findings regarding CSA probably resulted from the application of techniques (CT, ultrasound, anthropometry) that were not sensitive enough to changes in muscle CSA.

Higbie et al (1996)

In this previously mentioned study, eccentric training resulted in a slightly larger but significant quadriceps CSA increase (6.6%) compared to concentric training (5%). These differences were computed based on seven slices taken along a distance of 20–80% of the femur. In this study as well, it was clearly indicated that concentric conditioning was a sufficiently strong hypertrophying stimulus. However, it should be borne in mind that the exercise dose typical of maximal eccentric exercise (in work units) was higher than that which was obtained during its concentric counterpart. Therefore, comparison should have been made had, for instance, 100% effort of concentric contraction been compared to 75% of maximal effort eccentric contraction.

Hortobágyi et al (1996)

The morphological variations reported in this study were singular in pointing out, based on computerized digitometry, selective increase in type IIa and decrease in type IIb fibers. No significant change took place vis-à-vis type I (slow twitch) fibers. Moreover, type II fibers increased 10 times more due to eccentric compared to concentric training. Interestingly, one would have expected increases in concentric strength due to hypertrophy of type II fibers but such an increase failed to take place. The authors have attributed this phenomenon to 'activation pattern during concentric actions that failed to recruit hypertrophied larger units, leading to minimal increases in concentric strength'.

Seger et al (1998)

In one of the latest studies of its kind, morphological variations following concentric and eccentric isokinetic knee extension training at 90°/s were examined based on a protocol of $10w \times 3d \times 4s \times 10mr$, initially for the left leg followed by an identical protocol for the right leg. Measurements of CSA were accomplished using MRI and were supplemented by counting the number of fibers retrieved using muscle biopsy. Both morphological markers were largely unremarkable. The quadriceps CSA increased 3–4% reaching significance only with respect to training. No major changes in muscle fiber composition were apparent. These small changes do not agree with the abovementioned findings (Hortobágyi et al 1996) whose subjects evidenced close to 40% increase in type II fibers. Furthermore, against a drop in IIa fibers in this study, the Hortobágyi paper reported a drastic opposite trend. These interstudy variations remain to a large extent elusive although they may result from the measurement technique used.

Incompatibility of findings

The general picture emerging from these studies points to an increase in CSA and some changes in type II (particularly IIa) fibers. However these variations span quite a large spectrum reflecting differences in training protocols and analytical techniques. There is a clear dichotomy between the more conservative findings, which relied on biopsy-based histology, and those based on CT, which indicated significant changes. In the latter case the inclusion of connective tissue elements of a non-contractile nature, which are known to increase in size during training (Sale 1988), might possibly account for the difference. It should also be realized that often the initial phase of rehabilitation uses conditioning methods other than isokinetic, and it is reasonable to assume that morphological and neural adaptations are already in progress by the time isokinetic conditioning is initiated.

In addition, where concentric and eccentric actions are involved, a dilemma regarding the common denominator for comparison confounds the picture (Seger et al 1998). Specifically, since under the same conditions eccentric contractions produce higher moments, a direct comparison with their concentric counterparts is not valid. If in attempting to bring the magnitude of contractions to the same level the eccentric component is

limited to, for example, 90% of the concentric contraction (using a feedback module) then the level of neural activation in the latter mode is further lowered. To complicate matters even more, the net contractile-based moment in eccentric contractions is actually smaller than the apparent moment as part of the tension generated during this contraction is supplied by passive components. These factors that to a large extent are difficult or even impossible to control, render comparisons of conditioning protocols and particularly interpretation of the derived findings, exceedingly complicated.

PART 3
SPECIFICITY OF MUSCLE PERFORMANCE CONDITIONING

As mentioned earlier conditioning of muscle performance can be effected using the overloading principle in various contraction modes: isometric, concentric, eccentric, plyometric or combinations. For instance, for the purpose of conditioning of knee extensor performance, one may use single or multiple isometrics, concentric (non-isokinetic) resisted extension in single or multiple joint, angular or linear patterns, isokinetic concentric and/or eccentric, drop jumps from different heights (plyometrics), or combinations.

If a well-designed conditioning program is based on a single method of performance enhancement, postconditioning testing using the same method that was used for conditioning is likely to reveal significant gains in strength (and/or other performance parameters). The degree to which these gains are specific to the particular method but not revealed when tested using a different method is the essence of the principle of specificity. For example, if upon using a protocol consisting solely of isokinetic *eccentric* contractions the recorded gains are expressed exclusively during eccentric but not concentric testing, this means that subject to this protocol the eccentric mode is specific. If on the other hand the gains are generalizable to concentric effort, the meaning is the opposite.

Although absolute specificity may not exist, protocol constraints which consist of total available period of training, interset breaks and within-set intensity as well as factors associated with the measurement system's precision and accuracy, may suggest otherwise. Furthermore, how a conditioning-based variable should be classified – specific or general – depends on cutoff scores which have never been set. Specifically, not a single study employed a paradigm that systematically explored before and after variations in terms of test-retest design. With particular reference to small variations, using a b/b–a/a protocol (testing twice before and twice after training) would have helped in assessing the extent to which the observed post-training variations were in fact of a genuine nature. Until such a study is available, the following conclusions must be viewed with care.

- The degree of specificity is considered mainly with respect to mode of contraction (e.g. concentric versus eccentric), velocity (high versus low), the nature of the kinetic chain and bilateral effects.
- Isokinetic training using limited range of motion has been found to affect muscle performance outside the trained sector (McNair & Stanley 1996, Barak 2003); the main lessons of these studies will be discussed later in the text.

SPECIFICITY OF MODES OF CONTRACTION

Research data

The findings from a few studies which investigated this problem using non-isokinetic conditioning methods did not confirm specificity for any of them (see Petersen et al 1990). With isokinetic performance, the problem has been defined as either one- or two-way transfer of gains. Table 4.1 presents a sample of studies which have measured transfer from eccentric conditioning to concentric performance (Bishop et al 1991, Ryan et al 1991), from concentric conditioning to eccentric performance (Petersen et al 1990, 1991) or mutual transfer (Duncan et al 1989, Tomberlin et al 1991, Mont et al 1994, Higbie et al 1996, Hortobágyi et al 1996, Seger et al 1998). The data from these studies indicate that:

1. Compared to concentric training which demonstrates non-specificity, the evidence regarding eccentric training is equivocal although more studies point to some specificity. This difference may reflect a combination of neurophysiological as well as muscle related mechanisms.
2. Concentric conditioning is preferable for enhancement of concentric strength while eccentric conditioning is preferable for enhancement of eccentric strength.
3. Furthermore, eccentric conditioning may bring about greater improvement in eccentric strength compared to the concentric gains following concentric conditioning.

Since different protocols were employed in these studies the above indications must be viewed with caution; the scope of their interpretation is qualified because:

1. with the exception of possibly one study (Mont et al 1994) all studies were based on training and testing of knee region muscles, particularly the quadriceps. Activity of this muscle is pivotal to the functioning of the lower extremity. However, the relevance of conclusions drawn with respect to findings based on this specific muscle, should not be taken for granted.
2. most research designs applied a slow velocity of 60°/s. Although a study of contraction mode specificity as a function of conditioning velocity is not currently available, it is possible that gains from lower velocities might be more effectively transferable. This speculation arises from the principle of physiological overflow (see below); low conditioning velocities are closer to the 'transfer zone' from one contraction mode to the other. The study by Duncan et al (1989) may provide some evidence for this, as at least with regard to eccentric conditioning, the concentric gains were higher at the lower velocity.
3. none of the abovementioned studies was applied in a clinical setting and the extent to which one may generalize from findings based on healthy individuals must be qualified.

Table 4.1   Specificity of contraction mode in isokinetic conditioning protocols*

Source and subjects	Protocol Weeks × days × sets × maximal repetitions	Velocity	Muscles	Contraction mode	Transfer
Bishop et al (1991)					
n = 13	8 w × 3 d × 3 s × 6 mr	60°/s	Quadriceps + hamstring	Eccentric	Specific for quadriceps, not specific for hamstring
n = 15	8 w × 3 d × 3 s × 6 mr	180°/s	Quadriceps + hamstring	Eccentric	Negligible effect of pain in eccentric mode
Duncan et al (1989)					
n = 16	6 w × 3 d × 1 s × 10 mr	120°/s	Quadriceps	Eccentric	Highly specific
n = 14	6 w × 3 d × 1 s × 10 mr	120°/s	Quadriceps	Concentric	More general
					Negligible effect of pain in eccentric mode
Petersen et al (1990)					
n = 8	6 w × 3 d × 5 s × 10 mr	60°/s	Quadriceps	Concentric	Not specific
Petersen et al (1991)					
n = 14	12 w × 3 d × (2–3) s × (8–12) mr	60°/s	Quadriceps + hamstring and other muscles	Concentric	Not specific
Tomberlin et al (1991)					
n = 19	6 w × 3 d × 3 s × 10 mr	100°/s	Quadriceps	Concentric	Not specific
n = 21	6 w × 3 d × 3 s × 10 mr	100°/s	Quadriceps	Eccentric	Specific
Ryan et al (1991)					
n = 34	6 w × 3 d × 1 s × 15 mr	120°/s	Hamstring	Eccentric	Not specific
Mont et al (1994)					
n = 10	6 w × 3 d × 8 s × 10 sr	90, 120, 150, 180°/s	Shoulder internal and external rotators	Concentric	Not specific
n = 10	6 w × 3 d × 8 s × 10 sr	90, 120, 150, 180°/s		Eccentric	Not specific
Higbie et al (1996)					
n = 16	10 w × 3 d × 3 s × 10 mr	60°/s	Quadriceps	Concentric	Not specific
n = 19	10 w × 3 d × 3 s × 10 mr	60°/s	Quadriceps	Eccentric	Specific
Hortobágyi et al (1996)					
n = 8	12 w × 3 d × (4–6) s × (8–12) mr	60°/s	Quadriceps	Concentric	Not specific
n = 7	12 w × 3 d × (4–6) s × (8–12) mr	60°/s	Quadriceps	Eccentric	Not specific
Seger et al (1998)					
n = 5	10 w × 3 d × 4 s × 10 mr	60°/s	Quadriceps	Concentric	Not specific
n = 5	10 w × 3 d × 4 s × 10 mr	60°/s	Quadriceps	Eccentric	More specific

* All findings refer to gain in peak moment. mr, maximal effort repetitions; sr, submaximal effort repetitions.

Clinical implication

If indeed '[isokinetic] resistance training effects are not always as specific to the training mode as has been thought' (Petersen et al 1990), the clinical implication cannot be overlooked. Eccentric contractions are important for the performance of daily activities as well as for the induction of muscle hypertrophy, but can potentially damage muscle fiber (Stauber 1989). In addition, eccentric conditioning would not be desirable in the rehabilitation of previously inactive individuals (Peterson et al 1990). It should also be borne in mind that not every rehabilitation facility has access to an active dynamometer. Hence, it is significant that concentric conditioning can produce an increase in eccentric strength.

The magnitude of this increase is not negligible; it was about 20 and 15% in the studies of Petersen et al (1990, 1991), about 10% in the study of Tomberlin et al (1991) and less than 10% in the findings of Duncan et al (1989). Clearly, these transfers may not be sufficient in every case, necessitating either more vigorous exercising or ultimately the use of eccentric conditioning.

SPECIFICITY OF CONDITIONING VELOCITIES

The question of whether gains achieved during conditioning at a given velocity are transferable to other velocities has received much attention. The physiological rationale underlying the possible phenomenon of velocity specificity is the differential recruitment of muscle fibers. It has been suggested (see Ewing et al 1990) that fast twitch fibers could be selectively stressed (and hence 'conditioned') during high velocity conditioning and vice versa.

Practical implication of velocity transfer

In the field of isokinetic dynamometry, the undisputed stimulus to this debate was the option of controlling the angular velocity of the lever-arm. The need to assess the extent of velocity specificity is no less practical than theoretical. In isokinetic rehabilitation, the demands for reaching optimal muscle performance must be reconciled with the limited resources of time and equipment.

For instance, consider a unilateral muscular dysfunction and assume that 'optimal' means a bilateral parity in strength along the spectrum of velocities 30–300°/s. Further assume that this spectrum is represented by 10 velocities 30°/s apart. The question would then be: is it essential to exercise at each of these discrete velocities or will the use of two 'anchor point' velocities, low and high, be sufficient? The problem is really that of defining the optimal velocity differentials.

Research findings

The findings obtained in a number of representative studies which explored the phenomenon of velocity specificity are outlined in Table 4.2. It would appear that except for one study (Perrin et al 1989) all studies indicated the existence of a so-called 'physiological overflow', or transfer, which is the reciprocal of specificity. This lack of specificity acted both ways; conditioning at a certain velocity resulted in strength gains at velocities higher and lower than the said velocity.

In these studies, the range of overflow was 30–180°/s. One study included eccentric conditioning (Duncan et al 1989) where there was an up/down overflow of 60°/s. Obviously more research is needed in terms of velocity transfer gains using eccentric conditioning.

In other studies this phenomenon was analyzed in terms of a one-way effect and the data were generally of the same or even higher magnitude.

Using these findings it is not possible to determine whether the lack of specificity has some preferential directionality, i.e. whether the overflow should be associated more with higher or lower velocities. However, a velocity differential of 90°/s may confidently be used in isokinetic conditioning protocols.

SPECIFICITY OF ANGULAR ('OPEN KINETIC CHAIN') AND LINEAR PATTERNS OF ('CLOSED KINETIC CHAIN') CONDITIONING

The use of linear motion patterns (LMP, the so-called 'closed kinetic chain') effected using a

Table 4.2 Specificity of velocities in isokinetic conditioning protocol[a] (↑,↓ upwards, downwards transfer)

Source and subjects	Protocol — Weeks × days × sets × maximal repetitions	Muscles	Velocity	Transfer
Caiozzo et al (1981)				
n = 5	4 w × 3 d × 2 s × 10 mr	Quadriceps	96°/s	↑ to 240°/s
n = 5	4 w × 3 d × 2 s × 10 mr	Quadriceps	240°/s	↓ to 144°/s
Coyle et al (1981)				
n = 4	6 w × 3 d × 5 s × (6 or 12) mr	Quadriceps	60°/s	↑ to 180°/s
n = 4	6 w × 3 d × 5 s × (6 or 12) mr	Quadriceps	300°/s	↓ to 0°/s
Duncan et al (1989)				
n = 14	6 w × 3 d × 1 s × 10 mr	Quadriceps	120°/s	↑ to 180°/s C only
n = 16 (eccentric)	6 w × 3 d × 1 s × 10 mr	Quadriceps	120°/s	↑/↓ in E only: 60°/s
Esselman et al (1991)				
n = 5	12 w × 5 d × 1 s × (20 or 60) mr	Quadriceps	36°/s	
n = 5	12 w × 5 d × 1 s × (20 or 60) mr	Quadriceps	36, 108°/s	General ↑ and ↓ overflow
n = 5	12 w × 5 d × 1 s × (20 or 60) mr	Quadriceps	108°/s	
Ewing et al (1990)				
n = 10	10 w × 3 d × 3 s × (8–20) mr	Quadriceps	60°/s	↑ to 180°/s (peak moment and contractional power)
n = 10	10 w × 3 d × 3 s × (8–20) mr	Quadriceps	240°/s	↓ to 180°/s (peak moment and contractional power)
Jenkins et al (1984)				
n = 12	6 w × 3 d × 1 s × 15 mr	Quadriceps	60°/s	↑ to 240°/s
n = 12	6 w × 3 d × 1 s × 15 mr	Quadriceps	240°/s	↓ to 30°/s
Lesmes et al (1978)				
n = 5	7 w × 4 d × (2 or 10) s (30 or 6 s max)	Quadriceps	180°/s	↓ to 0°/s ↑ to 60°/s (contractional work)
	7 w × 4 d × (2 or 10) s (30 or 6 s max)	Hamstring	180°/s	↓ 120–0°/s ↑ to 60°/s (contractional work)

Study	Protocol	Muscle group	Velocity	Findings
Perrin et al (1989) n = 7	7w × 3d × 3s × 25mr	Quadriceps + hamstring	70°/s	No ↓ (at 180, 60°/s)
Petersen et al (1989) n = 15 n = 15	6w × 3d × (2–3)s (20s max) 6w × 3d × (2–3)s (20s max)	Knee extensors Knee extensors	180°/s 60°/s	↑ and ↓ (+60 and −30°/s) ↑ to 180°/s
Timm (1987) n = 30	8w × 3d × 1s (to 50% fatigue)	Knee extensors	180°/s	↑ 120°/s and ↓ 120°/s overflow (peak moment and contractional power)
Housh & Housh (1993) n = 12	8w × 3d × 6s × 10mr	Knee and elbow flexors and extensors	120°/s	↓ to 60°/s and ↑ to 180, 240 and 300°/s
O'Hagan et al (1995)[b] n = 6	20w × 3d × (3–5)s × (8–12)[c]mr	Elbow flexors	Approx. 30°/s	↑ to 120°/s
McNair & Stanley (1996) n = 14	8w × 3d × 3s × 8mr	Quadriceps	120°/s	↓ to 60°/s and ↑ to 180°/s
Seger et al (1998) n = 5 (concentric) n = 5 (eccentric)	10w × 3d × 4s × 10mr 10w × 3d × 4s × 10mr	Quadriceps Quadriceps	90°/s 90°/s	In both contraction modes ↓ to 30°/s

[a] All findings refer to gains in peak moment, and using concentric mode, except where indicated otherwise.
[b] Performed using quasi-isokinetic conditions.
[c] Coupled concentric–eccentric contractions.

multijoint approach has been gathering considerable momentum particularly with respect to rehabilitation of ACL pathologies. The advantages of this particular conditioning mode are both its more functional nature and, in some instances, a better load distribution within the joints that are spanned by the working muscles. Linear motion patterns such as the leg-press can be realized using linear or angular devices. Linear drive isokinetic dynamometers appear either as a stand-alone unit (e.g. Liftask by Cybex or the Linea by Lido) or in the form of a special attachment to an angular dynamometer (e.g. the linear attachment of Biodex).

Since LMP typically involve simultaneous contraction of several muscles for the purpose of executing a given task, it is possible that individual muscles would be denied the full effect of the overloading stimulus such as occurs during 'single' joint angular activity (the so-called 'open kinetic chain'). Hence, a well-balanced regime should incorporate both training modes. It is however imperative to assess the enhancement of single joint-based performance by multiple joint-based activity and vice versa, in order to design an optimal combination of the two variants. This, in other words, is a problem of specificity.

Currently, knowledge regarding this issue is almost non-existent. There is probably only one study where single joint (angular movement) training was applied in order to test its effect on non-isokinetic constant load cycling (Mannion et al 1992). The latter was chosen since it was a functional activity which put considerable demand on the knee extensors, but in a different coordination pattern from the conditioning (angular) maneuver. In this study, two experimental groups underwent bilateral quadriceps conditioning at 60 and 240°/s respectively, using the protocol: $16\,w \times 3\,d \times 6\,s \times 25\,mr$. The performance criteria were isometric knee extensor strength and power output during a 6-second all-out sprint on a bicycle ergometer. Findings indicated significant increases in the peak power output and peak pedal velocity during sprint cycling, with no difference between the two conditioning velocity groups. It was therefore concluded that the gains achieved in the course of angular isokinetic activity could be positively transferred to a non-isokinetic multijoint activity.

CROSS-EDUCATION (BILATERAL EFFECTS)

Some indications concerning cross-education during isokinetic concentric conditioning appear in the study by Esselman et al (1991). The experimental design included three subject groups, who trained the knee extensors of both limbs but with differing protocols (Table 4.3). The identical protocols of subgroups B and C (36°/s, 20 repetitions) and D and E (108°/s, 60 repetitions) enabled the analysis of cross-education.

The findings indicated that the increase in strength made by subgroup B was greater than that made by subgroup C, and those by subgroup D greater by 100% than E. It should be noted that in spite of an identical 'training dose' in both

Table 4.3 Cross-education effect due to isokinetic conditioning (Based on Esselman et al 1991)

Group	n	Velocity (°/s)	Repetitions	% increase	P
IA	5	36	60	129	<0.05
IB	5	36	20	126	<0.05
IIC	5	36	20	58	<0.05
IID	5	108	60	50	<0.05
IIIE	5	108	60	25	NS
IIIF	5	108	20	23	NS
Control				16	NS

NS, not significant.

subgroups B and C as well as D and E, the contralateral leg was trained differently, namely A versus D or C versus F respectively. In spite of the fact that direct comparisons cannot be performed (e.g. subgroups A and B did not train with the same number of repetitions), this study indicates that the tendency for the opposite lower extremity to respond similarly to conditioning, could be more important than the number of repetitions.

Later studies addressed this issue using different protocols. Housh & Housh (1993, see protocol in Table 4.2) have shown that the strength gains derived from a unilateral concentric training of the knee and elbow flexors and extensors could be transferred, with the exception of elbow flexors, to the untrained limb covering down and up velocity differences of 60 and 120°/s, respectively. Seger et al (1998) arrived at a more restrictive finding namely that cross-education was mode (concentric as well as eccentric) and velocity specific.

Another study (Hortobágyi et al 1997) examined the differential effect of concentric versus eccentric training on the untrained limb. Using a previously described protocol (Hortobágyi et al 1996) it was revealed that whereas concentric training improved the concentric capacity by 22% the respective effect of eccentric training on the eccentric contralateral limb was 77%. Furthermore, eccentric training was equally more potent in enhancing isometric strength. It was hence concluded that eccentric training was a more powerful stimulus for crossover muscle education.

Collectively, these studies indicate that performance gains due to muscle conditioning in one side are transferable to their unconditioned counterparts.

TRANSFER OF GAINS OUTSIDE THE TRAINED RANGE OF MOTION

Training using only a fraction of the available joint range of motion (ROM) has two main aims. First, muscular force vectors deriving from maximal efforts may result in the development of dangerously high stresses and strains either on joint surfaces or on associated structures. A typical case in point is the tension generated within the ACL when the quadriceps contracts concentrically and

forcefully near full extension of the knee. Hence, in partial tear of this ligament or after its reconstruction, great care must be taken in order to avoid excessive strains. The solution may be one of three:

1. to limit muscle force
2. to use configurations like leg-press which if performed isokinetically requires a linear dynamometer or a special attachment
3. to limit joint ROM to angular sectors well outside the problem zone, for instance 45–90° of knee flexion.

While the first option slows down muscle recovery, the second may be very costly. Thus the third option – applying limited ROM while maintaining maximal muscle capacity – is an effective one so long as gains within the untrained zone are ensured.

The second aim emerges in those cases where pain is present but is well located within a specific sector – the painful arch. Pain is a well known muscle strength inhibitor and therefore trying to increase muscle force may be negated by a reflexive shut-off. On the other hand, as long as the painful arch is not included within the trained sector, such an inhibition will be minimal. If gain overflow in the form of increased performance within the painful arch as a result of training outside it can occur, the therapeutic objective may be achieved in a more effective way.

That strength may be achieved outside the trained 'range' is well known when isometric training is applied (Kitai & Sale 1989). In other words when training statically at a given point in the joint ROM there is a carry-over effect to other points. However, whether a parallel transfer of gain principle applies when a *point* becomes a *range*, is not clear. In what was probably the first examination of this question, McNair & Stanley (1996) trained a group of 14 male and female subjects using a single velocity of 120°/s and the following paradigm: $8w \times 3d \times 3s \times 8mr$. A parallel control group consisted of a matched number of subjects. Maximal concentric isokinetic contractions of the quadriceps were performed between 45 and 90° of knee flexion. Baseline and post-training tests consisted of maximal contractions performed along a ROM from

90° to maximal extension (0°) using test velocities of 60, 120 and 180°/s. Significant increases were noted in the trained range across all angular velocities ranging from 10 to 13%. In the untrained range muscular work also increased over all velocities but reached statistical significance only at the training velocity, amounting to 11%. It is likely that this specific transfer reflects neural adaptation.

The effect of isokinetic concentric and eccentric conditioning of the quadriceps within a limited ROM (LROM) using more than one velocity on several mechanical parameters inside and outside this sector was recently examined by Barak (2003). Fifty-five young women were divided into four groups: concentric conditioning at 30°/s (group I) and 90°/s (group II), and eccentric conditioning at same angular velocities, groups III and IV respectively. All subjects trained at between 30 and 60° of knee flexion based on the following protocol: 6 w × 3 d × 4 s × 10 mr. For assessment of the training effect on gains achieved outside the LROM, criterion (pre/post) isokinetic and isometric tests were conducted at three individual sectors: 5–30° (the inner range), 30–60° (the trained range) and 60–85° (the outer range). The major findings of this study with respect to the gains and their transferability from the trained into the untrained ROM were:

1. The trained ROM was specific since the highest gains in work scores (significant at 13/16 of the cases and ranging from 8 to 34%) were achieved at those test modes that paralleled the training method, except for Ecc 90. In the latter case the gain in that velocity was second highest.
2. Eccentric training resulted in significantly higher gains compared to concentric training.
3. The outer ROM (60–85°) was characterized by even higher (and significant) increases compared to the trained ROM, in a similar number of instances (13/16 cases) and ranging from 18 to 48%. This trend was apparent with respect to all test conditions Hence, work gains were transferable from the middle to the outer range.
4. This was not the case in the inner ROM (5–30°) where in spite of an average increase

in work of 8.3% in most cases the recorded increases were not significant. Consequently work gains were generally non-transferable from the middle to the inner range.
5. Interestingly, isometric strength gains as well as the excitation frequency of the EMG increased significantly in the inner and outer ROMs. However, this EMG variation was significantly higher in the trained and outer range compared to the inner (5–30°) range.

It should be appreciated that in the study of McNair & Stanley (1996) the gain in the untrained range was a comparable 11% and limited to the conditioning velocity. Thus in spite of an ostensible variance, it is possible that both studies do in fact point to a limited benefit from training muscles in a region where they are relatively longer into a region where they are shorter. At least with respect to the more recent study, there is ground for attributing this effect to the limited EMG changes in the inner sector.

PART 4
PRINCIPLES OF ISOKINETIC CONDITIONING PROGRAMS (ICPs) IN CLINICAL REHABILITATION

In spite of more than 35 years' intensive use of isokinetic dynamometry, the body of clinical knowledge, especially research-based, concerning its use in rehabilitation leaves much to be desired. Some of the reasons for this have already been discussed with regard to conditioning studies in general. On the other hand, promotional material and courses offered by manufacturers, presentations given in user group meetings and, presumably, personal experience and sound clinical common sense, assist practitioners to extend the use of isokinetic systems beyond that of pure testing.

In the area of clinical rehabilitation, the great advantage of isokinetics lies in its capacity to accommodate the moment generated by the contracting muscle(s). Furthermore, it is possible:

1. to adjust the control parameters, particularly the upper limit of the muscular moment which may safely be generated, and

2. to visually display the trace of the strength curve in real time, sometimes for feedback to the subject.

These facilities enable clinicians to ensure that certain muscle/joint load values will not be exceeded. However, to the best of the present author's knowledge, these very values and their progressive modification during the course of rehabilitation, have never been systematically investigated and/or formulated. This is but one of a cluster of issues that makes the therapeutic use of isokinetics the most complicated of all topics discussed in this book. The final part of this chapter discusses some major problems associated with the therapeutic applications of isokinetics. These include:

1. isokinetics versus other performance conditioning methods
2. the objective of isokinetic conditioning programs (ICPs)
3. the timing of ICP introduction into the general rehabilitation program
4. protocol-related issues
5. selected protocols
6. delayed onset muscle soreness as a result of isokinetic conditioning programs.

ISOKINETICS VERSUS OTHER PERFORMANCE CONDITIONING METHODS

A compelling reason for employing isokinetic dynamometry in rehabilitation is its assumed superiority to other methods such as the isometric or isotonic. Only a handful of studies have tested the veracity of this assumption, and they cannot be compared with one another because of lack of consistency between studies on any variable.

Isokinetics versus weight- or self-training

Clinical evidence of the superiority of isokinetic conditioning comes from the illuminating findings of a study relating to quadriceps function by Grimby et al (1980). All the patients investigated had undergone surgery on the isolated anterior cruciate ligament (ACL), medial collateral ligament or a combination of both. During the post-operative period all were engaged in structured physical therapy programs and the athletes among them even resumed their activity.

Following a period of 14 months, on average, a comparative study of the effect of isokinetic conditioning versus weight training or self-training was undertaken. Preconditioning measurements had indicated a significant strength reduction in the quadriceps of the involved side. Histological findings had failed to indicate any significant bilateral differences.

The general regime was similar for the weight training and isokinetic methods: $6w \times 3d \times 3s \times 10mr$ with the latter performed at the low velocity of $42°/s$. The self-training program was somewhat different: $3w \times 6d$ $(25 \times 2–8kg) + 3w \times 6d \times (50 \times 2–8kg)$.

The results, based on testing at 0, 30, 42 and $120°/s$ are shown in Figure 4.2. A very important finding was that the isokinetic group showed a complete restoration of bilateral symmetry in strength at all velocities. Although all groups increased their quadriceps strength significantly, the highest gains were made by the isokinetic group. These gains were however significant only with respect to an isometric test. This is not very

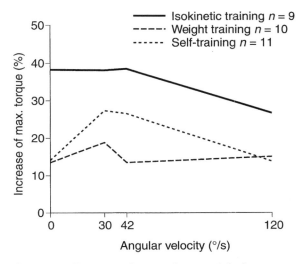

Figure 4.2 Percentage increase in strength for knee extension for three training groups. (From Grimby et al 1980.)

surprising since the conditioning velocity was low. The present author believes Grimby et al were correct in anticipating more significant improvement (over the other methods) had the conditioning velocity been higher. On the other hand, there was a conspicuous overflow effect, which is apparent from the relatively flat shape of the isokinetic curve.

A distinguishing feature of this study was the fact that all participants were pain free, with a reasonable ROM and already engaged in various athletic activities. This study indicates therefore that:

1. there is a need for a more systematized follow-up of patients with knee injury
2. spontaneous activity including athletic training may not suffice to restore muscular function
3. this insufficiency can be remedied very effectively using ICPs.

An epidemiological study

The most comprehensive study of this issue is epidemiological in nature and summarizes the postsurgical knee rehabilitation findings of more than 5000 patients, with a roughly equal gender division, during a period of 5 years (Timm 1988). The surgery involved a large variety of non-ACL procedures. The resumption of required activities without symptom recurrence, during the 5-year postoperative period, was defined as the criterion for success. This criterion was examined with respect to four methods of rehabilitation: no exercise, home exercise, isotonic exercise and isokinetic exercise.

Those patients who used isokinetic methods had a significantly shorter rehabilitation interval, 8.9 ± 3.7 weeks, compared to isotonic-based rehabilitation, 12.3 ± 6.1 weeks or home exercise, 10.0 ± 4.5 weeks. In addition an impressive correlation with success ($r = 0.92$) was recorded for patients comprising the isokinetic group compared with the isotonic and home exercise groups (0.48 and 0.09 respectively). Although these findings cannot be interpreted with the same confidence as those of a well controlled prospective study, they may indicate a 'general superiority' of isokinetics over other methods.

Effectiveness of ICPs

Consequently, in the light of the above studies it can legitimately be concluded that among the methods commonly employed for muscle performance enhancement in clinical and normal populations, ICPs are probably more effective, assuming equal resources. However, in the absence of other studies, this conclusion should currently be reserved for knee rehabilitation.

THE OBJECTIVE OF ISOKINETIC CONDITIONING

Progressive overloading

As with other methods of strength conditioning, isokinetics operates according to the mechanism of progressive overloading of the involved muscles. Muscle tension of the magnitude that is expected to develop during even submaximal isokinetic contractions is bound to have an effect on structures other than the muscle itself, i.e. the bones comprising the joint, the articular surfaces, the joint capsule and the ligaments. However, the extent to which isokinetic contractions are directly responsible for better proprioception, cartilage nourishment and the repair or growth enhancement of connective tissue is unknown. It is possible to generalize from other sources which have elucidated the important role which physical activity has in preserving the functional state of the abovementioned structures (Stone 1988). The objective of isokinetic conditioning is considered in this book to be related to the effect isokinetics has on its target organ: the skeletal muscle.

In terms of the control parameters, overloading refers to:

1. progressively increasing the active range of motion (ROM)
2. progressively raising the upper limit imposed on the generation of either the peak or the average moment (the former parameter is the almost universal criterion)
3. extending the range of angular velocities, concurrently with 1 and 2
4. the incorporation of isokinetic eccentric loading.

Optimization of muscle strength

Clearly since, with respect to either concentric or eccentric exertions, the moment levels that can be generated during isokinetic contractions span the full spectrum of muscle strength, the main objective of isokinetic conditioning is to optimize muscle strength through the induction of maximal gains at all angular positions of the available joint ROM and along a predetermined spectrum of angular velocities. It should be emphasized that:

1. Optimization rather than maximization defines the special advantage of an ICP. In theory it is possible to maximize strength gains through multiple angle isometric contractions. However, such a method demands the consumption of resources far in excess of those used in an ICP.

2. Enhancement of strength, rather than other performance parameters, is explicitly defined although the specificity of velocity studies, mentioned earlier, showed conditioning-based improvements in other performance parameters such as contractional work and power. These parameters, it should be remembered, are very closely correlated with the peak moment, the mechanical 'name' of strength. In addition, strength is the only parameter to which reference has been made in the few clinical studies of conditioning protocols.

3. The decision concerning the spectrum of velocities involved must rely on the patient's performance and functional requirements.

TIMING OF ISOKINETIC CONDITIONING

Leaving aside patient-linked factors such as compliance, the timing of the introduction of isokinetic conditioning into rehabilitation depends on two factors: the nature of the injury or dysfunction including its anatomical location, and the therapeutic approach – surgical or non-surgical. Postoperative isokinetic conditioning is by far the more complicated and more debated topic and therefore deserves particular attention. Where conservative treatment is concerned, the incorporation of isokinetics follows the general principles of progressive resistive exercise (PRE) or its

variants (see, for instance, Knight 1979), except, of course, where it is contraindicated.

Some models regarding the most suitable stage for introducing an ICP into postoperative rehabilitation have been proposed. Notably, none of the models was based on a methodical exploration of this problem and therefore should be viewed with caution; to quote Zarins et al (1985):

Not all patients are rehabilitated uniformly, and a great deal of variability exists following arthroscopic surgery … Therefore an arbitrary time frame for rehabilitation … is not recommended. Rather, each patient should progress from one stage of rehabilitation to the next, based on objective knee findings.

Hence, time per se should not serve as a criterion for introducing an ICP.

Quadriceps endurance as criterion

Sherman et al (1983) compared two methods of rehabilitation of patients following an open procedure for removal of the medial meniscus. The criterion for introduction of isokinetic conditioning was a level of quadriceps endurance which was equivalent to 8 sets × 10 repetitions of knee extension with 20 lb, using an NK table. The authors neither explained nor discussed the choice of this particular criterion which had been equally applicable to both experimental groups: one with knee immobilization and one without. Based on the above criterion, the ICP started 2 and 4 weeks after the operation, in the former and latter group respectively.

Phase of healing

A four-phase general rehabilitation program following surgery of the knee (Table 4.4) has been proposed by Zarins et al (1985). This program was also designed specifically for the rehabilitation of patients following open or arthroscopic meniscectomy, although the authors maintained that it was appropriate for other knee arthrotomy procedures.

According to this program, isokinetic conditioning may start as soon as early healing (phase II) is over. It should be noted that 'late healing'

Table 4.4 Phases of postoperative knee rehabilitation: the program of Zarins et al (1985)

Phase	Description	Characteristics	Exercises
I	Immediate postoperative period	Incision, bleeding, pain, quadriceps, inhibition	Quadriceps setting, straight-leg-raising, hamstring resistance, ambulation ± external support
II	Early healing	Less pain, effusion, muscles weak, 90° of motion	Active range of motion, continue isometrics, ambulate, cycle
III	Late healing	No pain, effusion ± weakness, 120° of motion	Walk, cycle, swim, functional exercise, high speed isokinetics
IV	Late rehabilitation and conditioning	Full range of motion, no effusion, muscle weakness, not returned to sports	Isotonic, functional activities, running, jumping, gradual return to sports, all speeds isokinetics

was characterized by less pain and effusion and hence less likelihood of quadriceps inhibition (De Andrade 1965). Thus the criterion for introducing isokinetic conditioning is clinical and subjective.

Clinical exercise progression of Davies (1992)

A general approach to clinical exercise progression has been proposed by Davies (1992). The principles of patient safety and overloading are the basis of this method. The program is conducted sequentially:

Stage I multiple-angle, submaximal isometrics
Stage II multiple-angle, maximal isometrics
Stage III short arc, submaximal isokinetics
Stage IV short arc, isotonics
Stage V short arc, maximal isokinetics
Stage VI full ROM, submaximal isokinetics
Stage VII full ROM, isotonics (if not contraindicated)
Stage VIII full ROM, maximal isokinetics.

According to this model isokinetic conditioning may be introduced fairly early and the criterion for its initial introduction is a safe performance of maximal, multiple-angle isometric contractions. The introduction of submaximal isokinetic before isotonic contractions is somewhat surprising, unless the former can be maintained at load values lower than the latter. Even more notable is the obscurity of the term 'submaximal'; its

quantitative significance is never spelled out, although the author maintains elsewhere that:

the minimum sub-maximal threshold to produce a training response with isokinetics is unknown at the present time. Therefore there is need for research in this area.

Another weakness of this model and of the others mentioned is the apparent omission of the eccentric model; it is not obvious whether 'isokinetics' refers to both contraction modes. The present author is not aware of any conditioning model that deals directly with this problem.

Suggested criteria for ICP introduction

To summarize, there are three general approaches to the timing of ICPs:

1. Use of predominantly clinical signs and estimation of the status of healing (Zarins et al 1985).
2. Use of a muscle performance criterion (Sherman et al 1983).
3. The sequential approach of Davies (1992).

Undoubtedly, where postoperative conditioning is concerned, the stage of tissue healing – which will reflect surgical procedure(s) – is the single most important criterion for deciding whether to refrain from, or initiate, an ICP. Obviously the exertion of high loads on an as yet unhealed tissue could set the healing process back or even undermine the surgical objective. On the other hand, a progressive build-up of stress is essential for healing. Hence the optimal stage for introducing an ICP can probably be determined using a combination of the three approaches.

Assuming normal tissue recovery, patient compliance and the availability of reasonable physical therapy, introduction of submaximal isokinetic conditioning should be based on isokinetic testing. Testing of the involved versus the contralateral sound structure(s) may be carried out when there is a reasonable level of healing (end of phase II as defined by Zarins et al) and after full active ROM is achieved. With these considerations in mind, the following procedures are suggested. Although based on postmeniscectomy conditioning, they may provide a convenient basis for future clinical exploration of this issue.

1. Testing should preferably be performed in a non-gravity plane.
2. Uninvolved side concentric and eccentric testing should be carried out to full capacity.
3. Involved side concentric-only testing should be performed at a submaximal level and an upper moment limit be set at 30% of the contralateral peak moment; this may be judged too low but it leaves a comfortable safety margin of 70%. This criterion incorporates the design of Sherman et al (1983) which was based on a 20 lb resistance load in an endurance test. Assuming a lever of 30 cm this load is equivalent to about 30 Nm. Normative values for knee extensor isokinetic strength (Freedson et al 1993) provide a basis for comparison. For example the extension moment at 180°/s, corresponding to the 50th percentile of the male age group 31–40 was about 110 Nm (120 nm and 100 Nm for the 21–30, 41–50 age groups respectively). Therefore the relative exertion here is $(30/110) \times 100 = 27\%$. This figure (27%) should also be valid for women.
4. At this level of exertion the level of pain, rated according to any common and applicable pain rating system, should be recorded; discomfort or other negative signs should also be recorded.
5. A pain level expressed by a statement such as 'it is really painful' (e.g. 5 on the Borg (1982) modified 0–10 pain scale) may signify that the tissues

are not yet ready to negotiate such a load and hence isokinetic conditioning should be deferred to a later date; the same logic applies to other signs.
6. Upon the positive completion of the test, a short conditioning protocol consisting of a single set of 10 repetitions may be attempted in order to assess the patient's ability to sustain these exertions satisfactorily, and an ICP may then follow.
7. Eccentric isokinetic conditioning may be introduced once the concentric peak moment has reached 50% of that of the sound side. This figure is based on an eccentric/concentric strength ratio of 1.33. This is a rough average of muscle performance at medium velocities (Albert 1991).

As mentioned, this procedure is but one way to rationally introduce isokinetic conditioning. Similar programs have to be worked out individually for specific therapeutic interventions.

CONDITIONING PROTOCOLS

This section deals with a number of problems concerning optimal isokinetic conditioning within the framework of a single set. These problems concern, for instance, the choice of high versus low velocity conditioning, or the use of a velocity spectrum design as advocated by Davies (1992). The scientific rationale for choosing an optimal protocol is virtually non-existent, a situation generally characteristic of isokinetic conditioning at large. The order of presentation of the following is not an indication of the relative importance of the problems.

Minimal initial contraction intensity for ICPs

This question may be phrased: what is the minimal magnitude of moment required to induce changes in strength? There are two approaches to this problem. One, proposed by Young et al (1985), maintains that the intensity of the neural drive, rather than the magnitude of the load, may represent the stimulus for increasing strength. The other states that the major determinant of the adaptive strength response is indeed the tension generated by the muscle. It seems, from the relevant literature, that the latter hypothesis prevails. For instance, it has been shown that at training loads below approximately 66% of the maximum, no increase in the maximal voluntary contraction (MVC) was obtained even if up to 150 contractions/day were used (McDonagh & Davies 1984). Though none of the available studies is directly relevant to isokinetics, they do provide a frame of reference.

Thus submaximal conditioning must on the one hand be limited by an upper moment value, and on the other, it must not fall below a certain minimum if change is to be induced. The present author suggests that an isokinetic endurance test, at a medium velocity, of the contralateral limb is carried out. The findings should be indicative of the desired potential of the involved muscles and/or associated structures. A reasonable initial 'performance ceiling' (non-surgical) would then be at a level of 50% of the above maximal force. Increases in this parameter should follow the usual course of PRE (see also below). This takes into consideration the fact that the patient is already well into the rehabilitation process.

High versus low velocity conditioning

This topic has been addressed in a clinical context by Thomee et al (1987) in a study of isokinetic conditioning following reconstruction (procedure unspecified) of the ACL. The ICP was initiated, on average, after a 6-month postoperative period, during which knee casts and conventional physical therapy had been used. Two patient groups participated in the study, one trained at 60°/s and the other at 180°/s. Both knee extensors and flexors were trained. The conditioning regimes were: $8w \times 3d \times (3–10)s \times 10mr$ and $8w \times 3d \times (3–10)s \times 15mr$ for the slower and faster velocity groups respectively. Compared with the contralateral limb, the increases in strength were from 56 to 74% and 78 to 102% for the quadriceps and hamstring respectively. However, upon testing along a velocity spectrum of 30 to 300°/s, no significant differences were noted between the two groups, although there was a slight tendency towards velocity specificity.

Considering the ACL surgical procedure as sufficiently representative of a number of knee interventions, in terms of soft tissue damage and intensity of rehabilitation, it can be concluded that if a concentric ICP is to be based on a single velocity, then a medium velocity is preferable to a low velocity. This has three benefits:

1. a shorter exposure time to the mechanical loads imposed due to the contraction force of the muscle(s)
2. a smaller contraction force as illustrated by the moment–angular velocity relationship
3. no loss of generality, because of an excellent downwards physiological overflow, which may extend isometric strength.

It should however be pointed out that if the patient finds it difficult to accelerate the distal segment forcefully enough to reach the preset velocity, adjusting the latter is necessary. Hence it may be beneficial to start at 120°/s and observe the angular sector of the ROM required to develop isokinetic conditions. If this takes up more than one-third of the ROM, it means that the patient is virtually performing a submaximal isotonic contraction. This in turn will require the use of an even lower velocity, 60–90°/s.

As indicated below, modern protocols involve more than one velocity yet the use of the medium/ higher end of the velocity spectrum, in the context of isokinetic conditioning (rather than testing), is still the more logical one.

Rest intervals and sets

The optimal numbers of repetitions and sets, and the length of rest intervals, are of prime importance to the design of an ICP, but there are few studies relating to these topics.

Number of repetitions

The optimal number of repetitions required for improvement of knee flexor and extensor total contraction work, contractional power, and endurance ratios was investigated by Davies et al (1985a,b). The study regime was: $6w \times 3d \times 3s$ with 5, 10, 15 or 20 repetitions at 180°/s. With respect to total contractional work and endurance ratios, it was found that the best results were obtained using 15 or 20 repetitions for the quadriceps (although 10 repetitions also yielded significant improvements), and 10 for the hamstring. The contractional power of both muscles increased maximally following a 10-repetition protocol.

The studies suggest that with these regimes, 10 repetitions overall is the optimal number. Although this is a very convenient parameter, a fixed number of repetitions is not essential.

Sherman et al (1982) proposed that the termination of an individual set should be decided by reference to a fatigue ratio, i.e. it should be ended when the peak moment of a contraction is only 50% of the initial moment. Although functionally it is a sounder parameter, technical difficulties prevent the wider use of this criterion.

Interset and intervelocity spectrum intervals

Ariki & Davies (1985) have studied the optimal intervals for interset and interspectrum time. The interspectrum time refers to the time period between two identical full spectra consisting of the velocities 180, 210, 240, 270 and 300°/s. The optimal interset and interspectrum time intervals were 90 s and 3 min respectively.

In his book, Davies (1992) claims correctly that a 90 s interval may be too long since a typical clinic may not have more than one isokinetic system. Therefore, unless the patient is uncomfortable or exhausted this period can be reduced to 30–60 s. On the other hand, a 3 min interspectrum period is appropriate.

Optimal number of sets

Determination of the optimal number of sets may be the most difficult question since this largely depends on the design of the protocol. However, a reasonable solution to this problem is to use the percentage reduction in peak moment as has already been suggested with regard to the number of intraset repetitions. Such a solution was indeed reported in a case study (Timm & Patch 1985) with respect to a full velocity spectrum program.

A reasonable way for establishing the number of sets is to have the subject perform a trial set of 10 repetitions and compare the mean of the peak or average moment (PM or AVM) of the last three (L) with the corresponding figure for the first three (F) repetitions. In the absence of pain the suggested rule is: if $L/F > 50\%$ proceed to the next set otherwise terminate conditioning.

Once the number of sets is determined, progression to the next phase should not be problematical.

Total contraction output

A study by Lesmes et al (1978) raised an important question regarding the total contraction output needed for an effective ICP. It was indicated that a significant improvement (5–25% in knee extensor and flexor force) could be derived from a protocol consisting of 4 min of conditioning per week! Therefore the relatively large volume prescribed for isokinetic conditioning in other methods is much in question.

Discharge from conditioning programs

Discharge from an ICP is based on achieving near or perfect bilateral parity. The 'near' approach is represented, for instance, by Tegner et al (1986), and indeed by most of the advocates of accelerated rehabilitation following ACL reconstruction (for a detailed discussion see Chapter 7). The 'perfect' approach, which has been advocated by Sherman et al (1982), may not be a realistic one, particularly with respect to ligament reconstruction surgery.

SELECTED PROTOCOLS

In theory, if not in practice, there is an infinite number of possible ICPs. Since the scientific and clinical bases of even the most commonly used ICPs have never been subjected to a rigorous comparative analysis, it is difficult to single out any particular ICP as a better, let alone the best option. As mentioned more than once, the variety of clinical situations, coupled with the individual differences among patients makes the selection of

Table 4.5 Protocols illustrating principles of isokinetic conditioning program (ICP) design

	Sherman et al (1982)*	Bennett & Stauber (1986)	Jensen & Di Fabio (1989)	Knutsson & Martensson (1991)
Objective	Rehabilitation after knee surgery (meniscectomy)	Rehabilitation of anterior knee pain	Rehabilitation of patellar tendinitis	Rehabilitation of spastic paresis
Muscles	Knee extensors and flexors	Knee extensors	Knee extensors	Knee extensors
Termination	Full strength parity	Pain relief	Time-based	Time-based
Protocol Weeks	Until termination criterion achieved	Until pain relief (usually 2–4)	8	6
Days/week	3–4	3	3	2
Sets	2	3	Week 1: 6 Weeks 2–8: 4 at each velocity	2 at submaximal followed by 5–15 at maximal intensity
Repetitions	Until peak moment is 50% of initial	10/set	5/set	10/set
Interset rest	3–5 min			
Effort intensity in contraction	Maximal	Patient-adjusted Maximal (pain-limited)	Maximal	Submaximal, maximal (see Sets)
Contraction mode	Con	Eco	Eco	Con in one, eco in contralateral
Velocities	Anchor: 60–120°/s (may be implemented immediately) 180, 240, 300°/s within 1–2 weeks	30, 60, 90°/s	Incremental: 30–70°/s Week 1 30°/s 2 30, 35°/s 3 30, 35, 40°/s 4 30, 40, 45°/s 5 30, 40, 50°/s 6 30, 45, 60°/s 7 30, 50, 65°/s 8 30, 50, 70°/s	30, 60, 120, 180°/s

	Connelly & Vandervoort (2000)	Mauer et al (1999)	Bast et al (1998)	Sharp & Brouwer (1997)	Schilke et al (1996)
Objective	Muscle performance enhancement in older adults	To evaluate the effects of isokinetic exercise vs patient education on pain and function in knee osteoarthritis	Muscle performance enhancement	Muscle performance enhancement in hemiparesis	Muscle performance enhancement in knee osteoarthritis
Muscles	Ankle dorsiflexors	Knee extensors	Humeral internal/external rotators and abductors	Knee extensors and flexors	Knee extensors and flexors
Termination	Time-based	Time-based	Time-based	Time-based	Time-based

Protocol (weeks × days × sets × maximal repetitions)	2 w × 3 d	8 w × 3 d × 3 s × 9 mr (at each velocity)	4 w × 3 d × 12 s × 10 mr	6 w × 3 d × 3 s × (at each velocity)
Effort intensity	Maximal	Maximal	Maximal	Maximal
Contraction mode	Con and Ecc	Con	Con and Ecc	Con
Velocities	30, 90, 180°/s	90, 120, 150°/s	60, 120°/s	30, 60, 120°/s
Special comments	Bears implications for improving functional mobility of the ankle joint	Effective and well tolerated for this pathology	Ecc training significantly more effective than Con/Ecc training	Gains in strength and gait velocity without concomitant increases in muscle tone are possible

Protocol (weeks × days × sets × maximal repetitions)	6 w × 3 d × 3 s × (6–8) mr (at each velocity)	8 w × 3 d × 6 s × 5 mr
Effort intensity	Maximal	
Contraction mode	Con	
Velocities	90°/s	
Special comments	Significant decrease in pain and stiffness, and a significant increase in mobility; significant decline in arthritis activity	

	Engardt et al (1995)	MacPhail & Kramer (1995)	Lyngberg et al (1994)	St Pierre et al (1992)
Objective	Muscle performance enhancement in stroke patients	To evaluate the effects of isokinetic training on functional ability and walking in cerebral palsy adolescents	Muscle performance enhancement in rheumatoid arthritis	Muscle performance enhancement after meniscectomy
Muscles	Knee extensors	Knee extensors and flexors	Knee extensors	Knee extensors and flexors
Termination	Time-based	Time-based	Time-based	Time-based
Protocol (weeks × days × sets × maximal repetitions)	6 w × 2 d × (5–7)'s × 10 mr	8 w × 3 d × 3 s × 5 mr	3 w × 3 d × 4 s × 12 mr	From (4–8) w × 3 d × 2 s × 5 mr to (4–8) w × 3 d × 2 s × 11 mr
Effort intensity	Maximal	Maximal	50% maximal	Maximal
Contraction mode	Con and Ecc	Con and Ecc	Con and Ecc	Con
Velocities	60, 120, 180°/s	90°/s	30, 60, 90, 120°/s	From 60, 120, 180, 240°/s to 60, 90, 120, 150, 180, 210, 240°/s
Special comments	Eccentric knee extensor training advantageous compared to concentric training in stroke patients	A significant number of subjects showed an increase in gross motor ability. However, walking velocity and walking efficiency were unchanged	Training effective and safe for patients with rheumatoid arthritis	Training in the early postoperative phase does not seem to improve recovery of strength

* Program initiated following phase I healing.
Con, concentric; Ecc, eccentric.

an appropriate ICP quite problematic. If in addition the issue of eccentric conditioning is considered, this problem becomes intractable.

Principles of ICP design

The principles governing ICP design have been laid out in this chapter. They are based on consideration of:

1. the nature of the pathology or dysfunction
2. the status of tissue healing and repair and the level of pain
3. the extent of the ROM of the joint(s)
4. the load intensity sustained by the joint(s) before initiation of the ICP
5. the correct application of the various phenomena associated with the specificity of muscle performance, particularly with regard to velocity and contraction mode
6. the correct integration of the abovementioned protocol-related issues.

The protocols shown in Table 4.5, which have been successfully applied (namely with significant enhancement of muscle performance) in clinical or other situations, are described in order to demonstrate the use of the above. The suitability of each may be judged according to the above points.

DELAYED ONSET MUSCLE SORENESS DUE TO ISOKINETIC CONDITIONING

This problem has been dealt with at length in a number of studies (Albert 1991). It was suggested that exercises of a predominantly eccentric character were more liable to cause delayed onset muscle soreness (DOMS) than concentric exercises. This assumption has been investigated by Fitzgerald et al (1991) using isokinetic dynamometry. The research design was based on two experiments, one in which subjects exercised at the same power level, and another in which they exercised at maximal effort level.

Findings indicated that there was no change in muscle soreness between pre- and postexercise periods with regard to the first experiment. Greater increases in muscle soreness were indicated by subjects in the second experiment. The result suggested intensity rather than contraction type was linked with soreness.

The significance of this study in this context cannot be overestimated. Eccentric action in itself is probably not responsible for the phenomenon of DOMS. Rather it is the intensity of eccentric contractions that overloads the muscle and contributes to the sensation of pain. Thus the setting of an upper limit for maximal eccentric effort could provide a solution.

REFERENCES

Akima H, Takahashi H, Kuno S Y et al 1999 Early phase adaptations of muscle use and strength to isokinetic training. Medicine and Science in Sports and Exercise 31: 588–594

Albert M 1991 Eccentric muscle training in sports and orthopaedics. Churchill Livingstone, New York

Ariki P, Davies G J 1985 Rest interval between isokinetic velocity spectrum rehabilitation sets. Physical Therapy 65: 733–734 (abstract)

Barak Y 2003 The effect of limited range of motion isokinetic strength conditioning on ipsilateral muscular performance and electromyographic activity within and outside the trained range of motion. Unpublished PhD thesis, Tel-Aviv University, Tel Aviv

Bast S C, Vangsness C T, Takemura J, Folkins E, Landel R 1998 The effects of concentric versus eccentric isokinetic strength training of the rotator cuff in the plane of the scapula at various speeds. Bulletin of the Hospital of Joint Diseases 57: 139–144

Bennett G J, Stauber W T 1986 Evaluation and treatment of anterior knee pain using eccentric exercise. Medicine and Science in Sports and Exercise 18: 526–530

Bishop K, Durrant E, Allsen P, Merrill G 1991 The effect of eccentric strength training at various speeds on concentric strength of the quadriceps and hamstring muscles. Journal of Orthopaedic and Sports Physical Therapy 13: 226–230

Borg G 1982 A category scale with ratio properties for intermodal interindividual comparisons. In: Geissler G H, Petzold P (eds) Psychophysical judgement and the process of perception. VEB Deutscher Verlag der Wissenschaften, Berlin

Caiozzo V J, Perrine J J, Edgerton V R 1981 Training-induced alterations of in vivo force–velocity relationship of human muscle. Journal of Applied Physiology 51: 750–754

Connelly D M, Vandervoort A A 2000 Effects of isokinetic strength training on concentric and eccentric torque development in the ankle dorsiflexors of older adults. Journal of Gerontology 55: B465–472

Costill D L, Coyle E F, Fink W F, Lesmes G R, Witzmann A F 1979 Adaptations in skeletal muscle following strength training. Journal of Applied Physiology 46: 96–99

Cote C, Simoneau J-A, Lagasse P et al 1988 Isokinetic strength training protocols: do they induce skeletal muscle fiber hypertrophy? Archives of Physical Medicine and Rehabilitation 69: 281–285

Coyle E F, Feiring D C, Rotkis T C 1981 Specificity of power improvements through slow and fast isokinetic training. Journal of Applied Physiology 51: 1437–1442

Davies G J (ed) 1992 A compendium of isokinetics in clinical usage. S & S Publishers, Onalaska, Wisconsin

Davies G J, Bendle S R, Wood K L et al 1985a The optimal number of repetitions to be used with isokinetic training to increase average power. Physical Therapy 65: 794 (abstract)

Davies G J, Bendle S R, Wood K L et al 1985b The optimal number of repetitions to be used with isokinetic training to increase total work and endurance ratios. Physical Therapy 65: 794 (abstract)

De Andrade J R 1965 Joint distension and reflex muscle inhibition in the knee. Journal of Bone and Joint Surgery 47A: 313–318

Duncan P, Chandler J, Cananaugh D, Johnson K, Buehler A 1989 Mode and speed specificity of eccentric and concentric exercise training. Journal of Orthopaedic and Sports Physical Therapy 11: 70–75

Engardt M, Knutsson E, Jonsson M, Sternhag M 1995 Dynamic muscle strength training in stroke patients: effects on knee extension torque, electromyographic activity, and motor function. Archives of Physical Medicine and Rehabilitation 76: 419–425

Enoka R M 1988 Muscle strength and its development: new perspectives. Sports Medicine 6: 146–168

Esselman P C, De Lateur B J, Alquist A D et al 1991 Torque development in isokinetic training. Archives of Physical Medicine and Rehabilitation 72: 723–728

Ewing J L, Wolfe D R, Rogers M A, Amundson M L, Alan Stull G 1990 Effects of velocity of isokinetic training on strength, power, and quadriceps muscle fiber characteristics. European Journal of Applied Physiology 61: 159–162

Fitzgerald G K, Rothstein J M, Mayhew T P, Lamb R L 1991 Exercise-induced muscle soreness after concentric and eccentric exercise. Physical Therapy 71: 505–513

Fleck S J, Kraemer J W 1987 Designing resistance training programs. Human Kinetics, Champaign, Illinois, pp 20–46

Freedson P S, Gilliam T B, Mahoney T, Maiszewski A F, Kastango K 1993 Industrial torque levers by age group and gender. Isokinetics and Exercise Science 3: 34–42

Grimby G, Gustafsson E, Peterson L, Renstrom P 1980 Quadriceps function and training after knee ligament surgery. Medicine and Science in Sports and Exercise 12: 70–75

Higbie E J, Cuerton K J, Warren G L, Prior B M 1996 Effects of concentric and eccentric training on muscle strength, cross-sectional area and neural activation. Journal of Applied Physiology 81: 2173–2181

Hortobágyi T, Hill J P, Houmard J A et al 1996 Adaptive responses to muscle lengthening and shortening in men. Journal of Applied Physiology 80: 765–772

Hortobágyi T, Lambert N J, Hill J P 1997 Greater cross education following training with muscle lengthening

than shortening. Medicine and Science in Sports and Exercise 29: 107–112

Housh D J, Housh T J 1993 The effects of unilateral velocity-specific concentric strength training. Journal of Orthopaedic and Sports Physical Therapy 17: 252–256

Housh D J, Housh T J, Johnson G O, Chu W-K 1992 Hypertrophic response to unilateral concentric isokinetic resistance training. Journal of Applied Physiology 73: 65–70

Jenkins W L, Thackaberry M, Killian C 1984 Speed-specific isokinetic training. Journal of Orthopaedic and Sports Physical Therapy 6: 181–183

Jensen K, Di Fabio R 1989 Evaluation of eccentric exercise in treatment of patellar tendinitis. Physical Therapy 69: 211–216

Kitai T, Sale D G 1989 Specificity of joint angle in isometric training. European Journal of Applied Physiology 58: 744–748

Knight K L 1979 Knee rehabilitation by daily adjusted progressive resistive exercise. American Journal of Physical Medicine 7: 336–340

Knutsson E, Martensson A 1991 The effect of concentric and eccentric training in spastic paresis. In: Eriksson E, Grimby G, Knutsson E, Thorstensson A (eds) Dynamic dynamometry in research and clinical work. Karolinska Institute, Stockholm, Sweden

Komi P V 1986 Training of muscle strength and power: interactions of neuromotoric, hypertrophic and mechanical factors. International Journal of Sports Medicine 7(suppl): 10–15

Lesmes G R, Costill D L, Coyle E F, Fink W J 1978 Muscle strength and power changes during maximal isokinetic training. Medicine and Science in Sports and Exercise 10: 266–269

Lyngberg K K, Ramsing B U, Nawrocki A, Harreby M, Danneskiold-Samsoe B 1994 Safe and effective isokinetic knee extension training in rheumatoid arthritis. Arthritis and Rheumatism 37: 623–628

MacPhail H E, Kramer J F 1995 Effect of isokinetic strength-training on functional ability and walking efficiency in adolescents with cerebral palsy. Developmental Medicine and Child Neurology 37: 763–775

Mannion A Q F, Jakeman P M, Willan P 1992 Effects of isokinetic training of the knee extensors on isometric strength and peak power output during cycling. European Journal of Applied Physiology 65: 370–375

Maurer B T, Stern A G, Kinossian B, Cook K D, Schumacher H R 1999 Osteoarthritis of the knee: isokinetic quadriceps exercise versus an educational intervention. Archives of Physical Medicine and Rehabilitation 80: 1293

McDonagh M J, Davies C T 1984 Adaptive response of mammalian skeletal muscle to exercise with high loads. European Journal of Applied Physiology 52: 139–155

McNair P J, Stanley S 1996 Quadriceps muscle training in a restricted range of motion: implications for anterior cruciate ligament deficiency. Archives of Physical Medicine and Rehabilitation 77: 582–585

Mont M A, Cohen D B, Campbell K R, Gravare K, Mathur S K 1994 Isokinetic concentric versus eccentric training of shoulder rotators with functional evaluation of performance enhancement in elite tennis players. American Journal of Sports Medicine 22: 513–517

Narici M, Roi V G, Landoni L, Minetti A E, Cerretelli P 1989 Changes in force, cross-sectional area and neural activation during strength training and detraining of the human quadriceps. European Journal of Applied Physiology and Occupational Physiology 59: 310–319

O'Hagan F T, Sale D G, MacDougall D J, Garner S H 1995 Comparative effectiveness of accommodating and weight resistance training mode. Medicine and Science in Sports and Exercise 27: 1210–1219

Perrin D, Lephart S, Weltman A 1989 Specificity of training on computer obtained isokinetic measures. Journal of Orthopaedic and Sports Physical Therapy 12: 495–498

Petersen S, Bagnall K, Wegner A et al 1989 The influence of velocity-specific resistance training on the in vivo torque–velocity relationship and the cross-sectional area of the quadriceps femoris. Journal of Orthopaedic and Sports Physical Therapy 12: 456–462

Petersen S, Wessel J, Bagnall K et al 1990 Influence of concentric resistance training on concentric and eccentric strength. Archives of Physical Medicine and Rehabilitation 71: 101–105

Petersen S, Bell G, Bagnall K, Quinney A 1991 The effects of concentric resistance training on eccentric peak torque and muscle cross-sectional area. Journal of Orthopaedic and Sports Physical Therapy 13: 132–137

Ryan L M, Magidow P W, Duncan P 1991 Velocity specificity and mode specificity of eccentric isokinetic training of the hamstrings. Journal of Orthopaedic and Sports Physical Therapy 13: 33–39

Sale D G 1988 Neural adaptation to resistance training. Medicine and Science in Sports and Exercise 20: S135–S145

Schilke J M, Johnson G O, Housh T J, O'Dell J R 1996 Effects of muscle-strength training on the functional status of patients with osteoarthritis of the knee joint. Nursing Research 45: 68–72

Seger J Y, Arvidsson B, Thorstensson A 1998 Specific effects of eccentric and concentric training on muscle strength and morphology in humans. European Journal of Applied Physiology 79: 49–57

Sharp S A, Brouwer B J 1997 Isokinetic strength training of the hemiparetic knee: effects on function and spasticity. Archives of Physical Medicine and Rehabilitation 78: 1231–1236

Shelbourne K D, Nitz P 1990 Accelerated rehabilitation after anterior cruciate ligament reconstruction. American Journal of Sports Medicine 18: 292–299

Sherman W M, Pearson D R, Plyley M J et al 1982 Isokinetic rehabilitation after surgery. American Journal of Sports Medicine 10: 155–161

Sherman W M, Pearson D R, Plyley M J et al 1983 Isokinetic rehabilitation after meniscectomy: a comparison of two

methods of training. The Physician and Sports Medicine 11: 121–133

Stauber W T 1989 Eccentric action of muscles: physiology, injury and adaptation. Exercise and Sports Science Review 19: 157–185

Stone M H 1988 Implications for connective tissue and bone alterations resulting from resistance exercise training. Medicine and Science in Sports and Exercise 20: S162–S168

St Pierre D M, Laforest S, Paradis S et al 1992 Isokinetic rehabilitation after arthroscopic meniscectomy. European Journal of Applied Physiology and Occupational Physiology 64: 437–443

Tegner Y, Lysholm J, Lysholm M, Gillquist J 1986 Strengthening exercises for old cruciate ligament tears. Acta Orthopaedica Scandinavica 57: 130–134

Tesch P A 1988 Skeletal muscle adaptations consequent to long-term heavy resistance exercise. Medicine and Science in Sports and Exercise 20: S132–S134

Thomee R, Renstrom P, Grimby G, Peterson L 1987 Slow or fast isokinetic training after knee ligament surgery. Journal of Orthopaedic and Sports Physical Therapy 8: 475–479

Timm K E 1987 Investigation of the physiological overflow effect from speed-specific isokinetic activity. Journal of Orthopaedic and Sports Physical Therapy 9: 106–110

Timm K E 1988 Postsurgical knee rehabilitation: a five year study of four methods and 5381 patients. American Journal of Sports Medicine 16: 463–468

Timm K E, Patch D G 1985 Case study: use of the Cybex II velocity spectrum in the rehabilitation of postsurgical knees. Journal of Orthopaedic and Sports Physical Therapy 6: 347–349

Tomberlin J P, Basford J R, Schwen E E et al 1991 Comparative study of isokinetic eccentric and concentric quadriceps training. Journal of Orthopaedic and Sports Physical Therapy 14: 31–36

Wilk K E, Andrews J R 1992 Current concepts in the treatment of anterior cruciate ligament disruption. Journal of Orthopaedic and Sports Physical Therapy 15: 279–293

Wojtys E M, Huston L J, Taylor P D, Bastian S D 1996 Neuromuscular adaptations in isokinetic, isotonic, and agility training programs. American Journal of Sports Medicine 24: 187–192

Young K, McDonagh M J, Davies C T M 1985 The effects of two forms of isometric training on the mechanical properties of the triceps surae in man. Pflugers Archives 405: 384–388

Zarins B, Boyle J, Harris B A 1985 Knee rehabilitation following arthroscopic meniscectomy. Clinical Orthopaedics and Related Research 198: 36–42

Medicolegal applications

INTRODUCTION

Ever since the invention of isokinetic dynamometry (ISD), its potential application to the field of impairment and disability assessment became a major source of interest. Indeed among the first to grasp the significance of *measurements* in the context of quantitatively based determination of the extent to which muscles became weak, either on a temporary or a chronic basis, were members of the bar. In later years it became apparent that another important issue relating to return to work status, could potentially benefit from quantitative assessment of muscle function. Doubtless the use of this technology in the medicolegal field could flourish only in those countries where the impairment rating and/or disability assessment systems recognized muscle strength (as a general representative of the muscle's mechanical output) as a relevant element. Whereas a comparative review of various legal–social codes is beyond the scope of this book, for the sake of this particular point and as an introduction to the complexity of this subject reference will be made to the American Medical Association's *Guides to the Evaluation of Permanent Impairment*, possibly the leading source in the field.

The following outlines how the subject of strength is presented by the Guides in the fourth and latest edition (1993) in the context of impairments of the upper extremity. Initially under the headings 'Motor Deficits and Loss of Power' it is stated:

Muscle testing including tests for strength, duration and repetition of contraction, and function, helps

Table 5.1 Grades of muscle strength and their associated impairment ratings

Grade	Description of muscle function	Motor deficit (%)
0	No contraction	100
1	Slight contraction and no movement	76–99
2	Active movement with gravity eliminated	51–75
3	Active movement against gravity only, without resistance	26–50
4	Active movement against gravity with some resistance	1–25
5	Active movement against gravity with full resistance	0

evaluate the motor function of specific nerves. Muscle testing rates one's ability to move a segment of the body through its full range of motion against resistance.

The Guides suggests that the motor function of individual muscles be tested and graded based on the technique of manual muscle testing (MMT), according to Table 5.1, as suggested by the UK Medical Research Council (1976).

The Guides proceeds under the heading 'Strength Evaluation' to argue that:

Because strength measurements are *functional tests* (italics, ZD) influenced by subjective factors that are difficult to control, and the Guides for the most part is based on *anatomic* impairment, the Guides does not assign a large role to these measurements. … In a rare case, if the examiner believes the patient's loss of strength represents an impairing factor that has not been considered adequately, the loss of strength may be rated separately … and *combined* with other upper extremity impairments. … Impairments due to motor deficits secondary to disorders of the peripheral nerve system and various degenerative neuromuscular conditions are evaluated according to [MMT]. It should be understood that weakness or loss of strength can occur without muscle atrophy.

In the opening paragraph of the section on grip and pinch strength the Guides states:

When evaluating strength, the examiner must have good reason to believe the patient has reached maximal improvement and that the condition is a 'permanent' one… This determination is based made with measurements taken over time… Many factors including fatigue, handedness, time of day, age, nutritional state, pain and the patient's cooperation, influence strength measurements. … Tests repeated at intervals during an examination are considered to be reliable if there is less than 20% variations in the readings [otherwise] one may assume the patient is not exerting full effort.

These words reflect in part the expert *medical* knowledge pertaining to muscle strength at the beginning of the 1990s. They raise a number of serious questions and reservations. First, in terms of muscle performance the Guides presents a conspicuous confusion of *impairment* and *function*, namely [dis]ability. Just because muscles are so intimately identified with the ability to move the body parts does not mean that they may not be impaired, namely become weaker in terms of either strength or endurance. Second, one cannot but wonder how only a decade ago an outdated and largely invalid system such as the MMT (Sapega 1990) could still serve as a guideline whereas the substantive advantages of modern instrumental techniques were never mentioned in the text. In particular the assumption that MMT can direct clinicians how to rate muscle strength when non-debilitating weakness is present, is absolutely unwarranted. Third, and no less troubling, is the fact that whereas grip strength plays an important role in hand impairment evaluation, strength deficiency in any other major muscle groups is accorded little to negligible value. Fourth, it is of interest to note that although the Guides adopts an anatomic approach, it recognizes that muscle weakness may not be associated with atrophy. Furthermore, despite this approach, the Guides does not, it seems, recognize trauma to muscles, such as tears, as a source of weakness known to have a direct and often drastic functional effect. Moreover, although the Guides refers explicitly to a number of factors influencing strength measurements it does not provide any tools for addressing them. Finally, while recognizing the problem of effort validation, the criterion suggested – namely consistency of effort within 20% – is not only vague but has been shown in recent years to be erroneous and misleading.

Grip muscles

Targeting grip muscles reflects a number of factors. First, grip constitutes a habitual activity of the hand and thus combines function with strength in perhaps the most intimate way. Second, the measurement is based on *isometric* contraction of several muscles and therefore does not require consideration of the elaborate system of parameters operating in dynamic measurements. Third, two of the major sources of error in dynamometry are readily solved by the instrument used in this measurement (the Jamar or Preston hand dynamometer). As far as *proximal stabilization* is concerned, by placing the thenar eminence against the instrument's frame and grasping the opposite adjustable handle by the various phalanges, no relative movement can take place. Moreover, as this configuration does not require rotational motion, no *axes alignment* is necessary. Fourth, these similar design instruments are accepted universally among hand specialists, not least because they are cheap, simple to use and are easily transferable instruments. Fifth, from the methodological point of view, grip strength findings have been shown to be highly reproducible and valid in the sense that they reflect known physiological relationships (length–tension), indicate bilateral differences in pathological situations and correlate with observed variations during the course of rehabilitation.

Sincerity of effort

Equally significant, the issue of sincerity of effort has occupied a considerable niche in grip strength assessment. In assessing strength impairment during grip, the Guides recommends that bilateral strength differences of up to 10% should not be considered an impairment. Differences of 10–30%, 30–60% and 61% and above should entitle the patient to 10, 20 and 30% impairment to the upper extremity, respectively. Clearly, the greater the weakness, the higher is the compensation awarded which potentially creates a motivation for performing at a reduced level. Hence maximal performance should not be taken for granted. Given the human ability to accurately modulate grip effort, the fact that grip strength testing is critically dependent on patient collaboration called for the development of procedures for ensuring that patients were indeed exerting a maximal effort. The existence of such procedures is in fact central to the validity of any performance test that incorporates active patient (subject) participation. In other words, if *full effort* (in the very broad sense of the word) cannot be confirmed, no inference or judgment may be made based on the measured trait (Polatin & Mayer 1992). This statement holds true irrespective of the modality that is being measured such as muscle strength and fatiguability, hearing or vision. Intensive research has indicated that with respect to grip, optimal effort could with some confidence be confirmed, a situation that was not applicable to other muscles until recently.

Other muscle groups

In comparison, impairment of other major muscle groups is not mentioned in the Guides (or for that matter in any other medicolegal corpus this author is aware of). This omission is particularly disconcerting regarding trunk musculature, especially the extensor apparatus. Comprehensive research (see Chapter 9) has repeatedly indicated that low back dysfunction (LBD) was closely associated with a significantly reduced level of trunk extensor mechanical output. Whether or not this observed impairment plays a role in disability is as yet an unsolved question. However, in view of the cardinal importance attributed to normally operating trunk muscles, reduction in their capacity to move the trunk as well as to stabilize it should have been viewed as a tangible impairment, albeit one that may be reversed. This omission can nevertheless be partly justified by the absence of standardized methods and firm normative databases.

In this chapter, an attempt is made to cover two interconnected issues. One relates to the so-called sincerity of effort, namely whether the patient is performing at optimal level. It has been argued that the term *sincerity* could be tainted with partiality and therefore the term *effort optimality* (EO) will henceforth be used. If the patient is judged to be exerting an optimal effort then in clinical terms the findings may lead to an interpretation whereas in legal terms they may be considered admissible. Admissibility enables determination of the severity of muscular dysfunction. What benchmark(s) should be applied in deciding that a muscular weakness exists, and how to interpret the isokinetic findings, form the core of the second issue.

EFFORT OPTIMALITY

The phenomenon of suboptimal effort (SE) is well recognized in the medical literature. In a review of methods applied for detecting effort optimality, Lechner et al (1998) state:

Some patients with known musculoskeletal dysfunction can give less than a full effort during physical evaluation for a variety of reasons. Pain, fear of pain, fear of reinjury, anxiety, depression, lack of understanding of instructions, lack of understanding of the importance of the test and secondary financial gain are some of the reasons underlying self-limiting behavior.

To these sources one could add difficulty in achieving adequate motor control which is expressed in extreme inconsistency among repeated tests as well as a similar expression in a patient suffering from post-traumatic stress disorder (PTSD).

Hence, avoiding the exertion of full effort does not necessarily reflect an intention to defraud. Indeed, failure to appreciate the extent to which other mechanisms are modulating SE may often leave the examiner with the impression that a so-called non-organic factor is operating. Furthermore, in spite of the well documented poor human ability in 'measuring'/detecting weakness (Sapega 1990) clinicians may still perceive findings derived from objective instrumental measurement as exaggerating the situation, giving rise to the impression that the reduction seen in strength is non-genuine. This trait is clearly reflected by the qualifying approach of the Guides. However, it seems that misrepresentation of impairment in order to gain unlawfully does exist (Fishbain et al 1999a). Moreover, it may be related not only to the abovementioned factors but to the sociocultural background of the patient. This

phenomenon – which among clinical circles is also known by such terms as *symptom magnification*, *exaggeration* or *malingering* – has been defined in another paper as the 'intentional production of false or grossly exaggerated physical or psychological symptoms, motivated by external incentives such as avoiding military duty, avoiding work [or] obtaining financial compensation' (Fishbain et al 1999a). In this context, it is essential to add the reservation put by Lechner et al (1998) concerning the use of the above terms. It is argued that since a *symptom* is a sensation experienced by the patient, no existing tool can measure the patient's true versus reported experience of sensation. Therefore when using terms such as magnification or exaggeration, one wrongly implies the ability to measure these sensations and compare them with individual reports.

Although this book focuses on the isokinetic method, isometric measurements, particularly of grip strength, have to a great extent shaped our understanding of the complex issue of EO. Four different methods for assessing EO during isometric grip tests have been reported and the application of one of them in particular, the coefficient of variation, has also been extended to the exploration of EO in other muscles systems. Due to the significance of a number of isometric exertions-based studies, their findings will first be introduced and then followed by more recent and promising research that used ISD.

Isometric methods

Coefficient of variation (CV)

As mentioned in Chapter 3, the CV is obtained by dividing the standard deviation of a set of repeated (within-session) measurements by their mean score. If multiplied by 100, this unitless index expresses in per cent the relative variability of these scores. The rationale for using the CV as a measure of EO stems from two sets of observations (Hamilton Fairfax et al 1997). First, a certain degree of strength output variability exists in any set of repeated trials irrespective whether the subjects are normal individuals (Young et al 1989) or patients (Andres et al 1988, Matheson et al 1988).

Second, this variability is greater where SE is exerted compared to its optimal counterpart (Bohannon 1987, Janda et al 1987, Bohannon & Smith 1988). Although several protocols were described for studying SE in grip strength, in most cases subjects were asked to exert a submaximal force that was equivalent to a percentage of their maximal (100%) force, for example 25, 50 and 75% (Chengalur et al 1990, Niebuhr & Marion 1990, Robinson et al 1993). Based on these repeated SEs, CV scores were computed.

Findings have indicated that in normal subjects the CV ranged between 5 and 20% depending on the joint–muscle system complexity (Tornvall 1963), gender (Matheson 1991), dominance (Niemeyer et al 1989) and presence of pain (Andres et al 1988). For instance isometric lifting strength was characterized by a CV of 13–18% (Harber & Soo Hoo 1984) whereas the corresponding values for elbow flexion (Saunders & Bohannon 1991) and knee extension (Robinson et al 1994) were $3.6 \pm 2.2\%$ and $4.2 \pm 2.8\%$ respectively. As for pain, it was indicated that its presence caused a considerable rise in the variability (Finsterbush et al 1983). However, in spite of repeated suggestions, no particular CV-based cutoff could be identified which effectively separated optimal from simulated weakness.

In one of the important studies in the field Birmingham et al (1998) have studied the test-retest reproducibility of the CV obtained from peak maximal and submaximal isometric knee extension both performed in two separate sessions. It was revealed that although the maximal effort (ME)-based CV were significantly smaller than their submaximal counterparts (3.5% versus 11.3%) there was a considerable overlap between the sincere and feigned efforts. As a precise cutoff distinguishing between the two levels of effort could not be identified and in view of the day-to-day variability of the CV it was recommended that the CV be used with caution and only in conjunction with other clinical tests. In another study (Hamilton Fairfax et al 1995) the reproducibility of the CV was examined in normal subjects who were asked to exert 100 and 50% of grip effort on two occasions. It was revealed that the test-retest intraclass correlation coefficients

(ICCs) were close to zero. Furthermore, applying CV = 7.5% as a cutoff in at least one test would have misclassified 97% of the women and 64% of the men. Therefore, applying a single CV cutoff to a mixed sample of subjects appeared to unfairly discriminate against women.

Perhaps the leading source in this regard is a study by Simmonsen (1995) in which 270 consecutive patients, 124 women and 146 men aged 19–62, were referred for functional capacity evaluation (FCE). The reasons for the FCE were typically assessment before work hardening program, determination of status at the conclusion of physical therapy, before returning to work and before disability rating. The tests consisted of eight different isometric lift/push/pull tasks and the forces exerted by the patients were recorded by an instrumented load cell. Each subject completed three trials of each task. The results have indicated that the CV was similar in all pathologies with an overall mean (SD) of $8.83 \pm 4.05\%$. There were significant differences among the task-based CVs ranging approximately between 6% (pull at shoulder height) and 125% (lift at ankle height). Significantly, the correlation matrix of the CV X task yielded very low scores (0.166–0.284). Based on the assumption that patients would perform suboptimally in all tasks the results indicated therefore that the CV could not be a reliable predictor of subject effort. Furthermore, in discussing an appropriate cutoff score for the CV, the authors have used the mean CV + 2SD. However, as stated in the paper, individual cutoffs may confound the interpretation even further. For instance:

- How should one apply the cutoff when multiple tests are at stake?
- How should a standard apply if a subject exceeds it (i.e. is suspected of SE) in a single test?
- How many 'positive SEs' are required before a subject is judged as a suboptimal performer, or should the overall CV be used instead?

None of these questions could reliably be answered.

On the other hand and in spite of this void, it was shown that the entire patient population exceeded the cutoff (mean + 2 SD) on 75% of the individual tests ($n = 1$) and 50% when $n = 2$. The presence of pain was implicit in each test: patients were instructed to do their best without hurting themselves and therefore their motor responses could not possibly be compared with subjects performing without such hints. It was concluded that the CV could not be used independently to make an objective assessment of EO.

Finally, the relationship between psychological factors and isometric effort variability has been the subject of a study of a clinical population made up of 98 chronic LBD patients performing the lumbar extension test (Robinson et al 1992a,b). These patients were classified using various personality tests/questionnaires which aimed at assessing psychological distress, disability, flexibility, pain and symptom magnification. Contrary to previous studies, psychological distress, tendency to report symptoms, and pain were negatively correlated with measures of torque variability. However, most of the correlation coefficients were low and not significant. It was therefore concluded that there was little support for the use of test-retest isometric strength variability as a means for detecting SE.

The 5-rung 'length–tension' test

This approach for testing EO is based on the physiological relationship between a muscle's strength and its length. It is well established that for most instances maximal strength is achieved at a length corresponding to a point within the joint range of motion rather than to one of its ends. Therefore, the strength (torque)/angular position curve typically assumes an 'inverted U' or 'bell' shape. The 5 rung (5R) hand dynamometer allows measurement of grip strength at successive muscle lengths (of all involved muscles) and hence upon exertion of ME the resulting curve should normally peak at rungs 2–4. It was hence argued that deliberate SE should be expressed by a flat curve. However, the degree of flatness indicative of SE remained an open issue. Stokes (1983) suggested literal flatness whereas others were less restrictive (Niebuhr & Marion 1987) thus permitting a larger number of false positives. This issue

has been further studied by Hamilton Fairfax (1996) using various paradigms. It was concluded that EO in grip could not be reliably interpreted from flatness of the strength curve. Rather, a flattened curve signified weakness but at the same time called for further investigation.

The rapid exchange grip (REG) test

This method is based on rapidly passing the dynamometer between the hands and recording the strength scores during a series of contractions. It is introduced for two reasons. One relates to the fact that it is based on physiological principles – the assumption that modulation of submaximal output requires time which is dedicated to a 'carefully controlled mixture of recruitment and rate coding, developed in response to feedback from the periphery' (Hamilton Fairfax et al 1997). The rapid exchange of the dynamometer between the hands means that the time available for the feed-forward and feed-back signals is so short that the operation of the above neurophysiological mechanisms is seriously frustrated. As a result the ability to repeat SEs is reduced and strength rises towards the real maximum. Hence if the subject exerts an ME during both the criterion slow-paced 5-rung Jamar test and the REG test, the differences between the two should be minimal. However in case of SE, the REG scores are expected to exceed those of the criterion. As indicated later in this chapter this method has some implications with regard to the dynamic methods of assessing EO.

The second reason for introducing REG relates to the employment of a cutoff score that effectively separates ME from SE. Similar to the CV approach, unless such a cutoff exists, the method is without merit. Although initial research has been promising (Hildreth et al 1989), indicating success in 14 out of 15 subjects, later studies became less optimistic (Joughin et al 1993). Significantly, it has been shown by Hamilton Fairfax (1996) that the REG method had an overall accuracy of only 56–63% which under no circumstances could be accepted as a valid indicator. Furthermore, feigned mild weakness could not be differentiated from feigned severe weakness and as a result the REG approach was not recommended for general clinical use.

Together with a few other studies and excepting that of Chengalur et al (1990), the abovementioned research indicates that with current isometric exertion-based techniques optimal effort cannot be effectively differentiated from SE. In particular, use of the CV, REG and 5R demonstrates that neither statistically based nor physiologically based indices were sufficient for this task. This result may reflect in part the poverty of data associated with this type of muscle contraction.

Isokinetic methods

As just a handful of studies dealt with dynamic non-isokinetic methods of testing EO, and then with little success, this section will be devoted to the use of isokinetics for identifying submaximal effort. The structure of this section is similar to that of the previous in that it first explores the application of consistency parameters and later describes the evolution towards the incorporation of and reliance on physiological principles.

Consistency parameters

A number of studies examined the utility of using consistency of performance through the use of either the CV or another index as a criterion for EO and practically all concluded that consistency was a poor measure. One of the first attempts that focused on trunk effort was carried out by Hazard et al (1988). Normal subjects were asked to exert ME and 50% ME in angular (trunk extension/flexion) and linear (lift) configurations. Visual assessment of the torque curves failed to provide any clear hint, misclassifying 25% of the cases. The authors have expanded their analysis by introducing complex discriminant analysis which increased the sensitivity of the procedure to 85–90%. It was correctly argued that this method was not only impractical in the clinic but biased towards yielding the most optimistic possible outcome (Newton & Waddell 1993). The latter group used another consistency index – the average point variance (APV, Newton et al 1993). The APV is calculated based on the difference

between the highest strength score of four consecutive tests and their mean value at each degree of movement along the tested arch of movement. It is expressed as a percentage and the suggested cutoff differentiating between ME and SE was 15%. Comparison of the APV in normal subjects and in patients with chronic low back pain (CLBP) failed to substantiate its relevance. Specifically, in a study comparing low-back-injured and non-injured workers, both groups have shown mean APV values of as much as 20% (Mandell et al 1993). The authors have suggested that '... APVs significantly greater than 20% should be present before determining that an individual is not putting forth maximum effort'. Moreover, it was argued that the use of the APV could '... clearly have significant negative consequences if incorrectly applied in medicolegal evaluations'.

Another attempt by Reid et al (1991) was based on visual inspection of consecutive isokinetic curves of a group of control subjects and patients with CLBP (Fig. 5.1). The authors have not explained the criteria of curve classification but argued that those who were categorized as subperformers had an inverted extensor/flexor (E/F) torque ratio. Specifically, whereas in both normal subjects and optimal effort CLBP patients this ratio was greater than unity (E/F > 1) it was less than unity among those patients who were classified as SE performers. Quite surprisingly the authors maintained that 'based on the group giving a maximal effort it would be reasonable that the submaximal group would also exhibit a true weakness' which clearly undermines their hypothesis.

Yet another approach for assessing EO using consistency indices was reported by Luoto et al (1996). Trunk extension and flexion strength was compared between normal subjects and two groups of mild and severe CLBP patients. All participants were instructed to exert ME and 50% ME. The CV of the peak moment was classified as low (0–10%), medium (11–20%) and high (>20%). In spite of a trend towards higher CVs in the SE (50% effort) this index did not reach significance. There was a conspicuous grouping of subjects, control as well as patients, into medium CV. The authors concluded that only those efforts that

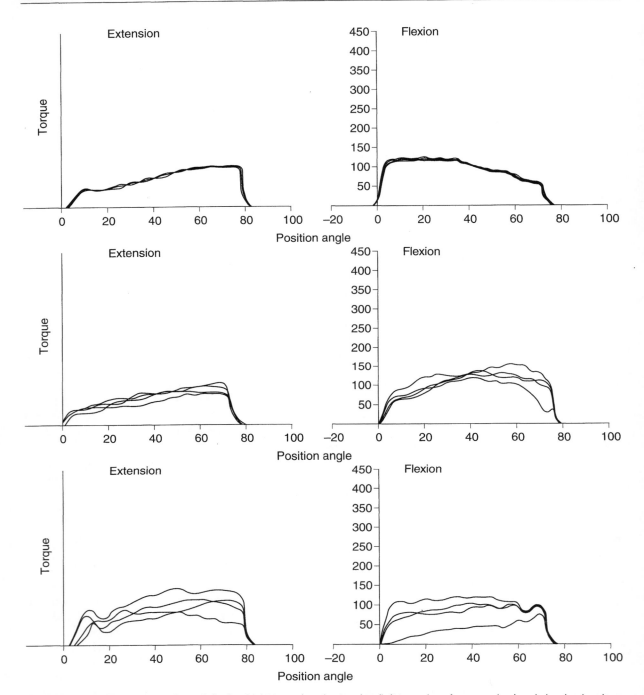

Figure 5.1   Isokinetic concentric trunk flexion (right traces) and extension (left traces) performance in chronic low back pain patients. Upper traces, maximal effort pattern; middle traces, 'gray zone' pattern; lower traces, submaximal pattern. (From Reid et al 1991 with permission of Lippincott Williams & Wilkins.)

corresponded to CV < 10% could safely be classified but in the absence of a more advanced statistical analysis this conclusion could not serve as a guideline.

Perhaps the most comprehensive study of the CV in the context of isokinetic testing of EO was conducted by Birmingham et al (1998). The importance of this study derives from the fact that it explored the reproducibility of the criterion, the CV. As stated by the authors 'knowledge about the range of scores the CV may assume, simply due to measurement error, is required before any cutoff value can be used confidently to make decisions regarding individual efforts'. The experimental paradigm consisted therefore of a test-retest of maximal effort and feigned weakness during concentric knee extension at 60°/s. Although the feigned weakness CV scores were significantly greater than the maximal effort scores, 15.0 ± 9.2% versus 3.9 ± 2.5%, there was a considerable overlap between the frequency distributions of the two effort levels as seen in Figure 5.2. For instance, although 95% of the maximal distribution lay below a cutoff of 8%, this came at the expense of having 25% of the SE

performers under this figure. Furthermore, an individual CV could vary by ± 3.1% as a result of the measurement error. Thus, the range of CV in which an individual scoring a CV of 8.0% might be expected to lie was between 4.9% (8 − 3.1) and 11.1% (8 + 3.1). In other words the true score could lie on either side of the 8.0% score just due to the measurement error.

To demonstrate the effect variation of the CV has on the *specificity* (the percentage of MEs correctly identified as maximal, i.e. true negative) and the *sensitivity* (the percentage of SEs correctly identified as submaximal, i.e. true positive) the receiver operator characteristics (ROC) curve was constructed (Fig. 5.3). This curve permits assessment of the interplay between these two variables. The overall *accuracy* of the detection technique is calculated based on the area under the curve. For this particular case the accuracy was 87.5%. As evident from the illustration, lowering of the cutoff causes a reduction in the specificity but the sensitivity rises. For example a cutoff of 2% means that many of those who were performing at their optimal output would have been falsely classified as SE performers just because they could not be as precise in reproducing their effort as the cutoff had dictated. On the other hand, for exactly the same reason the likelihood of classifying an SE performer as an optimal (false negative) one is equally negligible and stands according to this presentation at around 10%.

The extension of this analysis is as follows: consider a patient with a CV of 3% based on three consecutive repetitions of knee extension at 60°/s. At a 95% level of confidence his true CV could be as high as 6.1% (3 + 3.1). From the ROC curve, one could state with 95% certainty that less than 20% of a young *healthy* male population could produce such a low CV while feigning weakness of the knee extensors. This, it should be recognized, is still a considerable margin, resulting ultimately from the serious deficiency the CV has as an identifier of effort. While suggesting an improvement in the form of a larger number of strength variability measures and a larger number of repetitions, the authors conceded that the measurement error of the CV coupled with the great difficulty in setting a precise cutoff value

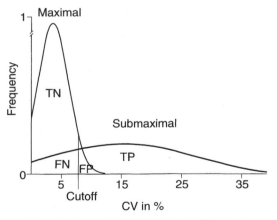

Figure 5.2 Idealized distribution of the coefficient of variation (CV) in maximal effort (ME) versus submaximal effort (SE). The means (SD) of the CV SD for ME were 3.7(2.6)% for ME and 15.6% for SE. Note the large overlap between the ME and SE distributions resulting in 25% of the subjects being classified as maximal performers, i.e. a false positive rate of 25%. FN, false negative; FP, false positive; TN, true negative; TP, true positive. (From Birmingham et al 1998.)

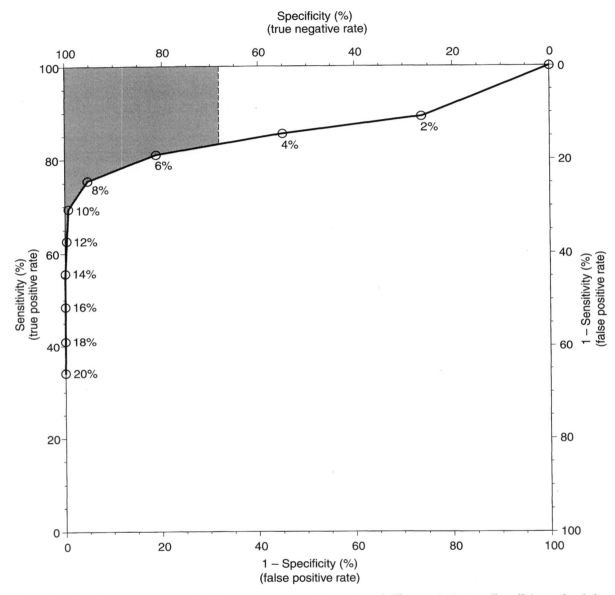

Figure 5.3 Receiver operator characteristics curve illustrating the accuracy of different criterion cutoff coefficients of variation (CV) (%) in identifying submaximal effort. The shaded portion corresponds to the range of CV scores in which the true score associated with an individual's observed score of 8% can be expected to vary as a result of measurement error (i.e. 95% CI = ±3.11%) and illustrates the range in corresponding specificity and sensitivity values. (From Birmingham et al 1998.)

rendered this index inefficient for this particular objective. It should also be recognized that this study was limited to normal subjects so that extension into clinical realms may not be allowed.

An often quoted study by Lin et al (1996) used the knee extensors as a model. Normal subjects

were asked to exert ME and 50% ME in five repeated contractions performed either isometrically or isokinetically, the latter consisting of two angular velocities: 60 and 180°/s. The indices used were CV of the peak moment, CV of the average moment and slope to the peak. The rationale for

Table 5.2 Differentiation of maximal effort (ME) from submaximal effort (SE) using consistency (CV) and recruitment rate (slope) variables

Index	Isokinetic 60°/s		Isokinetic 180°/s		Isometric	
	ME	SE	ME	SE	ME	SE
CVam	8.71 (4.3)	19.3 (9.2)	5.63 (2.1)	16.4 (8.5)	6.5 (4.1)	10.7 (6.6)
CVpm	6.26 (3.3)	14.6 (10.0)	4.27 (1.8)	15.9 (9.4)	4.4 (2.2)	10.0 (5.5)
Slope	39.6 (18.1)	17.0 (9.8)	53.8 (21.7)	21.7 (14.5)	10.2 (5.6)	9.6 (7.7)

CVam, coefficient of variation of the average moment (in %); CVpm, coefficient of variation of the peak moment (in %), ME, maximal effort, SE, suboptimal effort; Slope, to peak moment (in kgm/s).

incorporating the slope as a criterion derives from the theory governing the REG test, namely modulation of submaximal output (Hamilton Fairfax et al 1997). As mentioned above SE requires a period of time for processing of the feed-forward and feed-back signals that is unavailable when an all-out effort is performed. The results relating to the three indices are summarized in Tables 5.2–5.4.

All SE efforts, irrespective of their type, had a significantly higher CV compared to their optimal counterparts. To achieve a zero rate of false positives (namely misclassifying of ME as SE) the cutoffs shown in Table 5.3 were determined. The way these cutoffs translated into detection rate (in %) is outlined in Table 5.4.

As evident from Table 5.4 the static condition is totally unsuitable for identifying the effort level. On the other hand, dynamic muscle contraction is a significantly more powerful option resulting in a detection rate of 84% based on a combination of the CV of the average moment (CVam) and the slope, with or without the CV of the peak moment (CVpm). One of the main difficulties in interpreting the results of this and several other studies is the absence of confidence intervals relating to the degree of certainty with which a statement concerning the level of effort may be made.

In a later study the use of the CV in the context of SE identification was described in relation to grip effort (Dvir 1999a). This study compared static and isokinetic grip strength in normal subjects who were asked to exert maximal effort and to feign weakness of grip due to imagined accident in order to gain unlawfully (see also below).

Table 5.3 Suggested cutoffs for knee extension effort

Condition	CVam	CVpm	Slope*
180°/s	>10	>10	<20.62
60°/s	>19	>16	<18.27
Isometric	>18	>11	<3.74

* in kgm/s; CVam, coefficient of variation of the average moment (in %); CVpm, coefficient of variation of the peak moment (in %).

Table 5.4 Identification of power (in %) of the various indices in the three experimental conditions

Index	180°/s	60°/s	Isometric
CVam	75	53	16
CVpm	59	31	38
Slope	59	63	13
CVam + CVpm	78	56	41
CVam + Slope	84	84	22
CVpm + Slope	75	75	41
CVam + CVpm + Slope	84	84	44

CVam, coefficient of variation of the average moment (in %); CVpm, coefficient of variation of the peak moment (in %); Slope, to peak moment (in kgm/s).

Concentric and eccentric strength scores derived from two angular velocities were compared to 5R Jamar-based scores obtained at the optimal rung. The findings indicated highly significant differences between the two levels of effort. On the other hand attempts to use the CV as an identifier were unsuccessful in terms of the three different contraction modes, resulting in very low accuracy.

Physiologically based indices

Two approaches have been adopted in recent years: one led by Birmingham & Kramer (1998) and Fishbain et al (1999b) who applied various indices and another by Dvir & David (1996), Dvir (1997a,b, 1999b), Dvir & Keating (2001, 2003) and Dvir et al (2002) who used the DEC (difference between eccentric and concentric ratios) index in a series of papers dedicated to several joint–muscle systems.

Birmingham & Kramer. Birmingham & Kramer (1998) used a novel criterion: the difference obtained from subtracting isokinetic concentric knee extension strength scores obtained at 60°/s from their isometric counterparts. In outlining the criterion score used for the analysis, the authors state that 'the concept of distinguishing SE from ME on the basis of a difference score derived from absolute strength measures may be useful if the relationship between these measures is more difficult to maintain during submaximal efforts'. The SE instruction given to subjects was based on a self-selected submaximal effort in an attempt to feign weakness. Three contractions were performed at each contraction mode and at each effort level. The study consisted of two testing sessions completed between 1 and 7 days. The findings indicated that although the difference score in the ME was significantly greater than in the SE ($33 \pm 29\,Nm$ versus $13 \pm 30\,Nm$ respectively) the test-retest reliability was modest with a range of scores within which an individual's true score might be expected to lie being $\pm 25\,Nm$ and $\pm 37\,Nm$ for ME and SE, respectively. Since the mean difference in scores in the maximal effort was $33\,Nm$ this means that the true score was expected to lie within $8-58\,Nm$, doubtless a large range. This result renders the use of this particular difference score ineffective.

In discussing their findings the authors have not explained the reason for choosing 60°/s as the criterion velocity. Indeed, the likelihood of obtaining better results by raising the velocity to 120–180°/s is pretty tangible. Under concentric conditions, higher velocities translate into lower strength scores thus further increasing the difference with the isometric scores. Moreover, they allow a shorter contraction time thus enhancing the impact of the limited time factor in modulating SE. In such cases, it has been observed by the author of this book, that the normal appearance of the strength curve was often distorted in a way which was expressed by high frequency components. This factor could be incorporated as an additional indicator in a logistic model of SE.

Fishbain et al. In a study by Fishbain et al (1999b) normal subjects were asked to exert maximal effort and then feign weakness while performing a 'closed kinetic chain' exercise consisting of six reciprocal continuous shoulder-press and pull-down effected using a linear isokinetic apparatus. A subgroup of the performers was retested 2 months later for assessing the predictive validity. This is a rather unusual design in terms of movement pattern and particularly in the light of using a series of contractions instead of a single effort. No *single* parameter could effectively separate the levels of effort. Using a discriminant analysis yielded different combinations of parameters for women and men which could optimally differentiate between ME and SE. These parameters were:

- Women:
  — average power up
  — 40% of the repetition down
  — duty cycle up
  (91% correct classification, 100% sensitivity, 81% specificity)
- Men:
  — duty cycle down
  — work/weight down
  — peak value up
  (77% correct classification, 89% sensitivity, 65% specificity).

Based on the subgroup, the validity of this protocol was reflected in a classification rate of 75% with 83.3% sensitivity but 66.7% specificity. Thus a fairly large proportion of the feigned efforts would have been classified as optimal, namely the protocol led to an unacceptable rate of false negatives.

The authors have argued that interpretation of the instructions to perform maximally but particularly the subjects' interpretation of what should be construed as feigned weakness, introduced substantial confounding factors. It should be realized that the clinical relevance of this study is limited because:

1. the movement pattern was not particularly functional
2. in multijoint–muscle configurations it is difficult to isolate the primary source for the variation
3. the parameters used for differentiation were unique to this system and probably required time-consuming analysis.

On the other hand this is probably the only study of its kind to prove the efficacy of an isokinetic protocol relying on concentric contractions exclusively.

Dvir et al. The other method for the verification of EO is based on the incorporation of concentric and eccentric contractions. This method has been tested in a variety of muscles groups and in both genders: knee extensors (Dvir & David 1996, David et al 1996), flexors of the elbow (Dvir 1997a), extensors of the trunk (Dvir 1997b, Dvir & Keating 2001), grip muscles (Dvir 1999b) and flexors of the shoulder (Dvir et al 2002). Application of this method to clinical populations composed of patients with shoulder, knee and hand (grip) disorders has been recently described (Dvir 2002). Likewise, CLBP patients were tested for EO (Dvir & Keating 2003).

The physiological rationale for the method derives from the different mechanical output of eccentric and concentric contractions, especially when performed at a submaximal level. When maximal effort is produced, muscle strength is governed by the moment–angular velocity (M–ω) ('force–velocity') function. According to this function, which has been observed in all muscle groups, in concentric effort, strength is generally reduced with increase in the angular velocity of the relevant joint(s). On the other hand, the strength produced in eccentric contractions tends to change only slightly with the majority of studies reporting an increase in strength when the angular velocity increases. Consequently in healthy subjects, the eccentric to concentric (Ecc/Con) strength ratio which is defined with respect to the same velocity is in principle greater than 1 under all isokinetic test conditions. If the test velocity is very low – namely approximating isometric conditions – the Ecc/Con ratio approaches unity and in some instances, invariably indicating the presence of some disorder, it may be even less than 1.

These relationships are much accentuated when subjects are instructed to produce SE, irrespective of the nature of instruction (although not necessarily to the same extent). It seems that the ability to control muscle tension under SE differs significantly between the two contraction modes reflecting, most probably, the effect of distinct neurophysiological demands. Whereas concentric contractions bring about the required motion, eccentric contractions are inhibitory and defensive in nature, operating in order to restrain motion. This specific activity means by necessity a significantly reduced precision in tension production compared to the level of control exercised during concentric contractions. Moreover, a higher joint angular velocity is probably interpreted as a more threatening situation resulting in a larger motor unit pool recruitment and greater muscular tension. Indeed neurophysiological studies indicate that eccentric activity may even be modulated by different brain structures (Enoka 1996).

The variations in response pattern to increased joint velocity are well reflected upon comparison of SE and ME. As far as concentric activity is concerned, when subjects are asked to perform submaximally the difference between their strength output at low and high velocities is quite considerable. In contrast, the drop in eccentric output is rather moderate. These differences are demonstrated in Figures 5.4 and 5.5 which depict the strength curves obtained from a subject exerting ME and SE during isokinetic grip.

The general shape of the M–ω function during exertion of ME is depicted in Figure 5.6. These curves are based on protocols consisting of two angular velocities which were set at a gradient that was typically 1:4 (e.g. 20 and 80°/s or 10 and 40°/s). Figure 5.7 depicts the same functional relationship but in SE. The much sharper fall-off in the concentric exertions versus a moderate drop in the eccentric counterparts is clearly evident.

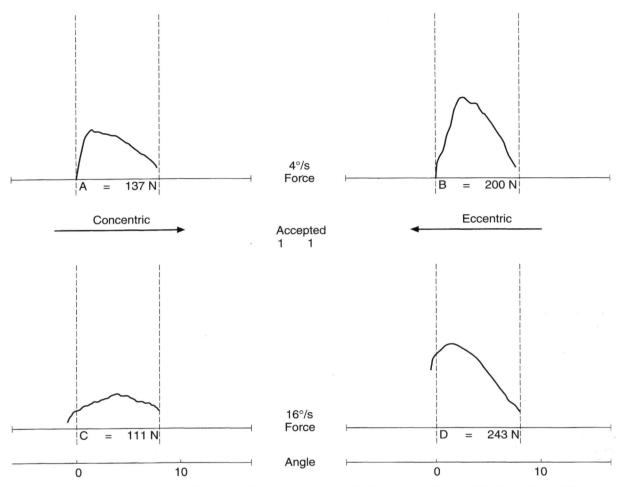

Figure 5.4 Maximal isokinetic grip effort curves. Upper traces, test at 4°/s; lower traces, test at 16°/s. (From Dvir 1999b.)

Based on these variations it was suggested that by comparing Ecc/Con ratios related to velocities that are set a sufficiently large gradient, one could potentially differentiate between ME and SE. As a result a parameter termed DEC (difference between Ecc/Con ratios) has been defined by the following formula:

$$DEC = \left[\frac{Ecc}{Con}\right]_{high} - \left[\frac{Ecc}{Con}\right]_{low}$$

where the 'high' and 'low' refer to the test angular velocities. The gradient employed, 1:4, was not arbitrary but in most of the cases, corresponded nominally (in terms of °/s) to half and twice the joint range of motion (ROM) for the 'low' and 'high' velocities, respectively. For example, for a ROM of 50° the 'low' and 'high' velocities are 25°/s and 100°/s, respectively. Likewise a ROM of 12° leads to 'low' and 'high' velocities of 6°/s and 24°/s. It has also been observed that a reduction in the ROM necessitated a greater gradient in order to retain a comparable efficiency of differentiation between ME and SE (Dvir et al 2002).

In a series of studies exploring the differentiation capacity of the DEC, subjects were asked to exert ME and then to perform submaximally according to different instructions. In the initial

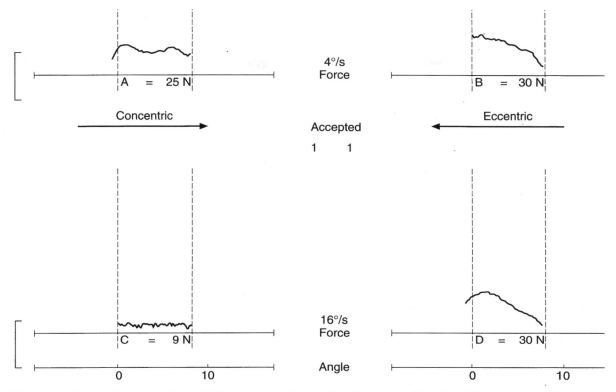

Figure 5.5 Same subject as in Figure 5.4 feigning isokinetic grip effort. Note drastic flattening of the curve at the higher velocity concentric effort. (From Dvir 1999b.)

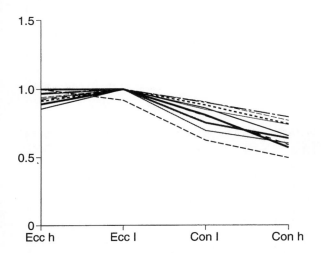

Figure 5.6 Moment–angular velocity (*M*–ω) curves during maximal effort. Curves are based on performance of various muscle groups. X axis: Ecc, eccentric; Con, concentric; h, high velocity; l, low velocity. Y axis: moments normalized relative to Ecc l. (From Dvir 1997a,b, 1999b, Dvir & Keating 2001, 2003, Dvir et al 2002.)

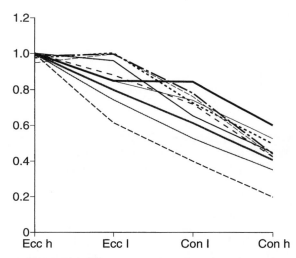

Figure 5.7 Moment–angular velocity (*M*–ω) curves during submaximal effort. Curves are based on performance of various muscle groups. X axis: Ecc, eccentric; Con, concentric; h, high velocity; l, low velocity. Y axis: moments normalized relative to Ecc l. (From Dvir 1997a,b, 1999b, Dvir & Keating 2001, 2003, Dvir et al 2002.)

studies the instructions related to a percentage of effort or to what the subjects perceived as a level of effort they could best reproduce (Dvir & David 1996, Dvir 1997a,b). In later studies (Dvir 1999b, Dvir & Keating 2001, Dvir et al 2002) subjects were presented with a vignette describing a fictitious injury. They were instructed to attempt to convince the examiner that this injury was still affecting them in the form of muscle weakness. In all studies there was a highly significant difference between the strength levels recorded in ME and SE. However more importantly, the DEC scores differed in an equally significant way. Using tolerance intervals – a statistical tool which allows establishment of cutoff values – it was possible to state at a given level of confidence if the effort was maximal or submaximal.

Table 5.5 outlines the findings of the DEC-related studies in terms of the acceptance/rejection zones. In other words, if based on a given protocol the DEC score is *below* the cutoff value, the effort is deemed maximal at the stated level of confidence. For example, if using a ROM of 20° (10° of flexion to 10° of hyperextension) and two angular velocities (10 and 40°/s; Dvir & Keating 2001) the DEC score of a male CLBP patient is 0.34, his performance is considered optimal at the 95% level of confidence (LoC). This decision is based on a cutoff value of 0.69 (Table 5.5). In another example, a female patient is complaining of weakness of grip following fracture of the base of the proximal phalanx of the third finger. Using a ROM of 8° and angular velocities of 4 and 16°/s

the DEC is 4.02. In view of a cutoff of 2.12, it may be stated with a 95% LoC that this patient is not exerting an optimal effort.

It should be realized that three LoCs may be used: 90, 95 and 99%. Depending on the strength with which a claim may be accepted or rejected these benchmarks will classify claims according to different sensitivities and specificities. For instance, consider a patient who performs submaximally but whose DEC score falls in between the cutoffs corresponding to 95 and 99% LoCs. Since the cutoff at 99% is greater than at 95%, this patient will be classified as exerting an SE at the 95% LoC but will 'pass' the test at 99%. Thus applying the previous cutoff (95%) will yield a true positive result but application of the latter (99%) will falsely classify this patient as an optimal performer (false negative). In other words, applying a higher LoC means accepting claims that may be rejected at a lower LoC or increasing the rate of false negatives. Which LoC should be applied is a question that is beyond the scope of this book. However since the biomedical standard of $\alpha = 0.05$ is quite universally accepted, a 95% LoC could be a reasonable benchmark (Dvir 1999a). Obviously the 99% would be indicated if a more conservative approach is taken.

The efficiency of the DEC in terms of retaining its differentiating power over time has been tested on normal male and female subjects using ME and feigned weakness in trunk extension (Dvir & Keating 2001). Findings have indicated that neither DEC_m nor DEC_s, corresponding to ME and SE

Table 5.5	Average KinCom-based DEC scores for ME and SE and the corresponding cutoff values: normal subjects				
Joint/movement	ROM	Velocities (gradient)	Mean DEC in ME	Mean DEC in SE	Cutoff: 95%
Trunk/extension[1]	40°	20°/s:60°/s (1:3)	0.21	1.23	1.01
Trunk/extension[2,a]	20°	10°/s:40°/s (1:4)	0.13	0.83	0.75
Trunk/extension[2,b]	20°	10°/s:40°/s (1:4)	0.075	1.09	0.69
Elbow/flexion[3]	60°	20°/s:60°/s (1:3)	0.034	1.68	1.14
Elbow/flexion[3]	30°	20°/s:60°/s (1:3)	−0.007	1.40	1.02
Grip[4]	8°	4°/s:16°/s (1:4)	0.68	3.40	2.12
Shoulder/flexion[5]	80°	40°/s:160°/s (1:4)	0.48	5.35	0.99
Shoulder/flexion[5]	16°	8°/s:32°/s (1:4)	0.11	0.68	0.36

[a] women; [b] men; DEC, difference between Ecc/Con ratios; ME, maximal effort, SE, suboptimal effort.
[1] Dvir 1997b; [2] Dvir & Keating 2001; [3] Dvir 1997a; [4] Dvir 1999b; [5] Dvir et al 2002.

respectively, have changed significantly between two test sessions spread over a period of 1–2 weeks. Moreover, in men the DEC could differentiate correctly 100 and 93% of the cases in the first and second testing sessions, respectively. In women the results were lower at 82 and 70%, respectively. Under the prescribed protocol, these results rendered the DEC particularly effective in normal men.

The applicability of the DEC concept in clinical subgroups has also been examined in two studies. In one study, 34 patients with shoulder, hand and knee problems were tested (Dvir 2002). Normal subject-based cutoffs at 95% LoC were used. All patients were at least 1 year post-injury and already claiming compensation. In all cases except one, the DEC confirmed that optimal effort was exerted. In another study, 44 well recovered CLBP patients were tested using the abovementioned ROM (20°) and velocities (10 and 40°/s). At a LoC of 99%, normal subject-based cutoff revealed that 89% of the patients performed optimally. Lowering the benchmark to 95% resulted in 84%. The reason for applying a more stringent benchmark (99%) was due to the outstanding complexity of factors taking part in trunk testing and the great care that ought to be exercised in interpreting the results.

The DEC-based cutoff system is probably the only one of its type to be systematically explored. It is not however free of limitations:

1. All data were collected on KinCom dynamometers, models II, 500H and 125E+ (whether the cutoffs apply equally to tests using the same protocols but different dynamometers requires further research).
2. Gender has an effect on the DEC and not all studies included both.
3. It is not clear to what extent age plays a role in the Ecc/Con ratios and therefore in the numerical value of the DEC.

However, since the eccentric mode is integral to all modern isokinetic systems, testing concentrically and eccentrically using a comparable velocity gradient should pose little difficulty, as well as providing a decisively more comprehensive muscle profile. Moreover, not only does the on-line

data and results screen allow instant calculation of the DEC, this easily interpretable parameter nullifies the need to resort to complex statistical analyses (Hazard et al 1988, Fishbain et al 1999b).

The last issue which confounds EO analysis concerns the effect of instructions given to the subject. There is some evidence that instructions may change performance level (Matheson et al 1992). At least seven different types of instruction have been identified (Dvir 2001):

1. Feign effort without specific instructions (Fishbain et al 1999b)
2. Feign an SE perceived to be the best reproducible on repeated contractions (Dvir & David 1996, Dvir 1997a)
3. Feign an SE perceived to be a percentage of the maximal effort (Luoto et al 1996, Robinson et al 1991)
4. Use a self-selected SE (Birmingham & Kramer 1998, Birmingham et al 1998)
5. Simulate injury (Robinson et al 1992b)
6. Simulate injury in order to gain (Dvir & Keating 2001)
7. Simulate pain (Ayalon et al 2001).

Invariably, the protocols applied in these studies have used maximal performance as the baseline to which its submaximal counterpart was compared; in most studies, ME preceded SE. Furthermore, in the majority of cases the subjects were normal individuals rather than patients. Although instructions of the types 1–4 may lead to different submaximal scores compared to those corresponding to types 5–7, no comparative study of the differential effect of instruction was available. On the other hand, slight differences were noted between a percentage-based (e.g. 50% of maximal effort) and a so-called best reproducible SE (Dvir & David 1996). The nature of instruction is of course very critical when applied to patient populations. Obviously, in order to establish clear cutoffs, it would be necessary to compare ME with SE in these groups as well. Although some research has been done using a percentage of effort as a cognitive anchor it is quite clear that the ultimate anchor is in fact straightforward feigning of effort in order to gain unlawfully. For ethical reasons administration of such instructions to patients may not be permitted by institutional review boards.

DETERMINATION OF IMPAIRMENT

This section refers to two principal subjects. The first outlines a list of substantive issues relating to the medicolegal assessment of muscular weakness. The other is more technical and refers to the actual test and method by which weakness and its associated impairment may be quantified.

Medicolegal assessment of muscular weakness

The ways various legal codes view personal injuries and their indemnification is profoundly versatile and a description of these is absolutely beyond the scope of this book. However, professionals involved in medicolegal assessment of motor deficits should be aware of the following:

1. Muscular weakness relates to reduction in the capacity to produce tension in a single or a limited number of repetitions, namely strength. This weakness should not be confused with reduction in mechanical power (the time rate of work produced by a muscle group) or with a lesser endurance capacity/fatiguability.

2. Strength is the sine qua non parameter for determination of muscular weakness. The use of strength as *the* criterion is correct not only as it is the most tangible and readily measurable of all parameters (e.g. work or power) but because it is linearly and strongly correlated with the others, or at least so with work.

3. From the purely clinical point of view, muscular weakness is an *impairment*. However, this weakness does not necessarily lead to or result in *disability*. Too often the lack of visible disability leads to a conclusion that the claimant is performing submaximally. This in turn may result in stigmatizing. Clinicians who are involved in the diagnosis and treatment of motor deficiencies are well aware of the enormous capacity to compensate and adapt in the face of very weak or even paralyzed muscles. This capacity should not deprive patients of their right to compensation.

4. In spite of (3), weakness is not universally recognized as an impairment.

5. No general agreement exists with respect to the question: which type of strength (strength testing) should serve as the criterion for determination of weakness – isometric, concentric or eccentric? As each of these modes of contraction and techniques may lead to a different outcome, this question is of prime importance.

6. No general agreement exists regarding test protocols, appropriate time for testing and EO procedures necessary to establish a clinically valid decision.

7. No general agreement exists concerning the question: when does a measured strength loss become an impairment although Sapega (1990) has certainly offered an interesting and methodologically sound criterion (see below).

8. In spite of a common acceptance of bilateral comparisons as a basis for assessing impairment and with the exception of grip strength (under the AMA's *Guides to the Evaluation of Permanent Impairment*, 1993), no mechanism exists for correlating the severity of bilateral differences with the rating of impairment.

9. In spite of its widespread use in various medical specializations (rehabilitation, orthopedics, neurology and sports medicine) as well as in physical therapy, exercise physiology and ergonomics, ISD is still not universally considered the standard instrument for measuring muscular dysfunction.

Among these, issues 5–7 may be addressed in the light of existing knowledge.

Instrumental testing

As for the appropriate mode of contraction that should be used as a criterion for assessing the percentage of strength loss, instrumental isometric techniques (e.g. hand-held dynamometry, HHD) offer two technical advantages over isokinetic measurements. First, in all respects they are much simpler and cheaper to apply. Second, they relate to a single 'angular velocity' (0°/s). On the other hand, it should be borne in mind that with the possible and qualified exception of grip, in most motor tasks muscles work dynamically. Therefore from the physiological and functional points of view, the correct way to assess deficiency is according to the way muscles operate. Moreover, research strongly indicates that confirmation of EO cannot be accomplished using isometric techniques. Other disadvantages of HHD concern the problem of testing strong subjects (particularly when the tester is weaker in comparison) as well as the great difficulty in measuring selected groups of muscles like trunk extensors and flexors.

As the so-called 'isotonic' methods cannot measure the maximal output throughout the range of motion, the only method for measuring muscle strength and confirmation of EO is ISD. Using this technology as the tool of choice results however in a number of questions that have never been properly addressed. For instance, research has indicated that concentric and eccentric strength losses were not equal (Reinking et al 1996, Dvir et al 2003) which naturally begs the question which of the two is more appropriate. There is a general consensus that concentric testing should continue to serve as the main criterion since it is this mode of contraction that normally produces the desired motion, invariably against the force of gravity. It is also compatible, at least partly, with the still commonly employed MMT technique whose cornerstone principle with respect to grades 3–5 is the ability to move a body segment against gravity with or without the effect of gravity.

On the other hand, the growing knowledge regarding eccentric contractions, especially their functional significance and role in EO testing, renders them no less appropriate for this purpose. Although no large scale statistical analysis has ever been published concerning the difference between concentric and eccentric deficiencies of the same muscle (group), a currently underway study based on medicolegal assessments of unilateral muscle weakness indicates that in the vast majority of cases the concentric deficiency was *greater* than the eccentric deficiency (Dvir 2003). Since eccentric efforts are less voluntarily controllable than their concentric counterparts, it could be argued that they reflect in a more accurate way the true capacity (weakness) of the relevant

muscles. Hence the eccentric rather than the concentric capacity should serve as the criterion. Clearly, whereas the concentric effort-based deficiency serves the claimant in a better way the eccentric effort-based deficiency is more favorable to the compensating body (e.g. insurance companies, social security). As a result averaging of the concentric and eccentric deficiencies is a possible solution that deserves systematic exploration. Moreover, the employment of a single criterion test velocity versus two test velocities (or their average score) is a major problem as invariably the calculated imbalances are not identical, particularly when the velocities are well spaced out. A possible solution is to include all four test conditions necessary for computing the DEC and consider the average score as the representative percentage of strength loss.

Time of testing

With respect to appropriate time of testing, an assessment aimed at estimating impairment may not be conducted unless a chronic state has been achieved. Whether or not this benchmark period is appropriate, depends on the type of damage, treatment (conservative or invasive), rehabilitation procedures, etc. Therefore the common approach is to consider 1 year as an acceptable period of time for strength loss, if any, to stabilize.

Degree of impairment

Another cardinal problem concerns the degree of weakness that may already be considered an impairment. In principle, any bilateral difference should be considered an impairment. However due to the measurement error, test results may be as much as 20% off the true score (see Chapter 3). Moreover, this error margin relates to measurements performed on the *same* muscle group; there is still a deep void regarding the behavior of bilateral isokinetic indices in normal individuals and especially in specific clinical groups. Given this situation, one has to resort, still, to a combination of the available knowledge and sound empirical observations. Quite coincidentally it has been suggested in one of the classical reviews on muscle performance evaluation (Sapega 1990) that in expected weakness (e.g. following injury) a bilateral difference of 10–20% is possibly abnormal whereas a difference of 20% or more should be considered as 'almost certainly pathological'. The author of this book fully supports this benchmark.

Acceptance of this criterion leads finally to the question: how should the severity of the loss be viewed? Although this is strictly a social–economical–legal decision there may be some creative venues for solving this problem. An appropriate authority in this regard is the Guides' policy of equivalence between percentage loss of grip strength and percentage impairment. This approach may, by analogy, be extended to cover other muscle groups in the following manner:

- Any bilateral difference up to 20% should not be recognized as an impairment.
- The remaining 80% can be subdivided into two halves: between 20 and 60% and between 60 and 100% (the upper boundary – 100% – is equivalent to grade 3 strength).
- A 20–60% loss of strength would be considered a moderate impairment whereas any loss in excess of 60% should be considered a severe impairment.
- A finer subdivision could lead to the classification: 20–50% (light), 51–75% (medium) and >76% (severe) impairment.

Quantifying impairment – test and method

The other major topic of this section refers to the actual administration of a medicolegal test for assessing muscle dysfunction and the calculation of strength loss. Clinicians involved in this type of testing are advised to:

1. have a complete medical record of the patient
2. confirm that the record provides a prima facie basis for muscular dysfunction
3. confirm that at least 1 year has elapsed since the initiation of the dysfunction
4. confirm that the patient is capable of performing the isokinetic test and is not suffering from any condition that may cause dangerous exposure (e.g. cardiovascular conditions). In this regard, pain is a relative

contraindication in the sense that severe pain should be absolutely avoided. However a tolerable degree of pain that does not interfere with initiating and completing a full protocol and that is not detrimental for later recovery, is permissible

5. explain as thoroughly as possible the objective of the test prior to the actual testing, confirm that the patient understands the explanation and can follow the instructions and is not apprehended by the actual testing. Refer explicitly to the fact that the test is very sensitive and therefore patients are expected to cooperate as fully as possible.

Ostensibly, in the absence of a standard method of testing, any rigorous protocol may fulfill the objective. However as confirmation of EO is essential the protocol must include a mechanism for this particular purpose. If EO is rejected, the test is invalid for estimating impairment, otherwise determination of strength loss depends on the tested muscle group. There are three situations:

1. a unilateral impairment of an upper or lower extremity muscle group
2. a bilateral impairment of the same muscle group
3. an impairment of axial skeleton muscles, typically of the trunk extensor or flexor apparatus.

In the most typical case (1) the loss of strength is determined according to the following formula in which SUS and SIS stand for strength of the unimpaired side and strength of the impaired side, respectively:

$$\% \text{ strength loss} = \frac{\text{SUS} - \text{SIS}}{\text{SUS}}$$

The decision whether to use a single or multiple testing modes (see above) rests with the examiner.

In the case of bilateral involvement there are two options. One is to compare the scores of both muscle groups to reference data but this is rather problematic for obvious reasons: type of dynamometer, protocol, gender, age, etc. This incidentally would also apply when the patient does not have a functional bilateral group for reason of palsy or amputation. The other option is to identify which of the two bilateral groups is less compromised and consider it as the unimpaired side.

In the case of trunk extensors (in particular) and flexors, comparison to reference data is the only venue. However, in contrast to extremity muscles, perhaps with the exception of knee and shoulder muscles, available databases relate to normal subjects as well as to CLBP patients. This allows a more reliable and systematic comparison.

REFERENCES

American Medical Association 1993 Guides to the evaluation of permanent impairment, 4th edn. AMA, Chicago

Andres P L, Finison L J, Conlon T, Thibodeau L M, Munsat T L 1988 Use of composite scores (megascores) to measure deficit in amyotrophic lateral sclerosis. Neurology 38: 405–408

Ayalon M, Rubinstein M, Barak Y, Dunsky A, Ben-Sira D 2001 Identification of feigned strength test of the knee extensors and flexors based on the shape of the isokinetic torque curve. Isokinetics and Exercise Science 9: 45–50

Birmingham T B, Kramer J F 1998 Identifying submaximal muscular effort: reliability of difference scores calculated from isometric and isokinetic measurements. Perceptual and Motor Skills 87: 1183–1191

Birmingham T B, Kramer J F, Speechley M, Chesworth B M, MacDermid J 1998 Measurement variability and sincerity of effort: clinical utility of isokinetic strength coefficient of variation scores. Ergonomics 41: 853–863

Bohannon R W 1987 Differentiation of maximal from submaximal static elbow flexor efforts by measurement variability. American Journal of Physical Medicine 66: 213–217

Bohannon R W, Smith M B 1988 Differentiation of maximal and submaximal knee extension efforts by isokinetic testing. Clinical Biomechanics 3: 215–218

Chengalur S N, Smith G A, Nelson R C, Sadoff A M 1990 Assessing sincerity of effort in maximum grip strength tests. American Journal of Physical Medicine and Rehabilitation 69: 148–153

David G, Dvir Z, Mackintosh S, Brien C 1996 Validity of a novel test protocol for the identification of submaximal muscular effort. Isokinetics and Exercise Science 6: 139–144

Dvir Z 1997a An isokinetic study of submaximal effort in elbow flexion. Perceptual and Motor Skills 84: 1431–1438

Dvir Z 1997b Differentiation of submaximal from maximal trunk extension effort: an isokinetic study using a new testing protocol. Spine 22: 2672–2676

Dvir Z 1999a Coefficient of variation I: maximal and feigned static and dynamic grip efforts. American Journal of Physical Medicine and Rehabilitation 78: 216–221

Dvir Z 1999b Identification of feigned grip effort using isokinetic dynamometry. Clinical Biomechanics 14: 522–527

Dvir Z 2001 Commentary. Isokinetics and Exercise Science 9: 51

Dvir Z 2002 Clinical application of the DEC parameter in assessing optimality of muscular effort: a report of 34 patients. American Journal of Physical Medicine and Rehabilitation 81: 178–183.

Dvir Z 2003 Concentric vs. eccentric strength deficiencies. An isokinetic study of patients with chronic knee, shoulder, ankle, hand and trunk compromise. Submitted.

Dvir Z, David G 1996 Suboptimal muscular performance: measuring isokinetic strength of knee extensors with a new testing protocol. Archives of Physical Medicine and Rehabilitation 77: 578–581

Dvir Z, Keating J 2001 Identification of feigned isokinetic trunk extension effort: an efficiency study of the DEC. Spine 26: 1046–1051

Dvir Z, Keating J 2003 Trunk extension effort in chronic low back dysfunction patients. Spine 28: 685–692.

Dvir Z, Steinfeld-Cohen Y, Peretz C 2002 Identification of feigned shoulder flexion weakness in normal subjects. American Journal of Physical Medicine and Rehabilitation 81: 187–193

Dvir Z, Shabbat S, Niska M, Steinfeld-Cohen Y 2003 Ankle inversion and eversion strength in patients with unilateral malleolar fractures: a post-operative measurement of concentric, eccentric and isometric efforts. Submitted.

Enoka R 1996 Eccentric contractions require unique activation strategies by the nervous system. Journal of Applied Physiology 81: 2339–2346

Finsterbush A, Frankel V, Arnon R 1983 Quantitative power measurements of extensor hallucis longus: a simple objective test in evaluation of low back pain with neurological involvement. Spine 8: 206–210

Fishbain D A, Cutler R, Rosomoff H L, Rosomoff R S 1999a Chronic pain disability exaggeration/malingering and submaximal effort research. Clinical Journal of Pain 15: 244–274

Fishbain D A, Abdel-Moty E, Cutler R, Rosomoff H L, Rosomoff R S 1999b Detection of 'faked' strength task effort in volunteers using a computerized exercise testing system. American Journal of Physical Medicine and Rehabilitation 78: 222–227

Hamilton Fairfax A 1996 An examination of methods used to discriminate between maximal and submaximal muscular exertions. PhD Thesis. Faculty of Health Sciences, University of Sydney

Hamilton Fairfax A, Balnave R, Adams R 1995 Variability of grip strength during isometric contractions. Ergonomics 38: 1819–1830

Hamilton Fairfax A, Balnave R, Adams R 1997 Review of sincerity of effort testing. Safety Science 25: 237–245

Harber P, Soo Hoo K 1984 Static ergonomic strength testing in evaluating occupational back pain. Journal of Occupational Medicine 12: 877–884

Hazard R G, Reid S, Fenwick J, Reeves V 1988 Isokinetic trunk and lifting strength measurements: variability as an indicator of effort. Spine 13: 54–57

Hildreth D H, Breidenbach W C, Lister G, Hodges A D 1989 Detection of submaximal effort by use of the rapid exchange grip. Journal of Hand Surgery 14A: 742–745

Janda D H, Geiringer S R, Hankin F M, Barry D T 1987 Objective evaluation of grip strength. Journal of Occupational Medicine 29: 569–571

Joughin K, Gulati P, MacKinnon S E et al 1993 An evaluation of rapid exchange and simultaneous grip. Journal of Hand Surgery 18A: 245–252

Lechner D E, Bradbury S F, Bradley L A 1998 Detecting sincerity of effort: a summary of methods and approaches. Physical Therapy 78: 867–888

Lin P, Robinson M E, Carlos J, Oçonnor P 1996 Detection of submaximal effort in isometric and isokinetic knee extension tests. Journal of Orthopaedic and Sports Physical Therapy 24: 19–24

Luoto S, Hupli M, Alaranta H, Hurri H 1996 Isokinetic performance capacity of trunk muscles. Part II: Coefficient of variation in isokinetic measurements in maximal effort and in submaximal effort. Scandinavian Journal of Rehabilitation Medicine 28: 207–210

Mandell P J, Weitz E, Bernstein J I et al 1993 Isokinetic trunk strength and lifting strength measures. Differences and similarities between low-back-injured and noninjured workers. Spine 18: 2491–2501

Matheson L N 1991 Work capacity evaluation: systematic approach to industrial rehabilitation. Employment and Rehabilitation Institute of California, Anaheim

Matheson L N, Carlton R, Niemeyer L O 1988 Grip strength in a disabled sample: reliability and normative standards. Industrial Rehabilitation Quarterly 1: 1–7

Matheson L, Mooney V, Caiozzo V et al 1992 Effect of instruction on isokinetic trunk strength testing variability, reliability, absolute value and predictive validity. Spine 17: 914–921

Medical Research Council 1976 Aids to the examination of the peripheral nervous system, Memorandum no. 45. MRC, London, UK

Newton M, Waddell G 1993 Trunk strength testing with iso-machines. Part I: Review of a decade of scientific evidence. Spine 18: 801–811

Newton M, Thow M, Somerville D, Henderson I, Waddell G 1993 Trunk strength testing with iso-machines. Part II: Experimental evaluation of the Cynex II back testing system in normal subjects and patients with chronic low back pain. Spine 18: 812–824

Niebuhr B R, Marion R 1987 Detecting sincerity of effort when measuring grip strength. American Journal of Physical Medicine and Rehabilitation 66: 16–24

Niebuhr B R, Marion R 1990 Voluntary control of submaximal grip strength. American Journal of Physical Medicine and Rehabilitation 69: 96–101

Niemeyer L O, Matheson L N, Carlton R S 1989 Testing consistency of effort: BTE work simulator. Industrial Rehabilitation Quarterly 2: 1–7

Polatin P B, Mayer T G 1992 Quantification of function in low back pain. In: Turk D C, Melzack R (eds) Handbook of Pain Assessment. Guilford Press, New York

Reid S, Hazard R G, Fenwick J 1991 Isokinetic trunk strength deficits in people with and without low back pain: A comparative study with consideration of effort. Journal of Spinal Disorders 4: 68–72

Reinking M F, Bockrath-Pugliese K, Worrell T et al 1996 Assesment of quadriceps muscle performance by hand-held, isometric and isokinetic dynamometry in patients with knee dysfunction. Journal of Orthopaedic and Sports Physical Therapy 24: 154–159

Robinson M E, MacMillan M, O'Connor P, Fuller A, Cassisi J E 1991 Reproducibility of maximal versus submaximal efforts in an isometric lumbar extension task. Journal of Spinal Disorders 4: 444–448

Robinson M E, O'Connor P, MacMillan M et al 1992a Physical and psychosocial correlates of test-retest isometric torque variability in patients with chronic low back pain. Journal of Occupational Rehabilitation 2: 11–18

Robinson M E, O'Connor P, MacMillan M, Fuller A, Cassisi J E 1992b Effect of instruction to simulate back injury on torque reproducibility in isometric lumbar extension test. Journal of Occupational Medicine 2: 191–199

Robinson M E, Geisser M, Hanson C S, O'Connor P D 1993 Detecting submaximal efforts in grip strength testing with the coefficient of variation. Journal of Occupational Rehabilitation 3: 45–50

Robinson M E, O'Connor P D, Riley J L, Kvaal S, Shirley F 1994 Variability of isometric and isotonic leg exercise: utility for detection of submaximal effort. Journal of Occupational Rehabilitation 4: 163–169

Sapega A A 1990 Current concepts review: muscle performance evaluation in orthopaedic practice. Journal of Bone and Joint Surgery 72A: 1562–1574

Saunders N E, Bohannon R W 1991 Can feigned maximal efforts be distinguished from maximal efforts? Journal of Human Muscle Performance 1: 16–24

Simmonsen J C 1995 Coefficient of variation as a measure of subject effort. Archives of Physical Medicine and Rehabilitation 76: 516–520

Stokes H M 1983 The seriously uninjured hand – weakness of grip. Journal of Occupational Medicine 25: 683–686

Tornvall G 1963 Assessment of physical capabilities. Acta Physiologica Scandinavica 58: 30–93

Young V L, Pin K, Kraemer B A, Gould R B, Nemergut L 1989 Fluctuation in grip and pinch strength among normal subjects. Journal of Hand Surgery 14A: 125–129

6 Isokinetics of the hip muscles

In the field of isokinetic research, the hip is probably the most neglected among the major joint systems, after the elbow. A search of the literature yields only a handful of papers relating to testing procedures and representative values, and offering little of clinical significance. Considering the important role of hip muscles in locomotion and posture this poverty is rather surprising. Moreover, the suggested contribution of the hip extension mechanism to the initial phase of lifting (see Chapter 9) could have been expected to stimulate considerable research into the relationship between hip and trunk extension functions.

This short chapter, therefore, mostly concerns procedures. As will be shown, these are far from definitive, and this may be a reason for the tardy development of a comprehensive database for hip muscle performance under isokinetic conditions.

PART 1
ISOKINETIC TESTING OF HIP JOINT MUSCLES

The hip joint affords lower limb movement about three independent axes, resulting in sagittal, frontal and axial motions. Isokinetic measurement of the performance of the muscles involved in executing these motions must take into account:

1. the tested range of motion (ROM)
2. positioning and stabilization
3. alignment of the biological and mechanical axes
4. positioning of the force pad
5. the test angular velocities.

The significance of these elements is discussed in the context of the three types of motion.

SAGITTAL PLANE MOTION

Range of motion

Movement in the sagittal plane is normally described in terms of flexion and extension. There are considerable discrepancies concerning norms for hip joint ROM in all planes. For instance whereas in one study the norm for extension was 10° (Boone & Azen 1979) in another it was 50° (Dorinson & Wagner 1948).

In one of the first instrumented analyses of hip muscle strength, Jensen et al (1971) indicated that, from multiple-point isometric measurements, the peak of the force versus angular position curve was located at an angle of about 30° of flexion, for flexion and extension alike. The curve was approximately symmetrical for extension, with the recorded forces diminishing very rapidly towards the initial (dependent lower limb) and final position (at about 80°). In flexion there was a comparable reduction in force towards the initial position but a much milder decline up to 90° of flexion.

In the most comprehensive study of hip musculature available to date (Cahalan et al 1989) the authors suggested that 45° should be a standard angle for isometric testing in the upright position. Consequently for strength measurements the recommended tested ROM in the upright position (see below) is 60–75° from the neutral (dependent) lower limb position.

The upright position

Sagittal, and also frontal motion testing, should be performed with the subject in the upright position, for two reasons:

1. Most of the functional activities involving the hip, like walking, running and stair climbing, are performed while the body is in the upright position. It also means that the activation patterns of the muscles which take part in these movements will basically be maintained during the test.

2. The gravitational factor in any other position, particularly supine, is quite considerable, and it is likely that some subjects will find it difficult or even impossible to generate sufficient moment to lift the lower limb.

Stabilization

Stabilization in the upright position requires a special attachment, whose potential bulk may be the reasons why the non-physiological supine or side-lying testing positions are recommended by a few manufacturers of isokinetic systems. Failure to properly stabilize the subject in the upright position is likely to result in poor reproducibility.

Cahalan et al (1989) designed a fixed special attachment for a Cybex II dynamometer, which allowed stabilization of the upper limbs and pelvis. Figures 6.1 and 6.2 show positioning for hip flexors and extensors testing respectively. The subject stands on a special platform designed by the author (not shown) which is compatible with the specific dynamometer in use. To prevent substitution the subject is strapped at various levels, including the contralateral shank and thigh as well as the upper pelvis.

Knee position, particularly when full extension is maintained throughout the test, is important for two reasons:

1. The resulting gravitational moment of the shank is higher than in testing where flexion is allowed.
2. Rectus femoris contraction, because of the combined hip flexion–knee extension, may result in variations in the strength curve of either the flexors or extensors.

Therefore it is suggested that when hip sagittal motion is tested the knee should be allowed to flex passively, i.e. as a result of gravity.

Axes alignment and force pad position

Alignment of the biological and mechanical axes is achieved by placing the axis of the actuator

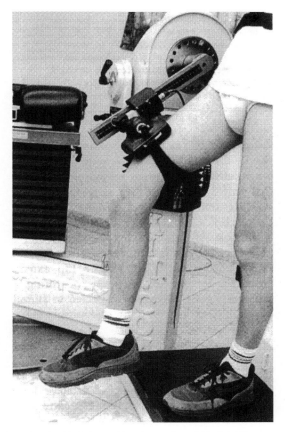

Figure 6.1   Upright position for testing of hip joint flexors.

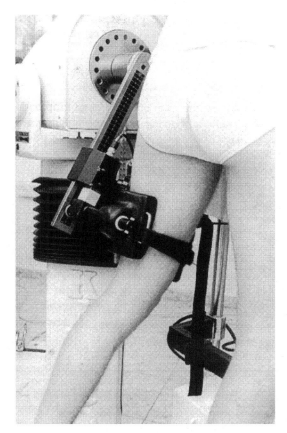

Figure 6.2   Upright position for testing of hip joint extensors.

against the greater trochanter which serves as the anatomical marker for the hip joint axis.

The resistance pad should be placed slightly above the superior pole of the patella.

Angular velocities

There is a lack of information regarding the most appropriate angular velocities for hip muscle testing, although the work of Cahalan et al (1989) is an important reference. There is a temptation to use velocities derived from walking or running but these are, par excellence, activities where conditions are not isokinetic.

As patients may find that lifting the lower limb through a ROM of 60–75° involves considerable effort, concentric testing may be more comfortably performed at slow velocities. Indeed two studies which concentrated on hip flexion and extension strength chose to stay at this end of the spectrum. Burnett et al (1990) used 30 and 90°/s as their test velocities (supine position) and found that the strength of extensors, flexors, abductors and adductors was similar at both velocities. Tis et al (1991) used 20°/s as the test velocity (upright position) but did not compare it with other velocities.

On the other hand, Cahalan et al (1989) studied a spectrum of velocities consisting of 30, 90, 150 and 210°/s. These authors indicated that the moment curves at the two higher velocities were characterized by overshoot inconsistencies, and hence recommended testing only at 30 and 90°/s.

The use of 60°/s as a single test velocity, or 30 and 90°/s as more comprehensive performance indicators is therefore recommended.

FRONTAL PLANE MOTION

ROM in the frontal plane

Movement in this plane is described in terms of abduction and adduction. The accepted ROM for abduction is 45°, whereas for adduction there is a very wide variation among different sources; however 25° may be considered a representative ROM (Miller 1985). The tested ROM may be much smaller, depending on both the position of peak moment (Donatelli et al 1991) and the functional demands. In the case of side-lying testing there is also a mechanical block, which prevents an adduction angle of more than 5° in the contra-lateral direction.

Upright position in frontal plane testing

Although testing in the supine or side-lying positions has been reported, the upright position is preferred for frontal plane testing, as with the sagittal plane, and for the same reasons. Figure 6.3 shows upright positioning during abduction/adduction testing.

Test ROM   The test ROM of abduction in this position is 0–30°.

Positioning and stabilization   Stabilization is centered on the contralateral hip region since there is a conspicuous tendency particularly during abduction to laterally flex the trunk towards the tested side. This tendency, which results from movement of the iliac crest towards the femur because of gluteus medius activity, causes a protrusion of the greater trochanter of the contralateral side, which detrimentally affects the length–tension relationship of this muscle. The opposite applies to adduction testing where the pelvis tends to move towards the tested side. The knee joint should be kept passively at full extension as only negligible motion is afforded in the frontal plane.

Alignment of axes   This is performed by placing the actuator axis opposite the hip joint at a coronal level about 1 cm medial to the anterior superior iliac spine.

The resistance pad   This should be placed on the lateral side of the thigh at the same level as that for sagittal testing.

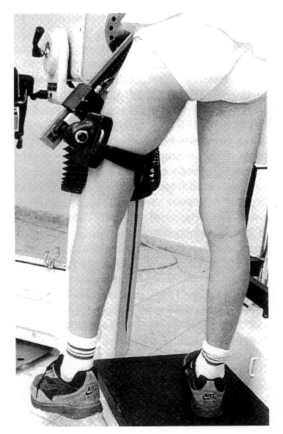

Figure 6.3   Upright position for testing of hip joint abductors.

Side-lying position

Though the supine position has been employed in one study (Olson et al 1972) its applicability seems limited. However, testing in the side-lying position, as reported by Burnett et al (1990) and Donatelli et al (1991), is more popular.

Positioning and stabilization   The single most important advantage of this position is the stabilization provided by the plinth, although strapping of the waist, pelvis and the untested lower limb is necessary (Fig. 6.4).

Resistance pad position and alignment of axes   These are similar to those of upright testing. Prevention of discomfort, or even slight improvement in moment generation, may be accomplished using a dual, thigh–shank pad as described in Donatelli et al (1991).

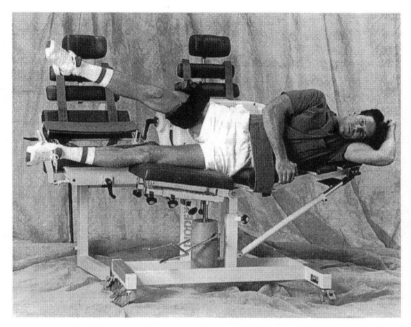

Figure 6.4 Side-lying position for testing the hip joint abductors.

Angular velocites in the frontal plane

Those employed in frontal plane testing have ranged from 30 to 210°/s (Cahalan et al 1989) but in two other papers velocities of 30, 60 and 90°/s (Burnett et al 1990, Donatelli et al 1991) were regarded as adequate. In view of the very limited functional ROM it is suggested that one velocity, i.e. 30°/s, may suffice for demonstrating frontal strength values.

AXIAL MOTION TESTING

Range of motion

Internal and external rotation of the hip joint are considered by most sources to span equal ROMs of 45° (Miller 1985). However, isokinetic testing of the muscles responsible for these movements can reliably reflect their major performance parameters using a much shorter arc. Although this arc has not been explicitly defined, it does seem that a ROM of 30°, from 5° of internal rotation to 25° of external rotation, is sufficiently comprehensive.

Positioning and stabilization

The most reliable source concerning positioning in axial motion testing of the hip is a study by Lindsay et al (1992). This reported the comparison of three distinct positions: seated with knee flexed at 90°; supine with knee flexed to 90°, and supine with knee extended. In all three positions stabilization was provided by straps around the distal thigh, across the pelvic crests and across the chest.

Findings indicated that the seated position was associated with the highest internal and external rotation strength scores, followed by the abovementioned second and third positions respectively. Figure 6.5 depicts the seated position and stabilization as recommended in this paper.

Alignment of axes and resistance pad positioning

Alignment of axes was carried out with reference to the long axis of the femur in the study of

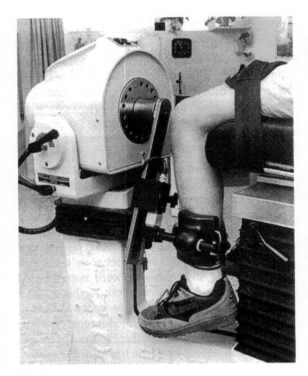

Figure 6.5 Seated position for testing of hip joint rotators.

Lindsay et al. The resistance pad was placed immediately above the lateral malleolus.

Angular velocities

The test velocity which was used by Lindsay et al was 60°/s, whereas Cahalan et al (1989) have reported their axial strength findings using a spectrum of velocities.

The recommended testing velocity is either 30 or 60°/s depending on the degree of compliance of the patient.

TESTING OF ECCENTRIC MODE

It should be noted that although most of the sources quoted in this section refer to concentric testing, the eccentric activity of hip muscles is conspicuous, notably in the walking cycle. Hence if an active dynamometer is available testing in eccentric mode is essential.

PART 2
REPRODUCIBILITY OF HIP PERFORMANCE

The dearth of information regarding hip muscles is reflected in reproducibility studies. Furthermore, no single study has incorporated all movements of the hip joint; such a study is obviously very much needed.

Studies of normal subjects

Three studies have dealt with reproducibility of normal subjects. Burnett et al (1990) tested the strength of the flexors, extensors, abductors and adductors in a group of children 6–10 years old. There were two testing sessions, one week apart, using the velocities of 30 and 90°/s. Testing was conducted in supine and side-lying positions for sagittal and frontal movements respectively. Intraclass correlation coefficients (ICCs) were employed to determine reproducibility, which was found to be acceptable (ICC = 0.84) only for the extensors at 90°/s. The corresponding ICCs for the other muscle groups were consistently lower, particularly in the case of abductors and adductors, where the range was 0.49–0.59. Some procedural factors, such as a definite lack of similarity between the conditions for testing and retesting, were mentioned as potential sources for the low reproducibility.

The major implication of this study is that, at present, there is no evidence for the reproducibility of test findings relating to the flexors, extensors, abductors and adductors of the hip joint in children. Consequently, follow-up measurements of muscle performance status in specific pathologies, such as Duchenne muscular dystrophy, cannot be relied upon.

In a study of the axial rotator muscles (Lindsay et al 1992) it was indicated that intrasession reproducibility was very good, exceeding 0.90 at each of the three positions employed, and for both internal and external rotation. However, as pointed out in Chapter 4, intrasession reproducibility does not provide a sufficiently strong basis for predicting intersession variation.

The third study was carried out by Emery et al (1999) and focused on reproducibility of concentric and eccentric adduction and flexion in normal subjects. Except for an acceptable ICC score for eccentric adduction (0.83, range 0.68–0.93) the reproducibility for concentric adduction and concentric and eccentric flexion was poor.

Study of arthritic individuals and controls

In a study of knee flexors and extensors and hip flexors in control and arthritic individuals (Giles et al 1990) it was found that the intersession reproducibility of the hip measurements, as expressed by the coefficient of variation, was greater than that of the knee. In this instance, hip flexors were tested in the supine position without the incorporation of a gravity correction. The authors have suggested that change may be inferred if there is a variation beyond the very wide margin of 20%.

Conclusion

Taken as a whole, these findings do not establish a general reproducibility for hip testing which gives rise to real concern after close to 40 years that this technology has been in existence. Moreover, given the significance of hip musculature, particularly at the older age, serious effort must be undertaken to rectify this situation. From the studies mentioned above, it will be seen that unless new evidence proves otherwise, it would be wrong to make any clinical inferences based on isokinetic testing of the hip muscles. The only exception is when a single examination reveals bilateral differences of at least 30%.

PART 3
REPRESENTATIVE VALUES FOR HIP STRENGTH

The database relating to hip muscles is particularly poor. For instance, the largest uniform sample consisted of 42 male subjects (Donatelli et al

1991), and other studies have based their findings on between 15 and 30 subjects. On the other hand, a growing awareness regarding the adoption of strict protocols of testing has been demonstrated in recent years. This is reflected in very acceptable reproducibility scores for groups of subjects (Lindsay et al 1992), which means that findings based even on small samples may sometimes serve as excellent guidelines. Attention should however be given to the type of dynamometer used to collect the test information.

The following tables outline strength values, means and standard deviations, of the six principal movements of the hip joint.

Flexion and extension

Table 6.1 refers to flexion and extension and is solely based on findings obtained by Cahalan et al (1989).

Unfortunately further flexion and extension findings by Tis et al (1991) were expressed in force (N) rather than moment (Nm) units and hence cannot be compared with those of Cahalan et al. However, two findings of Tis et al are worth mentioning:

1. The mean force in extension was only slightly higher than that in flexion. The discrepancy between this finding and the significant variations found by Cahalan et al probably resulted from different stabilization used by Tis et al.

Table 6.1   Hip flexor and extensor concentric strength*, based on Cahalan et al (1989)

Motion and angular velocity	Women		Men	
	20–40 years	40–81 years	20–40 years	40–81 years
Flexion				
30°/s	91 (24)	67 (21)	152 (50)	113 (21)
90°/s	70 (26)	46 (17)	126 (50)	84 (21)
Extension				
30°/s	110 (37)	101 (27)	177 (42)	157 (22)
90°/s	97 (41)	70 (26)	163 (49)	132 (32)

* Mean (SD), in Nm.

Table 6.2 Hip adductor and abductor concentric strength*, based on Cahalan et al (1989) and Donatelli et al (1991)

Motion and angular velocity	Women			Men		
	20–40 years	21–32 years[†]	40–81 years	20–40 years	21–32 years[†]	40–81 years
Adduction						
30°/s	82 (26)		63 (17)	121 (26)		99 (18)
60°/s		146 (28)			207 (63)	
90°/s	62 (32)		44 (19)	103 (32)		83 (28)
Abduction						
30°/s	66 (19)		48 (14)	103 (26)		75 (18)
60°/s		58 (9)			86 (20)	
90°/s	54 (20)		38 (13)	79 (20)		63 (19)

* Mean (SD), in Nm.
[†] Based on Donatelli et al (1991).

2. The eccentric/concentric ratios, which are unit independent, were 1.13 and 1.19 for hip extension and flexion respectively.

Another study (Emery et al 1999) has reported flexion strength scores that were very similar to those of Cahalan et al. Specifically, for men aged 21–43 the concentric peak moment at 60°/s was 157.2 (55.9) Nm whereas the eccentric peak moment was 171.3 (69.5) Nm.

Abduction and adduction

Table 6.2 incorporates findings obtained by Cahalan et al (1989) and Donatelli et al (1991), regarding abduction and adduction. The significant variations noted between these two sources arise from the use of different positions and stabilization, and different measurement systems, Cybex and Merac respectively. The findings by Emery et al (1999) for concentric and eccentric peak moment at 60°/s were 167.2 (52.2) and 188.6 (70.4) Nm, respectively. These figures are substantially higher than those reported by Cahalan et al and reflect different dynamometer and test position.

Internal and external rotation

Table 6.3 shows findings by Cahalan et al (1989) and Lindsay et al (1992) for internal and external

rotators. In this case also, there are significant variations which may be explained by different stabilization methods as well as the differing measurement systems, Cybex II and Cybex 340 respectively.

Strength ratios

The reciprocal strength ratios for frontal and axial movements are shown in Table 6.4.

PART 4
INTERPRETATION OF HIP ISOKINETICS

BILATERAL COMPARISONS

The integrity of function of the muscles moving the involved hip joint may be judged primarily against the performance of their contralateral counterparts. This assumes that performance, which hitherto was confined to strength measurements (i.e. no parameters other than strength, such as contractional work or power, was calculated), is generally equal on both sides. Surprisingly, there is only incidental reference to this issue, apart from in the study by Lindsay et al (1992), where axial rotations were compared. In the seated position with the knee flexed at 90°,

Table 6.3 Hip internal and external rotator concentric strength* based on Cahalan et al (1989) and Lindsay et al (1992)

Motion and angular velocity	Women			Men		
	18–30 years[†]	20–40 years	40–81 years	18–30 years[†]	20–40 years	40–81 years
Internal rotation						
30°/s		47 (13)	34 (9)		72 (17)	61 (21)
60°/s	87 (16)			139 (21)		
90°/s		36 (14)	22 (7)		53 (19)	41 (16)
External rotation						
30°/s		43 (13)	32 (11)		65 (24)	50 (15)
60°/s	53 (10)			84 (16)		
90°/s		31 (12)	21 (8)		49 (24)	38 (12)

*Mean (SD), in Nm.
[†]Based on Lindsay et al (1992).

Table 6.4 Reciprocal strength ratios: frontal and axial motions

	Women	Men
Adduction/abduction		
Donatelli et al (1991)	2.46	2.09
Lindsay et al (1992)	1.64	1.65
Internal/external rotation		
Cahalan et al (1989)		
30°/s	1.08	1.11
90°/s	1.16	1.09

the bilateral difference in both internal and external rotation was less than 1%. In the other two positions (supine with knee flexed to 90°, and supine with knee extended) the bilateral difference was less than 3%. One may reasonably assume that with proper positioning and stabilization, these figures apply for other hip muscle groups, though it should be clear that this is not completely certain.

Clinical findings

In an early study (Nicholas et al 1976), thigh muscle weakness was studied in relation to various unilateral pathological states of the lower extremity, including disorders of the knee (patellofemoral, intra-articular, ligamentous and arthritic); ankle and foot (chronic sprains and anatomical abnormalities), and the back. The strength of hip flexors, abductors and adductors, and knee flexors and extensors was assessed bilaterally.

It was found that significant weakness in abduction and adduction was associated with ankle and foot disorders. Significant weakness of the hip flexors was associated with patellofemoral disorders. The latter finding could be attributed to a possible inhibition of the rectus femoris which operates simultaneously in the movements of hip flexion and knee extension.

Total leg strength

In addition to investigation of single muscle groups, the total leg strength, which is the composite score of the individual strength of knee extensors and flexors and hip flexors, adductors and abductors, was compared between the affected and unaffected sides. It was indicated that in all those lower limb pathology groups which consisted of a sufficiently large sample, there was a highly significant total leg strength deficiency in the affected side. Table 6.5 outlines the results of this analysis.

Further findings

In an extension of the study of Nicholas et al (Gleim et al 1978) it was indicated that there

Table 6.5   Total leg strength scores (Nm) in various pathologies (Nicholas et al 1976)

Pathology	n	Mean total leg strength (Nm)		Deficit
		Affected side	Unaffected side	
Ankle and foot disorders	14	431	576	26*
Back	19	462	515	10*
Ligamentous instability	23	518	602	14*
Intra-articular defects	14	496	557	11*
Patellofemoral disorders	16	462	523	12*
Arthritis	5	405	492	18

*$p < 0.01$.

was a definite deficit in muscle strength, which amounted to more than 5%, when the affected and unaffected sides were compared in the above disorders. However these deficiencies were not limited to the affected side. Often a weakness associated with a single muscle group also appeared in the contralateral side. However in most subjects, the total leg strength was deficient in the affected side. It was also observed that large standard deviations were characteristic of single muscle groups, whereas for the total leg strength they were much smaller. The authors suggested that, in view of these findings, 5 and 10% could be considered a significant deficit in total leg strength and single muscle groups respectively. Given the lack of evidence concerning the reproducibility of hip muscle testing, this conclusion must be re-evaluated.

TESTING OF OTHER MUSCLE GROUPS

If hip muscle testing is indicated, there is a good reason to proceed with knee and, perhaps, even ankle testing. The global or total leg strength may reveal whether the deficiency is confined to the hip or whether it affects other areas as well. Conversely, particularly where the ankle complex is concerned, frontal plane hip testing may be justified.

THE STRENGTH ORDER OF HIP MUSCLES

Consideration of the strength order of hip muscles is likely to assist in interpreting findings. As highlighted by Cahalan et al (1989) the order, from the strongest to the weakest, is: extensors, flexors, adductors, abductors, internal rotators and external rotators. This order was strictly preserved throughout the spectrum of test velocities used in this study.

Therefore, a relative 'within-side' deficiency may be brought to light upon testing the entire musculature of the hip joint. Such testing is not difficult to apply in the upright position and using the stabilizing frames mentioned earlier. Hence, testing at the initial phase (preoperative, or at the beginning of treatment, or for general assessment) and the final phase should include the three principle planes of the hip.

REFERENCES

Boone D C, Azen S P 1979 Normal range of motion in male subjects. Journal of Bone and Joint Surgery 61A: 756–759

Burnett C N, Filusch Betts E, King W M 1990 Reliability of isokinetic measurements of hip muscle torque in young boys. Physical Therapy 70: 244–249

Cahalan T D, Johnson M E, Liu S, Chao E Y S 1989 Quantitative measurements of hip strength in different age groups. Clinical Orthopaedics and Related Research 246: 136–145

Donatelli R, Catlin P A, Backer G S, Drane D L, Slater S M 1991 Isokinetic hip abductor to adductor torque ratio in normals. Isokinetics and Exercise Science 1: 103–111

Dorinson S M, Wagner M L 1948 An exact technique for clinically measuring and recording joint motion. Archives of Physical Medicine 29: 468–470

Emery C A, Maitland M E, Meeuwisse W H 1999 Test-retest reliability of isokinetic hip adductor and flexor muscle strength. Clinical Journal of Sports Medicine 9: 79–85

Giles B, Henke P, Edmonds J, McNeil D 1990 Reproducibility of isokinetic strength measurements in normal and arthritic individuals. Scandinavian Journal of Rehabilitation Medicine 22: 93–99

Gleim G W, Nicholas J A, Webb J N 1978 Isokinetic evaluation following leg injuries. Physician and Sports Medicine 6: 74–82

Jensen R H, Smidt G L, Johnston R C 1971 A technique for obtaining measurements of force generated by the hip muscles. Archives of Physical Medicine and Rehabilitation 52: 207–215

Lindsay D M, Maitland M E, Lowe R C, Kane T J 1992 Comparison of isokinetic internal and external rotation torque using different testing positions. Journal of Orthopaedic and Sports Physical Therapy 16: 43–50

Miller P J 1985 Assessment of joint motion. In: Rothstein J M (ed) Measurement in physical therapy. Churchill Livingstone, Edinburgh

Nicholas J A, Strizak A M, Veras G 1976 A study of thigh muscle weakness in different pathological states of the lower extremity. American Journal of Sports Medicine 4: 241–248

Olson V L, Smidt G L, Johnston R C 1972 The maximum torque generated by the eccentric isometric and concentric contractions of the hip abductor muscles. Physical Therapy 52: 149–158

Tis L L, Perrin D H, Snead D B, Weltman A 1991 Isokinetic strength of the trunk and hip in female runners. Isokinetics and Exercise Science 1: 21–24

CHAPTER CONTENTS

It may safely be claimed that, at one time, more than 75% of all papers which dealt with any aspect of isokinetics – theory, methodology or clinical applications – were based on a single joint system: the knee. In fact, during the early period of research in isokinetics and until the late 1970s, the relevant medical and physiological literature was strictly knee-related. This trend is still evident, although the knee no longer enjoys the same degree of exclusivity. Rather, research on knee isokinetics has come of age, in the sense that an increasing number of papers deal with the clinical aspects of this technology. This, among other things, is a reflection of the significant progress made in recent years in knee surgery and rehabilitation, conservative or postoperative. In addition, the basic design of isokinetic dynamometers (except for special purpose trunk units) has not changed since the original Cybex instrument became available in the late 1960s. This design is still better suited for knee testing and rehabilitation than it is for other joints.

Clearly, much of the voluminous literature on the knee is not directly relevant to this chapter. For instance, a large number of papers describe parameters of knee muscle performance in relation to general methodological problems such as reproducibility. Others relate to the athletic rather than the clinical setting. The main objective of this chapter is the description and critical analysis of topics of clinical relevance to knee isokinetics. However procedural issues and normative values are first discussed.

The issue of reproducibility has been covered in detail in Chapter 4.

PART 1
ISOKINETIC TESTING PROCEDURES FOR THE KNEE

As with the trunk and the shoulder, testing of the knee involves particular consideration of:

1. the alignment of the biological and mechanical axes
2. positioning and stabilization
3. position of the resistance pad, and
4. test angular velocities.

ALIGNMENT OF THE BIOLOGICAL AND MECHANICAL AXES

The knee has two major articulations, the tibiofemoral and the patellofemoral. However, since patellar motion per se is irrelevant in the context of isokinetic testing, tibiofemoral alignment only is discussed. For testing in the usual, sitting, position, assuming minimal femoral motion because of distal stabilization of the thigh, a convenient alignment axis extends through the lateral femoral epicondyle. However the center of rotation for sagittal tibial motion is not fixed on this axis. In fact it has been shown that for sagittal tibial motion, in a normal tibiofemoral joint, the center of rotation itself moves in the shape of an arc (Smidt 1973). This means that the length d_e (see Fig. 1.2) between the resistance pad and the center of rotation in the joint changes during the movement (Nisell 1985). The strength (maximal moment) of the quadriceps or the hamstrings can be obtained from the data, using the relationship, maximal moment = force registered × lever-arm length. However, calculation of the actual force developed requires an additional set of length parameters derivable from radiological analysis of the joint. This issue is even more significant when interpreting knee muscle forces in patients afflicted with unstable knees.

Alignment in the leg-press test

For multijoint lower limb testing, as exemplified by the leg-press test, the greater trochanter is used as a convenient marker for alignment. Although the quadriceps is a major contributor in this activity, its exact share in developing the force recorded by the dynamometer cannot, at the moment, be obtained from any of the available isokinetic dynamometers.

POSITIONING AND STABILIZATION

Three positions may be used for testing the knee joint: the seated (Fig. 7.1), the supine and the prone. The first position is by far the most common.

The seated position

With the back slightly reclined, the subject sits with the thighs well supported by the seat. In this position, the knee is tested along a range of motion

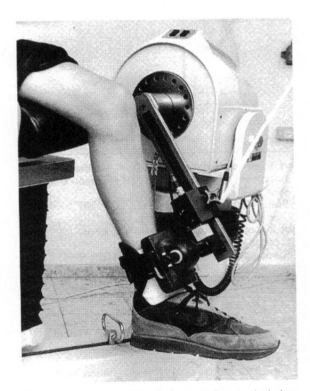

Figure 7.1 Seated position for knee testing, particularly for quadriceps performance.

(ROM) which extends from 75 to 90° of flexion, towards maximal allowable extension.

The angle of recline

It has been indicated that the angle of recline has a differential effect on the strength of the quadriceps and the hamstring (Bohannon et al 1986). While quadriceps strength was not significantly different between the upright and semireclined positions, hamstring scores were significantly higher in the upright position. Thus upright sitting (back at approximately 80°) is probably the optimal position for testing both the extensors and flexors, at least in terms of testing time.

Stabilization in the seated position

Though stabilization in the seated position is normally accomplished using femoral and pelvic strapping, the optimal set-up is probably more involved and has been the subject of a number of papers. Hart et al (1984) have shown that adding thoracic strapping improved quadriceps strength significantly.

Magnusson et al (1992) explored the effect of four stabilization methods on knee flexion and extension strength. Stabilization of the back and hands was compared with stabilization of the back, the hands and no stabilization. Findings revealed a significant effect of method: back and hands stabilization and no stabilization were associated with the highest and lowest scores respectively.

On the other hand, Hanten & Ramberg (1988) failed to find such differences while applying 'maximal' and 'minimal' stabilization. 'Maximal' stabilization consisted of thoracic, pelvic and femoral straps. In 'minimal' stabilization subjects were instructed only to grip the sides of the testing table. These authors concluded that with gripping, the subject's weight and backrest support were sufficient to ensure scores similar to those obtained in maximal stabilization.

The gripping of the table is therefore an important factor, and this had already been highlighted with respect to isometric testing (Currier 1977). Its effect is mainly explained by the counterforce that the handles exert against the forearm. Ultimately, this force works to stabilize the thorax. However, since gripping cannot be applied to all subjects with the same efficiency (Bohannon et al 1986) most isokinetic dynamometers do not offer this option. Therefore stabilization in sitting is normally confined to the pelvic and thigh segments.

The supine position

In the supine position stabilization should be provided at the pelvic level using straps. The contralateral (untested) knee should be maintained in the flexed position in order to reduce somewhat the stresses on the lumbar spine.

The prone position

In the prone position the subject is also stabilized with straps at the pelvic level. There is the added benefit that the table's surface helps prevent excessive thigh movement.

The prone position is particularly suitable for hamstring testing. A comparison between the supine and prone position (Barr & Duncan 1988) demonstrated that if gravity correction was performed, the moments generated by the hamstring in the prone position were significantly higher than in the supine position. In the study of Worrell et al (1990), hamstring strength was significantly higher in the prone, as compared to the sitting position. These authors suggested that the beneficial effect of the prone position could be attributed to a neurophysiological mechanism: the tonic labyrinthine reflex. This reflex is believed to increase flexor tone in both the iliopsoas and the hamstring, thus significantly amplifying the moment about the hip and knee.

In another study Worrell et al (1989) tested the hamstring and quadriceps in the seated and supine positions. Although the seated position yielded higher moments for both muscle groups, the authors suggested that the supine position should be used for testing. This was because, in the many athletic activities which involve running, the position of the hip is closer to that tested in the supine position rather than the seated. However, as one of the main objectives of isokinetic testing is to expose the maximal potential of a given muscle, the above proposal might not be followed.

The present author recommends that the hamstring is preferably tested in the prone position, or alternatively, in the less demanding seated position.

POSITION OF THE RESISTANCE PAD

In the testing of normal subjects, the resistance pad is normally placed at a level immediately superior to the medial malleolus. In a study of the optimal placement of the pad, more than 70% of the subjects, women and men, preferred this position most while the rest reported that a position at two-thirds of the usable leg length was more comfortable (Kramer et al 1989).

When using the selected location the examiner should ensure that the subject is free to maximally dorsiflex the ankle, and that the strap around the lower part of the shank is not overtight.

A number of studies have shown that variations in the site of the resistance pad may result in significant differences in the moment generated by knee muscles. Siewert et al (1975) indicated that the strength of both the extensors and the flexors became successively smaller as the resistance pad was placed nearer to the knee joint. This trend was apparent at all test velocities. In a later study, in which parallel findings were obtained, the authors (Taylor & Casey 1986) suggested that the reason for this phenomenon was compression of the soft tissues which in turn caused divergence of the knee axis away from the actuator's axis.

The latter argument was also supported by Kramer et al (1989) whose findings were similar. Moreover, it was argued that shortening of the dynamometer application arm increased the angle between the arm and the shank. These mechanical factors interacted with a number of neurophysiologic inhibitory mechanisms, such as reduced motor unit activation, discomfort or pain to account for the general reduction in quadriceps strength.

Consistency in the position of the resistance pad is therefore crucial both for bilateral and follow-up comparisons.

Anterior cruciate ligament deficiency and siting of the resistance pad

In patients with an anterior cruciate ligament (ACL) disorder, the resistance pad is positioned differently. In this case there is a need to reduce the anterior (translocating) force of the rotatory component of the quadriceps. To control this force, Johnson (1982) designed a dual pad (the 'anti-shear device'), which consisted of distal and proximal pads. Another version was described by Brown et al (1992). The proximal pad in Johnson's design supplies a compressive force component which balances off the abovementioned rotatory component.

The use of this accessory has been validated (Timm 1985), and its incorporation in testing and rehabilitation of patients after ACL repair/reconstruction, or those suffering from anterior laxity is strongly recommended.

TEST ANGULAR VELOCITIES

The hamstring and, even more, the quadriceps have been tested or conditioned using an extensive range of angular velocities. For instance, in a study of normative values of extension and flexion strength, Borges (1989) chose the extremely low value of 12°/s for one of the criterion velocities. On the other hand Ghena et al (1991) and Hall & Roofner (1991) tested subjects at velocities as high as 450 and 500°/s respectively.

Use of high angular velocities

It is debatable whether the use of high (greater than 180°/s) velocities, particularly for knee testing, yields findings that significantly enhance interpretation.

First, it is unclear whether a reasonable sector of the ROM is covered at a constant velocity. This may be determined only through the use of an objective external velocity measuring device. Such measurement is seldom undertaken, but one study which dealt with this problem (Kues et al 1992) showed that even at a velocity as low as 90°/s there was one case in which non-isokinetic conditions prevailed throughout the first and last 15° of the tested 90° of knee ROM. With a dramatic increase in the test velocities, the acceleration and deceleration phases would occupy such a large proportion of the ROM as to make the effort basically 'isotonic'.

Second, in their study, Ghena et al (1991) demonstrated only a very slight (3 Nm) and non-significant difference between the concentric strength of the hamstring at 300 and 450°/s. For the quadriceps, there was a significant decrease (33 Nm) in peak moment between these velocities, but it was small compared to the difference between 120 and 300°/s (74 Nm).

Third, the findings by Hall & Roofner (1991) reveal a moment–angular velocity curve which may easily be defined in mathematical terms and hence prediction of strength values at high velocities would be possible.

It seems therefore that in testing, very high velocities would provide no useful information, unless there was a good reason to believe that the main deficiency was associated with high speed muscle performance. Moreover, other than for professional athletes, high velocities do not seem to simulate any purposeful activity.

For muscle conditioning, a velocity of 450°/s may constitute a genuine stimulus, and this has indeed been recommended by Mangine & Noyes (1992). However, at the time of writing, no quantitative information concerning the use or validity of very high velocities was available.

Recommended range of test angular velocities

A reasonable and comfortable range for test velocities would be between 60 and 180°/s. It also seems to meet the essential requirement of test validity and the need for information about muscle performance at the functional range. An added benefit is the very wide usage of this range in numerous studies.

The use of the very low velocities mentioned earlier is contraindicated in ligamentous or patellofemoral disorders, unless the purpose of the test is the provocation of a specific reaction like a 'break' in the moment curve (see Patellofemoral dysfunctions section below).

PART 2
REPRESENTATIVE VALUES FOR THE KNEE

In view of the vast research on knee muscle testing, one could justifiably assume that much work had been done to determine performance norms. This however, is not the case. The establishment of norms requires a large database, consisting of subjects who share a number of 'descriptors'. These descriptors may be classed as subject-linked (gender, age, activity level, fiber types, health status, anthropometric factors), protocol-linked (contraction mode, angular velocities, testing procedures) and measurement-linked (measurement device, and the measured variables, i.e. peak moment, average moment, power, etc.). Given this variety of factors, it becomes almost impossible to provide a coherent and dependable normative framework.

NORMS ASSOCIATED WITH SPORTING ACTIVITIES

If the requirement of a large and age-stratified sample size is waived, numerous studies can provide some guidelines. These refer to specific sporting activities such as ice hockey (Smith et al 1981), football (Gilliam et al 1979), middle and distance running (Morris et al 1983), cross-country skiing (Davies et al 1980), ballet (Kirkendall et al 1984) and soccer (Constantin & Williams 1984).

Ghena et al (1991)

Since isokinetics is a very commonly used tool in the testing and rehabilitation of athletes, a 'normative' database for this group is highly desirable. A relevant database is found in a study by Ghena et al (1991) who based their findings on subjects representing various athletic branches. A total of 100 male athletes, aged 18–25, were tested using their dominant limb, for quadriceps and hamstring concentric strength at 60, 120, 300 and 450°/s, and eccentric strength at 60 and 120°/s. The findings are outlined in Table 7.1.

GENERAL POPULATION NORMS

Murray et al (1980)

With respect to the general population, one of the first reports of normative isokinetic values for the knee was by Murray et al (1980), dealing with flexor and extensor strength. A total of 72 normal men, aged between 20 and 86 years, without any neuromuscular or skeletal dysfunction, took part in the study. A single test velocity, 36°/s, was used and the strength findings, which were angle-based, related to three age groups. The use of a slow velocity, the relatively insensitive resolution and the absence of an acceptable performance parameter, such as the peak moment, limited the usefulness of this source.

Freedson et al (1993)

The most comprehensive study, at least in terms of the population size was by Freedson et al (1993) who tested 4541 subjects, 1196 women and 3345 men. Subjects were drawn from 20 companies which carried out medium to heavy physical work. All participants passed a standard physical examination and were considered free of injury at the time of evaluation. Tests used three angular velocities, and the peak moments of the extensors and flexors were recorded, apparently without gravity correction.

Findings for men and women are presented as percentiles and according to age, in Tables 7.2 and 7.3. There was a faster strength loss with age in women, as compared to men.

Table 7.1 Peak moments of knee extensors and flexors in male athletes, based on Ghena et al (1991)

Muscle group	Mode	Angular velocity (°/s)	Mean peak moments* (SD), Nm
Extensors	Concentric	60	260 (59)
	Concentric	120	219 (40)
	Concentric	300	146 (27)
	Concentric	450	113 (20)
	Eccentric	60	257 (36)
	Eccentric	120	260 (38)
Flexors	Concentric	60	142 (28)
	Concentric	120	126 (24)
	Concentric	300	88 (20)
	Concentric	450	92 (27)
	Eccentric	60	166 (40)
	Eccentric	120	168 (39)

* Rounded to nearest integer.

Table 7.2 Normative values (in Nm) of flexion (F) and extension (E) in men, for angular velocities of 60, 180 and 300°/s, based on Freedson et al (1993)

Angular velocity (°/s)	Percentile	<21 years		21–30 years		31–40 years		41–50 years		>50 years	
		F	E	F	E	F	E	F	E	F	E
60	90	163.7	255.2	171.5	267.8	163.5	256.3	159.3	240.0	143.7	222.0
	70	139.0	225.2	149.8	233.2	143.7	218.7	139.0	214.1	129.1	198.0
	50	126.1	203.4	133.6	209.5	130.2	196.6	125.2	189.8	111.9	171.9
	30	113.9	185.1	120.7	188.5	116.1	177.6	118.0	172.5	101.8	152.8
	10	101.8	156.3	103.7	162.7	98.9	152.3	97.1	148.5	88.1	126.9
180	90	114.9	150.5	118.0	153.2	111.2	142.1	109.7	133.6	94.4	115.7
	70	98.3	129.5	102.4	132.9	96.3	122.0	91.5	111.9	81.8	101.6
	50	89.5	116.6	92.2	118.7	87.5	108.5	83.0	99.7	71.9	90.9
	30	73.9	105.1	82.0	106.4	78.6	95.6	72.5	89.0	67.1	74.2
	10	67.5	90.9	69.2	90.9	63.1	79.3	61.7	73.9	53.3	59.0
300	90	97.2	107.4	96.7	108.8	90.2	101.0	85.4	92.9	76.3	86.5
	70	81.4	92.9	81.4	91.5	76.6	84.1	73.2	76.6	65.1	70.4
	50	71.9	82.0	71.9	80.7	67.8	72.5	64.4	65.8	59.0	60.7
	30	63.1	72.5	63.7	70.5	59.0	63.1	55.6	56.3	50.3	46.2
	10	51.3	61.0	52.2	58.7	47.4	50.9	43.4	45.4	40.0	34.6

Borges (1989)

In another comprehensive study of 280 subjects, the isokinetic strength of women's knee flexors and extensors was compared with that of men using a test protocol with three angular velocities (Borges 1989).

The data, which are outlined in Tables 7.4 and 7.5, revealed a significant decrease in strength between the ages of 20 and 30 years in men and between 40 and 50 years in women. There was another decrease in strength for both genders between the ages of 60 and 70 years. There were no significant differences between the right and left limbs. Most importantly, both isokinetic and isometric strength were not significantly different between moderately active and inactive subjects,

Table 7.3 Normative values (in Nm) of flexion (F) and extension (E) in women, for angular velocities of 60, 180 and 300°/s, based on Freedson et al (1993)

Angular velocity (°/s)	Percentile	<21 years F	E	21–30 years F	E	31–40 years F	E	41–50 years F	E	>50 years F	E
60	90	101.2	160.0	108.5	176.3	109.8	167.9	105.8	152.3	93.2	120.4
	70	90.2	144.4	94.2	149.8	94.1	148.2	91.8	129.5	77.0	109.7
	50	82.7	132.9	86.8	135.6	84.1	131.5	84.1	120.7	69.2	106.4
	30	74.6	120.0	79.3	123.4	76.6	118.7	73.9	109.6	55.5	91.8
	10	62.4	103.1	67.8	105.1	64.8	100.8	61.7	98.0	46.5	67.1
180	90	71.2	90.2	71.2	92.2	69.6	87.5	62.1	75.5	51.1	60.7
	70	60.3	78.0	64.4	80.4	60.3	73.9	55.6	63.7	47.7	51.8
	50	54.9	70.5	57.6	71.9	53.3	65.1	50.2	56.3	39.3	40.0
	30	48.1	65.1	51.5	63.1	47.9	57.0	45.4	50.2	30.4	35.0
	10	40.0	52.9	42.0	52.7	38.6	47.2	36.2	42.8	14.1	23.3
300	90	57.0	63.1	59.0	63.2	54.9	58.7	50.0	50.0	42.8	42.3
	70	48.8	52.9	50.2	53.6	46.6	47.5	44.3	40.7	39.5	32.5
	50	43.4	46.8	44.7	46.8	40.7	40.7	38.0	38.0	29.2	23.7
	30	37.3	41.4	38.6	40.7	35.9	34.6	33.2	29.8	25.1	19.0
	10	28.5	34.6	31.9	32.5	28.5	27.8	25.8	25.1	11.9	6.8

Table 7.4 Normative peak moments of knee extensors* (in Nm), at three angular velocities, based on Borges (1989)

	Age (years)	12°/s Right	Left	90°/s Right	Left	150°/s Right	Left
Women	20	183 (34)	172 (31)	143 (25)	137 (24)	110 (18)	106 (19)
	30	169 (34)	163 (30)	138 (22)	134 (20)	108 (19)	107 (15)
	40	172 (28)	161 (26)	134 (20)	131 (20)	105 (15)	102 (14)
	50	153 (30)	143 (26)	122 (18)	114 (17)	94 (16)	92 (14)
	60	145 (20)	126 (24)	113 (13)	99 (15)	84 (10)	79 (12)
	70	128 (28)	120 (25)	98 (17)	93 (15)	74 (12)	70 (11)
Men	20	289 (44)	269 (47)	231 (32)	217 (27)	180 (24)	179 (22)
	30	258 (45)	243 (47)	207 (38)	196 (35)	158 (34)	160 (28)
	40	248 (29)	238 (42)	203 (27)	197 (31)	158 (24)	155 (26)
	50	226 (51)	220 (45)	186 (36)	177 (32)	145 (27)	143 (30)
	60	223 (48)	212 (40)	179 (34)	169 (32)	142 (28)	136 (22)
	70	188 (36)	183 (37)	143 (24)	145 (30)	113 (22)	113 (21)

* Findings expressed as mean (SD).

Table 7.5   Normative peak moments of knee flexors* (in Nm), at three angular velocities, based on Borges (1989)

	Age (years)	12°/s		90°/s		150°/s	
		Right	Left	Right	Left	Right	Left
Women	20	100 (20)	95 (20)	68 (21)	66 (17)	49 (19)	46 (16)
	30	90 (18)	88 (18)	61 (15)	58 (13)	46 (14)	42 (12)
	40	93 (20)	91 (18)	62 (14)	61 (13)	46 (14)	46 (13)
	50	76 (24)	75 (20)	52 (13)	51 (13)	36 (13)	38 (11)
	60	77 (14)	74 (17)	53 (12)	47 (13)	38 (11)	35 (12)
	70	65 (12)	59 (13)	39 (13)	38 (13)	28 (8)	25 (9)
Men	20	155 (28)	144 (27)	122 (21)	113 (21)	96 (19)	91 (19)
	30	150 (28)	143 (35)	113 (23)	108 (29)	91 (26)	87 (25)
	40	149 (22)	144 (24)	112 (18)	106 (21)	87 (16)	83 (15)
	50	142 (32)	129 (30)	98 (24)	91 (25)	82 (23)	76 (25)
	60	130 (38)	133 (34)	95 (29)	86 (30)	78 (24)	75 (25)
	70	109 (30)	109 (32)	78 (26)	77 (23)	61 (23)	60 (26)

* Findings expressed as mean (SD).

for both women and men. This finding widens the applicability of these norms.

COMPARISON OF SWEDISH AND AMERICAN DATA

Though analysis of the findings from the comparable age groups in the Borges (1989) and Ghena et al (1991) studies already mentioned must be made with extreme caution, it is interesting to note that there is a significant measure of similarity. The youngest men's group in the Swedish study (Borges 1989), with an average age of 20 years, may be compared with the American group, whose mean age was 20.13 years. Weight and height, both of which are important factors in strength (Gross et al 1989) were also very similar: 75 and 76 kg and 180 and 182 cm for the Swedish and American groups respectively.

Since the velocities used were different, the average of the findings relating to 90 and 150°/s in the Swedish study (Tables 7.4 and 7.5) may be compared with the isokinetic findings at 120°/s in the American study (Table 7.1). Therefore, average quadriceps strength was 205 Nm in the general population (Swedish) and 219 Nm in athletes (American). The average hamstring strength was 109 Nm and 126 Nm respectively. The difference is hence about 6% in quadriceps and 14% in hamstring strength.

If this very simple analysis is any lesson, it indicates that strength may not be a primary differentiating factor between athletes and non-athletes and therefore the applicability of Borges's findings may be even wider.

PREDICTION OF INDIVIDUAL PERFORMANCE FROM NORMATIVE VALUES

In view of the growing interest in using high velocity knee testing and rehabilitation, the work of Hall & Roofner (1991) offers original information and a practical approach to determining individual performance from equations based on normative values. The authors used a sample of 60 normal subjects, 30 women and 30 men, of 20–62 years of age, and velocities of 60, 180, 300, 400 and 500°/s. The measured parameters included quadriceps strength (peak moment), average work and power.

It was suggested that the descriptive statistics obtained and the following equations enable the prediction of these performance parameters from age, weight and sex data. At 180°/s the latter

Table 7.6   Normalized strength at 50°/s of knee extensors and flexors* as a ratio of peak or average moment/bodyweight (Nm/kg), based on Highgenboten et al (1988)

Peak moment	Concentric		Eccentric	
	Extensors	Flexors	Extensors	Flexors
Women				
15–24 years	2.19 (0.51)	0.87 (0.16)	2.37 (0.90)	1.06 (0.26)
25–34 years	1.98 (0.49)	0.85 (0.18)	2.36 (0.77)	1.11 (0.28)
Pooled	2.12 (0.51)	0.85 (0.17)	2.36 (0.85)	1.06 (0.26)
Men				
15–24 years	2.98 (0.57)	1.21 (0.24)	3.09 (0.88)	1.44 (0.33)
25–34 years	2.49 (0.66)	1.08 (0.28)	2.67 (0.82)	1.37 (0.32)
Pooled	2.76 (0.66)	1.16 (0.26)	2.88 (0.86)	1.40 (0.33)
Average moment				
Women				
15–24 years	1.26 (0.30)	0.59 (0.12)	1.31 (0.53)	0.70 (0.22)
25–34 years	1.22 (0.37)	0.58 (0.12)	1.38 (0.51)	0.72 (0.21)
Pooled	1.25 (0.32)	0.58 (0.12)	1.34 (0.52)	0.70 (0.22)
Men				
15–24 years	1.78 (0.42)	0.85 (0.29)	1.87 (0.62)	1.01 (0.32)
25–34 years	1.48 (0.45)	0.73 (0.18)	1.71 (0.57)	0.95 (0.26)
Pooled	1.66 (0.45)	0.80 (0.26)	1.81 (0.60)	1.00 (0.29)

* Findings expressed as mean (SD).

factors may account for 80, 74 and 51% of the differences in quadriceps strength, average work and average power respectively.

Strength = $54.607 - (\text{age} \times 1.187) + (\text{sex} \times 32.905) + (\text{weight} \times 0.378)$

Average work = $113.534 - (\text{age} \times 1.617) + (\text{sex} \times 58.471) + (\text{weight} \times 0.371)$

Average power = $-1.107 - (\text{age} \times 2.102) + (\text{sex} \times 11.264) + (\text{weight} \times 1.296)$

where sex has the value 1 for men and 0 for women.

ECCENTRIC PERFORMANCE

Eccentric muscle performance was not widely reported until the late 1980s though its significance for knee activity is now firmly established.

A study by Highgenboten et al (1988) reported on the concentric and eccentric average strength of knee flexors and extensors in a group of 127 normal subjects, women and men, ranging in age between 15 and 34 years. Both knees were tested, and strength scores were pooled. The activity

status of the subjects was not specified. A single test velocity, 50°/s, was used and the units of strength were normalized for bodyweight (Nm/kg). Flexor strength was tested in the supine position. Table 7.6 outlines the findings.

The choice of hamstring test position, test velocity and units of measurement precludes comparison between the norms derived from this study and those mentioned earlier.

SUMMARY

Assuming that the required normative parameter is the concentric strength (peak moment) of the quadriceps and hamstring (tested in the seated position), the present author would recommend using the findings by Freedson et al (1993) or by Borges (1989) as general normative sources. For eccentric tests, the findings by Highgenboten et al (1988) may serve as an adequate source, providing one converts the units accordingly.

Users of these norms should however be aware that findings based on isokinetic dynamometers of different makes are not compatible (see Chapter 3 for detailed analysis). Consequently reasonable error margins should be used.

PART 3
SELECTED DISORDERS OF THE KNEE

The great majority of studies of isokinetic aspects of knee muscle dysfunction concern either ligamentous or patellofemoral disorders. Among the former, the anterior cruciate ligament has received almost exclusive attention, whereas interest in disorders of the posterior, medial and lateral collateral ligaments has been negligible. This reflects not only the major role of the anterior cruciate ligament in maintaining a normally functioning knee, and the incidence of partial or complete rupture, but also the dramatic progress made during recent years in anterior cruciate ligament reconstruction and rehabilitation.

'Patellofemoral dysfunctions' is a collective term for a number of pathologies.

Muscle involvement in other fairly common disorders of the knee, such as torn menisci, have been studied also, and relevant findings will be presented.

ANTERIOR CRUCIATE LIGAMENT DISORDERS

As mentioned above, work on the anterior cruciate ligament (ACL) comprises the lion's share of research into ligamentous disorders. A constructive approach to the testing of ACL patients and to the interpretation of findings emerges from consideration of the following questions:

1. At a given time, postinjury or postoperatively, how does the strength of the involved side compare with that of the sound side (bilateral comparison) and is there a general decline relative to the expected norm?
2. Will isokinetic performance parameters other than strength assist in interpretation of the findings?
3. What is the significance of the hamstring/quadriceps ratio (HQR)?
4. Is there an objective, isokinetically measurable goal at which rehabilitation or steady state performance should be aimed?

The answers to these questions depend to an extent on the history of the patient. Some will suffer from 'chronic' ACL deficiency, i.e. the torn ligament has not been surgically rectified, while others have undergone surgical repair of the ACL. Following loss of the ACL, in chronic patients, a steady state neuromuscular performance, at a lower level than previously, is normally achieved. The time span postinjury for reaching this plateau is not known, but is regarded as years rather than months.

BILATERAL COMPARISONS
Chronic ACL deficiency

Concentric and eccentric testing, at 30°/s, of chronic ACL patients who had declined surgery, was performed by Dvir et al (1989) approximately 1.5 years postinjury. Comparing data for the involved and uninvolved sides, concentric strength deficits were, on average, 21 and 14% for the quadriceps and hamstring respectively, whereas the corresponding eccentric deficits were 18 and 15%.

Tegner et al (1986) tested patients with 'old' tears of the ACL (the period postinjury was not specified). The group consisted of predominantly chronic patients and a few who suffered from instability in spite of an operation. Concentric isokinetic tests at 30 and 180°/s revealed that, compared to the sound side, the quadriceps strength deficiency was, on average, 21 and 16% at these velocites. The corresponding hamstring deficiencies were 8 and 4% respectively.

Bonamo et al (1990) studied various factors associated with conservative treatment of 59 active but non-competitive recreational athletes with ACL deficiency. Using isokinetic testing (60 and 240°/s), performed more than 4 years following injury, these authors reported quadriceps deficits of 11–14%, and deficits of 3–4% for the hamstring. It was however suggested that conservative treatment meant significant activity modification.

Kannus & Jarvinen (1991) tested subjects with partial tear of the ligament, 8 years postinjury. The tests revealed that except for a significant decrease in quadriceps strength at the low velocity of 60°/s there were no significant differences between the involved and sound knee.

Conclusions

These and other studies indicate therefore that in the chronic ACL patient:

1. in spite of conservative intervention, significant quadriceps strength deficits, of approximately 20%, exist during at least the first year following tear of the ligament
2. these deficits subside quite sharply in the longer term but a change in activities is sometimes inevitable
3. the effect of the tear on hamstring strength is significantly less conspicuous than for the quadriceps. Providing proper attention has been given to flexor function, full recovery of hamstring strength in the involved side may be expected.

Chronic partial tears and hamstring strength

Interestingly, in a group of patients with chronic partial tears of the ACL, with or without medial collateral ligament rupture, the hamstring strength was generally more compromised than that of the quadriceps (Kannus et al 1992). This trend was even more pronounced with an increase in the velocity.

Besides the possibility of a more selective atrophy of type II fibers, another explanation of this finding may be that a partially functioning ACL does not stimulate an increase in hamstring strength to the same extent that the absence of the ACL does.

Reconstructed ACL and bilateral comparisons

A different situation obtains where patients have undergone surgical repair of their torn ACL. For example, patients are expected to regain muscle function within a relatively short period of time. On the other hand, the particular operative technique and the rehabilitation regime especially are crucial factors affecting the rate of improvement. Although it is not the intention here to review the procedures and complexities associated with surgery of this ligament, Table 7.7 shows variables affecting rehabilitation after ACL reconstruction, as identified by Wilk & Andrews (1992).

Among these variables, the type of surgical procedure has been mentioned in connection with isokinetic performance of thigh muscles. For instance, Seto et al (1988) indicated that 5 years postoperatively, there was a significant correlation between the increase in quadriceps strength on the operated side and a return to functional activity, in patients with intra-articular, but not extra-articular, ACL reconstruction. However, this author is not aware of any comparative, systematic, long-range study that discusses surgical procedure and isokinetic performance in a satisfactory manner. Rather, most studies consider either the postoperative time span or the rehabilitation program (e.g. accelerated or non-accelerated) in relation to the isokinetic data.

Table 7.7 Variables influencing rehabilitation of patients after ACL reconstruction, based on Wilk & Andrews (1992)

1. Type of surgical procedure: Arthrotomy Arthroscopic assisted Endoscopic	5. Graft tensioning 6. Tourniquet time 7. Concomitant surgeries: Collateral ligament
2. Tissue type used: Patellar tendon Semitendinous Iliotibial band	Meniscal lesions Posterior cruciate ligament (PCL) injuries
3. Graft fixation: Screw Button Staple Suture	Condral lesions Surgical notchplasty Capsular deficiencies
4. Graft placement: Isometric Non-isometric	8. Patient variables: Size Alignment Activity level Compliance

Non-accelerated rehabilitation: up to 2 years postoperatively

Some studies have investigated the variations over a period of time in thigh muscle function following ACL reconstruction.

Murray et al (1984) compared patients who were treated conservatively with those who underwent reconstruction following 6 months of non-accelerated rehabilitation. Isokinetic tests were carried out bilaterally at 30 and 180°/s. Quadriceps strength deficits in both groups were significant: 17% for reconstruction and 7% for conservative treatment, but the difference was not statistically significant between the groups. Deficits in the hamstring were similar in the two groups, and generally less conspicuous than the quadriceps deficit.

Elmqvist et al (1989) increased the span of assessment, testing bilateral extensor function at 90°/s in patients before, and at 14, 20, 34 and 52 weeks after, ACL reconstruction (for technique see Marshall et al 1979). Following cast immobilization, patients underwent intensive non-accelerated rehabilitation. Preoperatively, there were significant strength (21%) and total work (27%) deficiencies. Figure 7.2 illustrates the variation in strength during the first year. Despite isometric or isokinetic conditioning administered during the first year after the operation, quadriceps strength of the involved knee was still approximately 20% lower than that of the contralateral knee.

Elmqvist et al (1988) also investigated quadriceps strength 2 years after ACL reconstruction. The findings were similar, i.e. there was a 20% deficit compared to the uninjured limb. These results are very similar to those of Murray et al (1984) though the operative procedures, rehabilitation protocols and testing velocities were not identical.

Lopresti et al (1988). Using the 'bone–patellar tendon–bone graft' procedure, Lopresti et al (1988) reported deficits of, on average, 12 and 20% in quadriceps strength in men and women respectively, at both 60 and 120°/s. There were no detectable deficits in hamstring strength.

Rosenberg et al (1992), who also used the central third of the patellar tendon, showed that 12–24 months postoperatively, there was still a quadriceps deficiency of 18% (measured concentrically at 60°/s) whereas hamstring deficiency stood at 10%.

Halperin & Dvir (1993). Finally, a 13% concentric deficit and a 4% eccentric deficit were found in the quadriceps and hamstring respectively 2 years after a semitendinosus and gracilis ACL reconstruction. It is worth noting that although a significant component of the hamstring was used for the reconstruction, the eccentric force of this muscle, which controls the anterior motion of the tibia, was regained in its entirety.

Conclusions. Therefore during a period of up to 2 years post-ACL reconstruction, and following a non-accelerated rehabilitation program, a quadriceps deficit of 15–20% compared with the uninvolved side should be expected. There is however a negligible deficit of hamstring strength.

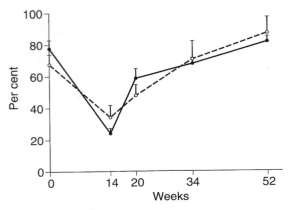

Figure 7.2 Relative strength (isokinetic strength as percentage of non-injured leg strength) at 90°/s of the quadriceps of the injured leg in 17 patients with ACL reconstruction. Patients trained either isokinetically (solid circles) or using isometrics and PRE (open circles). (From Elmqvist et al 1989.)

Non-accelerated rehabilitation: long-term results

Only a limited number of studies describe long-term postoperative results of ACL reconstruction (greater than 2 years) related to thigh muscle strength. Yasuda et al (1992), who used the bone–patellar tendon–bone graft technique, suggested that quadriceps strength of the operated side reached 85% of that of the sound side at final follow-up (3–7 years) in men and 70% in women, while hamstring strength was fully recovered.

Seto et al (1988) used a 5-year post-ACL reconstruction period. In the extra-articular reconstruction group, quadriceps deficiency at 120°/s was still a significant 14%, whereas hamstring strength was practically identical in both limbs. It should however be emphasized that a considerable extensor deficit, 33%, existed in the intra-articular group.

At a period of about 8 years post-ACL reconstruction Arvidsson et al (1981) found significant quadriceps strength deficits in two groups of patients whose functional capacity was rated as 'fair' or 'poor', but quadriceps strength was not significantly different from that of the sound side in the 'good' and 'excellent' groups.

Conclusions. The performance level of thigh muscles long after an ACL reconstruction is still characterized by a significant reduction in extensor strength. A reduced activity level and/or a permanent impairment to the extensor mechanism, due to harvesting of the graft, are probably the main factors behind this deficit.

Accelerated rehabilitation

The concept of accelerated rehabilitation was first introduced by Shelbourne & Nitz (1990). It is used following surgery based on an intra-articular bone–patellar tendon–bone graft. Two factors stimulated this change in rehabilitation after ACL reconstruction (De Carlo et al 1992).

1. Non-compliant patients made faster progress than patients who rigidly obeyed a traditional, non-accelerated protocol.
2. A certain percentage of patients experienced problems associated with quadriceps dysfunction when using a non-accelerated protocol.

Briefly, accelerated rehabilitation emphasizes early terminal extension, early weight bearing, and the exclusive use of closed kinetic chain efforts for reconditioning of the quadriceps.

Comparison of accelerated and non-accelerated rehabilitation. Using one of the most impressive databases ever reported in isokinetics-related research, De Carlo and his colleagues (1992) indicated that in terms of strength gains, and improved ROM, accelerated rehabilitation was significantly superior to non-accelerated. Some of the findings are outlined in Table 7.8, and a consistent pattern of higher quadriceps and hamstring strengths is evident.

The difference in time taken for rehabilitation is most important. For instance, quadriceps strength at 3 months in the accelerated group was similar to that at 6 months in the non-accelerated group. The more intensive rehabilitation therefore benefits the patient, allowing an earlier return to normal activity.

Moreover, compared with non-accelerated protocols, which after 1 year still result in an extensor deficit of about 20%, the accelerated regime brings the patient much closer to parity, with only a 13% deficit. Though the study of De Carlo et al

Table 7.8 The effect of accelerated vs non-accelerated rehabilitation on the postoperative strength variations in knee extensors and flexors (in percentage of strength of uninvolved side, at 180°/s) based on De Carlo et al (1992)

Postoperative time (months)	Extensors		Flexors	
	Non-accelerated	Accelerated	Non-accelerated	Accelerated
3	63.9 (2.3)	69.6 (0.5)*	79.4 (2.3)	92.7 (1.1)[†]
6	71.5 (1.2)	76.8 (0.5)[†]	91.0 (1.2)	97.8 (0.5)[†]
12	80.0 (1.5)	87.4 (0.9)[†]	95.1 (1.5)	98.7 (0.9)

*$p < 0.05$; [†]$p < 0.01$.

refers only to the first postoperative year, extrapolation based on other studies shows that, with other factors being equal, the trend towards a continuous improvement may not disappear.

Conclusion. For the special case of accelerated rehabilitation, during the first year post-ACL reconstruction a quadriceps deficit of 10–15% compared with the uninvolved side should be expected.

Margin of error

Variations for a given individual's scores may reach 5–10% within the same testing session. This margin of error should be used with the rehabilitation criteria (accelerated or non-accelerated) when judging whether a rehabilitation objective has been achieved.

OTHER ISOKINETIC PERFORMANCE PARAMETERS

The use of parameters derived from strength, other than those related to endurance, has not helped to interpret test findings, since these parameters are so closely related to strength. The point has been demonstrated in studies dealing with the significance of total work during a series of contractions (Kannus 1988a,b, Elmqvist et al 1989), and of angular impulse or average power (Kannus 1990) in ligamentous disorders of the knee.

Therefore, the strength of the quadriceps and/or hamstring is sufficient for describing the basic mechanical capacity of these muscles, and other variables derived from the strength curve are redundant.

It should be mentioned that other parameters such as the rise time of the moment of the hamstring may be relevant. However, these are correctly derivable from isometric rather than isokinetic strength functions.

THE HAMSTRING/QUADRICEPS RATIO

This parameter has attracted a great deal of interest and was used as an indicator of normal balance between the extensor and flexor function in the knee. It became evident that the ratio was velocity dependent: for low velocities the normal HQR was about 0.60, and for high velocities it was greater than one (Osternig et al 1983). However, the omission of a gravity correction in a number of studies means that their findings and conclusions must be viewed with reservation.

There has been some research on the role of the hamstring muscle group in controlling the unstable ACL-deficient knee, notably by Walla et al (1985) and Solomonow et al (1987). These authors have shown that instability is associated with increased reflex activity in the hamstring when the knee is exposed to extensor load.

The dynamic control ratio. Coactivation of the quadriceps and hamstring takes place through opposite contraction modes, the quadriceps contracting concentrically, and the hamstring eccentrically. Therefore in order to assess the balancing nature of the hamstring in the ACL-deficient knee the hamstring/quadriceps ratio should correctly be H_e/Q_c, i.e. the eccentric strength of the hamstring divided by the concentric strength of the quadriceps or the 'dynamic control ratio' (Dvir et al 1989).

However, almost all of the studies of the ACL-deficient knee and the HQR have been based on the concentric strengths of both muscles.

Kannus (1988a,b) studied the HQR in subjects with ACL-deficient knee 8 years after injury and found a high intersubject variability in this parameter of 23–205%. On the other hand, the HQR was significantly higher for the involved compared with the sound limb at the higher testing speed (180°/s).

Lopresti et al (1988) reported HQRs of 0.66 versus 0.75 in the involved and sound knees respectively and related the difference to a reduced quadriceps strength, as no detectable differences were indicated in the bilateral hamstring tests.

Dvir et al (1989) compared the values of the dynamic control ratio, H_e/Q_c, with the HQR, H_c/Q_c and H_e/Q_e at the test velocity of 30°/s. The findings indicated that whereas the same contraction mode ratios, HQR and H_e/Q_e, differed by no more than 3% between the involved and sound knees, there was a significant difference in the dynamic control ratio. A reduction of 11% in the concentric strength of the deficient side quadriceps accounted for this finding.

Interpretation of the HQR

It is therefore apparent that the hamstring/quadriceps ratio itself is a rather crude parameter whose relationship to ACL deficiency derives directly from the marked weakness of the quadriceps which is typical in this disorder. It is rather surprising that in the 'long chronic' patient, HQR still differs significantly between limbs (Kannus 1988a) since quadriceps weakness tends to diminish. However, the use of HQR for clinical inference may not be essential.

AN ISOKINETIC CRITERION FOR REHABILITATION IN ACL DISORDERS

There is a growing consensus among experts that the bilaterial ratio of quadriceps strength – the quadriceps/quadriceps ratio (QQR) – may serve as a milestone for rehabilitation or long-term performance in ACL dysfunction. On the other hand, the timing of the tests and/or the postoperative phase in which they are performed is still a matter of controversy.

Usefulness of bilateral comparison

With regards to the isokinetic parameter, it has been shown by Kannus (1988a,b) that what matters in the long run is the extent to which performance of the muscles of the involved knee approximates that of the uninvolved knee. For instance, regarding the relevance of the HQR, it was claimed that neither did this parameter correlate with the long-term outcome, and nor could an optimal magnitude of HQR be recommended generally as a target for rehabilitation (Kannus 1988a,b). Rather 'a suitable HQ ratio may be the HQ ratio of the patient's uninvolved knee'. Therefore, comparison with the uninvolved side provides a comfortable and a reasonable goal for the steady-state phase, either in the chronic or postoperative patient.

The performance of the extensor mechanism in patients with chronic ACL tear was assessed, among other parameters, relative to the bilateral strength ratio of the quadriceps at a test velocity of 30°/s (RQ30) by Tegner et al (1986). The authors suggested that the aim of rehabilitation should be to reach an RQ30 of 90% in view of the significant improvements in strength, performance, knee score and activity level associated with this value. The omission of any flexor component is notable.

Progression and discharge in rehabilitation

Another, perhaps more pressing problem is the decision whether to progress to a more advanced stage or to discharge a patient from rehabilitation following surgical correction of ACL tear. There are three commonly accepted mechanical parameters which guide clinicians in making such a decision: range of motion, knee joint stability and muscle performance. To these should be added the level of function which ultimately may be the most important.

Thigh muscle performance under isokinetic conditions can be measured very accurately and with acceptable reproducibility. Given that the choice of criteria is important for the success of the operation, it is tempting to rely upon isokinetically based standards when deciding to vary the rehabilitation regime.

Morever, bearing in mind the prevailing trends in medical malpractice litigation, the end-product of the testing – a clear, quantitative and graphical document which describes the performance of the patient throughout the rehabilitation process – may constitute a significant tool.

Use of the QQR in rehabilitation

Baseline measurements

Irrespective of the rehabilitation protocol, accelerated or non-accelerated, a preoperative test furnishes an important baseline (Elmqvist et al 1989). In the absence of any contraindication such a test should be performed.

Table 7.9 The effect of accelerated ACL rehabilitation methods on strength variations in knee extensors and flexors (as a percentage of the strength of the uninvolved side)*

Postoperative time (months)	Wilk & Andrews (1992)		DeCarlo et al (1992)	
	Extensors	Flexors	Extensors	Flexors
3	69	94	70	93
6	73	97	77	97
12	91	110	87	99

* Tests performed at 180°/s.

The QQR in a non-accelerated program

One of the most frequently quoted non-accelerated rehabilitation protocols was designed by Paolos et al (1983). This protocol was also used by De Carlo et al (1992) in a comparative study of accelerated and non-accelerated regimes. In this design isokinetic tests are initiated 6 months postoperatively, protecting the knee with the Johnson antishear device (1982) and blocking extension at 20°. The tests are carried out at medium to high velocities (180–240°/s). Tests should be performed, at monthly intervals, after the first one.

Return to normal activity levels is allowed when: the QQR reaches 80%; full ROM is gained; no pain or swelling is present, and successful completion of functional progression has been achieved.

Use of the QQR in accelerated programs

The accelerated rehabilitation regime used by De Carlo et al differed considerably from the non-accelerated, in the timing of the initial isokinetic test and the criteria applied. The first test was performed 5–6 weeks postoperatively under the same conditions as in the non-accelerated system. If the QQR was greater than 70%, more demanding activities such as lateral shuffles, cariocas and rope jumping were incorporated. At 10 weeks another isokinetic evaluation was made, adding a slow test velocity of 60°/s. At 16–24 weeks a QQR of 80% and successful completion of functional progression indicated return to sporting activities, including contact sports.

Wilk & Andrews (1992) have described another accelerated rehabilitation protocol which allows athletes to return to sporting activities within 5–6 months following a patellar tendon–graft reconstruction. The protocol, in many respects similar to the one described by Shelbourne & Nitz (1990), is nevertheless less aggressive, notably with regard to the initiation of isokinetic testing as well as the velocities employed. The first testing session takes place 12 weeks postoperatively and velocities of 180 and 300°/s are used. A test at 60°/s is omitted as this velocity results in a greater amount of tibial translation compared to 180 and 300°/s (Nisell et al 1989).

Wilk & Andrews do not regard a QQR of 70% as a criterion for progression to the next, 'light activity' phase even though it is implied that on average, such a score is indeed expected. The exact criterion for a 'satisfactory isokinetic test' is also not specified though at 6 and 12 months postoperatively QQRs of around 75 and 90% are envisaged.

The QQRs and the bilateral hamstring ratios, obtained using the accelerated rehabilitation regimes of Wilk & Andrews and De Carlo et al, are compared in Table 7.9. It should be noted that other than a slight difference in hamstring strength 1 year postoperatively, the two designs result in almost identical strength increases.

Conclusions

The current isokinetic criterion for either progression or termination of conditioning in ACL deficiency, chronic or surgically corrected, is the bilateral ratio of quadriceps strength, the QQR. Tests should preferably be conducted at the medium velocity of 180°/s, although addition of another test at 60°/s may sometimes reveal specific deficiencies.

Accelerated rehabilitation. Tests may be introduced as early as 5–6 weeks postoperatively, in which case:

- a QQR of 70% and above indicates progression to light functional activities.

Accelerated or non-accelerated rehabilitation. Assuming the scores representing other parameters (ROM, function, etc.) are satisfactory:

- a QQR of 80% indicates the resumption of normal activity.

For ACL insufficiency, following reconstruction or conservative treatment:

- a QQR of 90% may be required to ensure a satisfactory level of functioning.

DISORDERS OF THE COLLATERAL LIGAMENTS

Isokinetic research regarding the medial and lateral collateral ligaments (MCL and LCL) has been very limited in spite of the fact that damage to the MCL and medial capsular ligament may be the most common injury in sporting activities (Bergfeld 1979). However, the injury may not result in a complete rupture of the MCL (or LCL). In the latter cases, which are referred to as grade I and II, conservative treatment is exclusively prescribed, and it is sometimes used even for complete (grade III) rupture (Hastings 1980, Ballmer & Jakob 1988, Shelbourne & Porter 1992).

In systematic studies dealing with the collateral ligaments and thigh muscle performance, there is a conspicuous dearth of information regarding the short-term effects. Hence the extent of potential deficits and their significance cannot be specified.

On the other hand, the long-term effect of grade II (partial tear) insufficiency of the MCL, 8 years postinjury, was studied by Kannus & Jarvinen (1991). Tests were performed at 60 and 180°/s. Strength deficits were minimal: on average 4 and 2% for the quadriceps and hamstring respectively.

Systematically higher strength deficits were noted in the higher velocity indicating possibly greater atrophy in type II fibers.

In another study, the long-term effects of grade II and III (complete tear) of the LCL were studied (Kannus 1988b). The reduction in the quadriceps strength of the involved side, 8 years postinjury, was still significant, being between 10 and 13% (using the mean scores which appear in the paper). In other words the QQR was about 87–90%. Bilateral hamstring strength scores were almost identical.

Consequently, chronic collateral ligament injuries result in some strength deficit in the quadriceps but minimal deficit in the hamstring.

No research has been found which describes short-term variations in thigh muscle performance following isolated injuries to the collateral ligaments.

PATELLOFEMORAL DYSFUNCTIONS

Patellofemoral dysfunction (PFD) is one of the most common problems of the knee encountered by rehabilitation clinicians. It has been defined as 'pain, inflammation, imbalance and/or instability of any component of the extensor mechanism of the knee from congenital, traumatic or mechanical stresses' (Shelton & Thigpen 1991). It therefore encompasses a broad range of syndromes notably patellofemoral malalignment and pain, chondromalacia patella, patellar instability, plica syndrome, quadriceps and patellar tendinitis.

PFD has a particular significance in the physiotherapeutic setting since, unless there is an explicit indication otherwise, conservative management is generally accepted. Indeed, in an analysis of the results of extensor mechanism reconstruction, Cerullo et al (1988) suggested:

In dealing with a stable knee cap or so-called 'anterior knee pain', it is better to use conservative treatment, since the pathologic basis of the clinical syndrome is still obscure. In the absence of a diagnosis, the rationale for performing any operation is also suspect when the patient has all or some of the predisposing physical findings (high and lateral patella, vastus medialis obliquus dysplasia, increased Q angle) but has a stable patella.

Classification by cartilage damage

Pain is a very common consequence of many PFDs, though not necessarily of a magnitude commensurate with the degree of damage. In his classic paper on patellar pain, Insall (1981) described eight well recognized causes of patellar pain. His classification was based on the extent to which the articular cartilage was damaged.

General damage appears in grade I–III chondromalacia where the cause of pain is believed to be mostly increased pressure due to maltracking, though in some patients the pain arises directly from the pathology (basal degeneration). Osteoarthritis (grade IV chrondromalacia), direct trauma and osteochondral fracture and osteochondritis are the other causes typical of the general damage group.

Variable cartilage damage is associated with malalignment syndromes which may produce pain through overloading and incorrect fit.

Pain may also be provoked in knees with usually normal cartilage, due to overuse syndrome, sympathetic dystrophy, or peripatellar causes like plica and tendinitis.

Patellofemoral pain syndrome

Those PFDs associated with anterior knee pain where there is no disruption to the cartilage are often referred to collectively as patellofemoral pain syndrome (PFPS). The malalignment of the patellofemoral joint which probably accounts for PFPS results from a number of sources: abnormal anatomical architecture; extensor mechanism malalignment; retinacular restraints, and muscular imbalance and strength (Sczepanski et al 1991).

The muscular factors are of considerable importance as they are the basis of the conservative approach to the initial management of PFD. The mechanism by which conditioning the quadriceps alleviates the pain is not entirely clear, but its efficacy is unquestionable in a great number of cases (Insall 1981). An imbalance between the moments generated by the vastus medialis obliquus (VMO) and vastus lateralis (VL) has been suggested as a causative factor of patella maltracking (Mariani & Caruso 1979, Taunton et al 1987). Insufficiency of the VMO could lead to excessive lateral pull by the VL and exposure of the lateral facet of the patella, increased friction, erosion of the cartilage and pain. Additionally, lateral displacement of the patella could adversely affect the patellar retinacular structures, eventually leading to the need for surgical realignment procedures.

The nature of quadriceps atrophy

The nature and extent of quadriceps atrophy in PFDs, particularly in PFPS, has therefore theoretical as well as clinical implications. Current technology cannot show the individual contributions of the parts of the quadriceps. Consequently, the problem of imbalance between the VMO and VL has been studied semiquantitatively using electromyography. Though one study (Moller et al 1986) indicated that the quadriceps as a whole was weak in patients with PFPS, a yet older study (Mariani & Caruso 1979) and, particularly, a recent study by Souza & Gross (1991) showed that the VMO/VL ratio, as measured by integrated EMG, was significantly greater in normal subjects than in those with PFPS.

PFD AND QUADRICEPS PERFORMANCE
Dependence on test velocities

Studies of quadriceps performance, under isokinetic conditions, in patients with PFD show a definite dependence on the test velocity. This relationship is evident not only in the strength scores but also in the shape of the strength curve particularly at slow testing velocities (see below).

In a validation study of clinical (including isokinetic) parameters versus arthroscopy for diagnosis of chondromalacia (Elton et al 1985), the authors failed to reveal significant concentric strength differences between the affected and unaffected knee. The tests were carried out at 180°/s 'to avoid the risk of causing patellofemoral damage. This might account for [the] inability to find torque curve abnormalities in [the] subjects'.

In another study no significant differences in either the concentric or eccentric strength of the quadriceps were indicated upon comparing women with PFPS and a control group (MacIntyre & Wessel 1988). Again, the reason for this finding might have been the high velocity, 200°/s, at which the test was carried out.

The use of medium/high velocities means that:

1. the joint is exposed for a shorter time to the external resistance, leading to a lower load on the patellofemoral joint and hence reduced potential inhibition
2. the reflex arc may be too slow to react and inhibit the quadriceps.

On the other hand, concentric tests performed at the lower end of the velocity spectrum told a different story. Hoke et al (1983), using a test velocity of 30°/s, indicated quadriceps strength curve variations in patients with chondromalacia. In a prospective study of quadriceps strength, the pre- and postoperative scores were compared in patients who underwent advancement osteotomy of the tibial tuberosity due to patellofemoral chondromalacia and osteoarthrosis (Nordgren et al 1983). Tests were performed at velocities of 6, 12, and 60°/s. Table 7.10 outlines some of the findings:

1. Compared with matched normal subjects, both women and men demonstrated a highly significant reduction in strength. Considering the full spectrum of velocities, this reduction amounted to 34 and 22% in women and men respectively.
2. Quadriceps strength in the involved knee improved significantly following the operation (no significant differences were noted for the sound knee).
3. Using the averages quoted in the study, the estimated average preoperative QQRs were 66 and 59% for women and men respectively.

Contraction mode and QQR

In a later study, Dvir et al (1990) tested a mixed group of young women and men presenting with PFPS. Bilateral concentric and eccentric tests were performed at 30, 60 and 120°/s. Table 7.11 outlines the results, normalized for bodyweight. Compared with healthy subjects, women and men with PFPS had a reduction in strength of 35 and 27% respectively. In addition:

1. The reduction in eccentric contractions was larger than in concentric contractions: 44 versus 35% in women, and 41 versus 27% in men.
2. The average QQR was very stable at about 65 and 67% in women and men (concentric) and 60 and 62% (eccentric). (The close

Table 7.10 Pre- vs postoperative findings* for pain and knee extensor strength. Based on Nordgren et al 1983 copyright © Springer-Verlag

Angular velocity (°/s)	Peak moment (Nm)				Pain value (0–9 Lund scale)		
	n	Uninvolved	Involved knee		n	Preoperative	Postoperative
			Preoperative	Postoperative			
60							
Women	16	133 (31)	86 (36)	106 (36)	13	3.85 (2.00)	2.02 (2.03)‡
Men	11	228 (77)	131 (52)	186 (49)†	9	5.01 (1.63)	2.22 (2.20)‡
12							
Women	17	139 (32)	84 (34)	109 (38)†	13	3.71 (2.05)	1.92 (1.86)‡
Men	11	207 (94)	112 (38)	174 (38)‡	9	4.89 (1.41)	2.19 (2.05)‡
60							
Women	17	125 (23)	79 (32)	92 (31)	17	2.28 (1.72)	0.87 (1.29)†
Men	13	188 (73)	109 (31)	147 (41)†	9	3.40 (2.05)	1.78 (1.92)

* Shown as mean (SD); $^†p < 0.05$; $^‡p < 0.01$.

Table 7.11 Concentric and eccentric knee extensor strength (in Nm/kgbw)*: controls vs patients with patellofemoral pain syndrome (PFPS), based on Dvir et al (1990)

Group	Contraction mode	n	Angular velocity (°/s)		
			30	60	120
Women					
Control	Concentric	15	2.47 (0.49)	2.41 (0.47)	1.93 (0.37)
PFPS	Concentric	21	1.69 (0.40)	1.55 (0.79)	1.22 (0.90)
Men					
Control	Concentric	15	3.02 (0.51)	2.77 (0.52)	2.43 (0.41)
PFPS	Concentric	34	2.00 (0.49)	1.93 (0.60)	1.97 (0.44)
Women					
Control	Eccentric	15	3.39 (0.70)	3.23 (0.70)	3.20 (0.63)
PFPS	Eccentric	21	2.04 (0.73)	1.87 (0.70)	1.67 (0.72)
Men					
Control	Eccentric	15	3.80 (0.92)	3.65 (0.83)	3.66 (0.67)
PFPS	Eccentric	34	2.29 (0.64)	2.27 (0.60)	2.34 (0.62)

* Shown as mean (SD).

correspondence in the strength scores between this study and that of Nordgren et al is notable.)

Conclusions

Two principles thus emerge from the above analysis:

1. Slow test velocities, 30–60°/s, may be used for PFD testing.
2. Chronic PFPS may result in a significant reduction in the QQR, of greater than 30%.

Regarding the first point, although the policy of avoiding excessive pressure on the patellofemoral joint is entirely justified, the present author believes that a sounder interpretation of findings, based on low speed testing, can more than offset the potential risk from a set of 3–4 consecutive maximal contractions performed once every 2–3 weeks.

CORRELATION BETWEEN PAIN AND ISOKINETIC MEASUREMENTS IN PFPS

Clinical examination of patients suffering from patellofemoral pain frequently reveals that one of the most common mechanisms of avoiding pain is 'a reluctance, whether voluntary or involuntary, to initiate and maintain a strong quadriceps contraction' (Wild et al 1982). Both static and dynamic contractile activity may be avoided. Pain is probably the main obstacle to normal force generation when quadriceps strength in PFPS patients is measured. Moreover, improvement in the symptoms is often accompanied by an improved quadriceps performance; thus recording the pain level, as well as quadriceps strength, is of paramount importance in PFPS testing and rehabilitation.

Quadriceps strength and pain rating

The association of pain and patellofemoral stressing under isokinetic conditions was first reported by Nordgren et al (1983). Patients used the Lund 9-point scale to rate the pain perceived after each contraction, pre- and postoperatively. The significant reductions in anterior knee pain rating correlated with a significant increase in quadriceps concentric strength and the general functional level. In a later paper, Lysholm (1987) studied the combined effect of drug therapy and activity modification on quadriceps strength and knee pain in 25 subjects with patellar tendinitis.

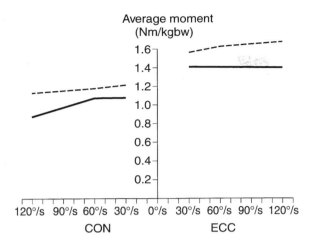

Figure 7.3 Normalized average moment–angular velocity curves in patients with patellofemoral dysfunction. (From Dvir et al 1991a Isokinetics and Exercise Science 1: 26–30, with permission of Butterworth-Heinemann.) CON, concentric; ECC, eccentric; solid lines, females; broken lines, males.

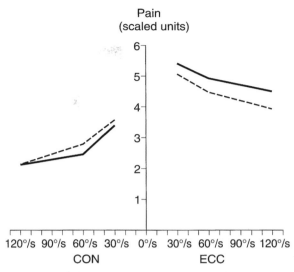

Figure 7.4 Pain scores during maximal knee extension effort in concentric and eccentric contractions. (From Dvir et al 1991a Isokinetics and Exercise Science 1: 26–30, with permission of Butterworth-Heinemann.) CON, concentric; ECC, eccentric; solid lines, females; broken lines, males.

A significant negative correlation was indicated between the pain, as measured by a visual analog scale, and peak moment. The negative correlation was more pronounced at 30 (-0.59) than at 180°/s (-0.40). The closer association between pain and strength at the lower velocity testing could mean that the pain magnitude reflected either the higher moment generated at 30°/s or the longer exposure during a slower test.

Contraction mode, load and perceived pain

In a recent study of patients with PFPS, the association between concentric and eccentric quadriceps strength and perceived pain was analyzed (Dvir et al 1991a). Pain was assessed using the 10-point Borg modified pain scale. Figure 7.3 shows the average moment–angular velocity relationship. Figure 7.4 shows that the variations in the pain scores did not correspond to variations in strength, at least with respect to eccentric efforts, as the levelling-off of the eccentric strength curve is not reflected in a similar shape for the pain curve.

Pain and load. However, variation in the load, or impulse, which is the product of two distinct variables, the magnitude of the moment generated by the muscle and the period of time the joint is exposed to the contractile activity, is closely correlated with changes in the pain (Fig. 7.5). Therefore, the pain perceived by patients with PFPS was predominantly dictated by the load on the joint.

Eccentric contractions and pain mechanisms. Eccentric contractions resulted in significantly higher pain ratings ($p < 0.005$) than concentric contractions. Two possible causes are suggested. Higher moments are generated during eccentric contractions which result in greater patellofemoral forces and therefore greater pain. The other mechanism lies in patellar kinematics. During concentric activity, the area of contact between the patella and the femoral notch diminishes with greater extension (Goodfellow et al 1976). On the other hand, during eccentric activity, the knee flexes and the contact area becomes larger. Although this may result in an improved pressure distribution, the total area exposed to friction increases, leading potentially to the greater intensity of pain. It is of interest that in a recent study no observable relationship between perceived pain and quadriceps force output was indicated (Conway et al 1992).

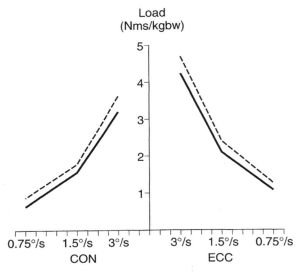

Figure 7.5 Impulse (load) versus angular velocity during maximal knee extension effort in concentric and eccentric contractions. (From Dvir et al 1991a Isokinetics and Exercise Science 1: 26–30, with permission of Butterworth-Heinemann.) CON, concentric; ECC, eccentric; solid lines, females; broken lines, males.

As shown above, such a relationship may indeed not exist unless load is used instead of moment and a spectrum of velocities rather than a single test velocity.

PFPS AND THE SHAPE OF THE QUADRICEPS MOMENT CURVE

Normally, an isokinetic moment curve which is derived from a perfectly sound joint–muscle unit should consist of a relatively smooth 'inverted-U' shape (Chapter 2). When there is either a sudden and considerable change in the muscle's lever or a 'shut-off' of its contractile activity this curve may assume an irregular shape. Here irregularity does not refer to common oscillatory phenomena (Hart et al 1985) but to single, sometimes double or triple, conspicuous 'dents' in the curve.

The 'break' in PFPS moment curves

Such an irregularity in the moment curve of the quadriceps is a striking expression of PFPS,

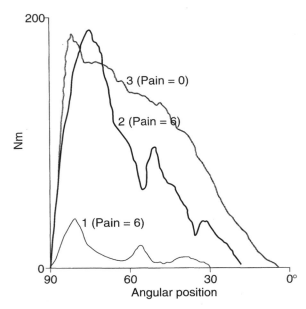

Figure 7.6 Maximal isokinetic knee extension strength in a woman with chondromalacia of the patella. 1, before the operation; 2, before the operation and after intra-articular anesthesia; 3, at the follow-up. Rating of pain was made according to the Borg–Lindblad scale. (From Nordgren et al 1983 copyright © Springer-Verlag.)

obtained during low velocity isokinetic testing. Nordgren et al (1983) were among the first to document this phenomenon. Figure 7.6 (Nordgen et al 1983) shows three different quadriceps moment curves from the same patient on three occasions: preoperatively, under intra-articular anesthesia and during (supposedly) a later rehabilitation phase. This irregularity which was termed 'break' by Grace et al (1984) was later mentioned in other papers (Bennett & Stauber 1986, Lysholm 1987).

In the first quantitative analysis of this phenomenon in patients with PFPS (Dvir et al 1991b) a break was defined as a perturbation in the curve which exceeded a drop of 10% or more in the magnitude of the prebreak moment (see Fig. 7.7 for explanation).

In this study, whose design has been described earlier (Dvir et al 1991a), breaks occurred exclusively during eccentric contractions. Nearly 50% of the subjects had at least one break during the series of tests.

The break was associated with a partial relief of pain in the patellofemoral joint, at about 45° flexion, close to the value reported by Hart et al (1985), but not at 75°, which has been calculated to coincide with maximal patellofemoral joint reaction force (Kaufman et al 1991, Nisell & Ericson 1992). Whether, therefore, a different pain mechanism operates during eccentric contractions is not known at present. However, since the concentric loads (which at 30°/s were greater than the eccentric loads at 60°/s) were not associated with breaks, one could speculate that the underlying reason for the breaks was not the load imposed on the joint. Breaks occurred predominantly during the 30°/s test, which had the longest exposure time.

To further analyze the pain–break relationship, the average pain scores in tests which showed breaks were compared with tests which did not. Though the former were consistently higher in both genders throughout the entire spectrum of velocities, the differences were not significant. On the other hand, using an alternative analysis, it was evident that the pain provoked during a 'break contraction' was most frequently perceived as the most intense among the eccentric tests. As already mentioned in this study, the break phenomenon occurred exclusively during eccentric activity, a finding which was in accordance with those of Hart et al (1985) and Bennett & Stauber (1986) but at variance with the finding of Nordgren et al (1983). The reason for this discrepancy is probably the very low test velocities employed in the latter study which led to exceedingly long exposures.

ISOKINETIC TESTING IN PFPS: A PRELIMINARY MODEL

A combination of the three factors – significantly reduced quadriceps strength, pain and the break phenomenon – has been utilized to set up a preliminary model for analysis and interpretation of PFPS based on isokinetic testing (Dvir & Halperin 1992). Each of these factors was assigned a positive or negative value according to certain criteria, so that every subject was classified according to the following triad: strength (+/−), pain (+/−) and

break (+/−). For instance, the description '+ + −' meant that the subject demonstrated significant strength reduction and pain but no break. A relatively high percentage of patients, 27%, were classified as negative on all factors but this might have reflected the stringency of the criteria (Sherman et al 1987). On the other hand, 24% of the subjects were categorized as '+ + +' and when those classed as '+ − +' and '+ + −' were added, the percentage of patients rose to about 40%. This value is on a par with the clinical tests employed, reflecting an empirical impression among clinicians that most of the accepted techniques in diagnosing PFD are no more powerful than this. This conclusion is however very tentative and much more research is required on the interdependence of morphological, pathological and functional variables, of which muscle strength, pain and irregularity in the moment curve form an important subset.

Need for pain assessment

But even without validation of the above, or other, models, clinicians are advised that testing patients with PFPS should be supplemented with some form of pain assessment. Considerably more may be learned, clinically and functionally, than from assessment of strength or pain alone. The location of breaks and attention given to their continued presence or disappearance, during a rehabilitation process, also significantly assists in judging outcome. Figure 7.7 provides a good demonstration of this practice.

MENISCAL DISORDERS

Meniscal disorders have been studied using isokinetics, particularly concerning the effect of the surgical technique. During recent years, arthroscopy has become exceedingly popular for treating some of the typical meniscal disorders. In order to prove its efficacy in terms of muscle function, isokinetic analyses of thigh muscles have been performed. One of the first reports (Patel et al 1982) indicated a QQR of 88% and a much smaller hamstring deficit of 5%, 1 month

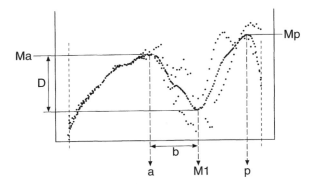

Figure 7.7 An example of the break phenomenon. Ma, value of the maximal prebreak moment; a, the angle at which Ma occurs; M1, value of the minimal within-break moment; b, the angular displacement from a to the angle at which M1 occurs; D, the difference between Ma and M1; Mp, the value of the maximal postbreak moment; p, the angle at which Mp occurs.

following meniscectomy. Hamberg et al (1983) studied the effect of open and closed (arthroscopic) meniscectomy and found that:

1. compared to the preoperative levels at the same side, there was a 40% decrease in quadriceps strength, 1 week following the operation, in patients who underwent partial or total closed meniscectomy; normal function was recovered 8 weeks later
2. open meniscectomy resulted in 70% loss of quadriceps strength at 1 week and recovery was not complete after 8 weeks
3. flexor function was recovered 1 month following the intervention.

Somewhat less drastic effects but showing the same trends were reported by Prietto et al (1983). Mariani et al (1987) reported a QQR of better than 90% only 2 weeks after arthroscopic meniscectomy for medial bucket-handle tears. Flexor strength remained at preoperative levels throughout rehabilitation. The differences between the studies of Patel et al and Mariani et al, and between those of Hamberg et al and Prietto et al, may be explained by the nature of the cases involved and differing rehabilitation procedures. However, according to the available sources:

1. arthroscopic meniscectomy is significantly less detrimental to quadriceps function compared with the open approach

2. with the closed technique, the immediate and sharp decrease in QQR should be recovered within a period of 4–8 weeks
3. flexor function should not be compromised.

PART 4
ISOKINETICS FOR KNEE MUSCLE CONDITIONING

Most of the published literature concerning the isokinetics of the knee concerns muscle testing. Less has been written concerning the application of isokinetics to muscle conditioning in clinical situations. The principles governing this aspect of isokinetics – namely submaximal versus maximal muscle tension, pretensioning and grading of velocities – were described in detail in Chapter 4. This section will therefore concentrate on the use of a specific modality, eccentric conditioning, which has been studied with particular respect to PFPS. The treatment, as opposed to the testing, of ACL deficiency increasingly uses functional activities. Correspondingly, there is a growing emphasis on the use of closed kinetic chain exercises involving multiple joint efforts, which has only recently been recognized by manufacturers of isokinetic systems. An attachment for this purpose (leg-press) is illustrated in Figure 7.8.

ECCENTRIC MODE TRAINING
Rationale

A novel approach to the treatment of anterior knee pain was described by Bennett & Stauber (1986). The basic tenet of their approach was that:

Errors in control of muscle function during the performance of negative work (expressed as depressed muscle forces during muscle lengthening activities) might cause varying degrees of soft tissue trauma, especially in those situations where no well-defined orthopaedic disorder could be identified.

According to this theory, a (neurophysiological) deficiency existed and its removal could alleviate the pain.

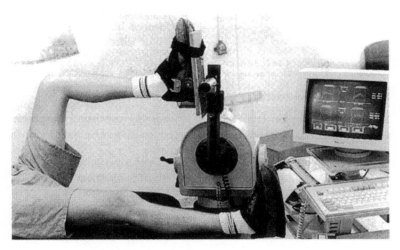

Figure 7.8   The leg-press attachment and testing position.

Patient selection and protocol

The clinical basis for selection of patients, other than the presence of anterior knee pain, was vague. The isokinetic criterion was moment-based strength, measured at 30°/s. The eccentric moment of the muscle, Q_{ecc}, was compared with its concentric counterpart, Q_{con}, and only those with a score of 85% or less for the ratio Q_{ecc}/Q_{con} (at any point throughout the tested ROM) were admitted to the study group. The rehabilitation program was based on eccentric training which consisted of three sets of 10 repetitions at each of the velocities 30, 60 and 90°/s, with three sessions per week until pain was relieved.

Results

Figure 7.9 shows the relative moment–position curve for the uninvolved knee; Figure 7.10 the findings for the symptomatic knee, pretreatment, and Figure 7.11 the postreatment symptomatic knee findings. A success rate of 93% was claimed by the authors with a full reversal of the eccentric deficiency.

Although the authors were not able to offer a rigorous explanation for their findings, it was suggested that the rapid reversal of the symptoms pointed to an 'error' in the use of the eccentric component of the vastus medialis. Though the

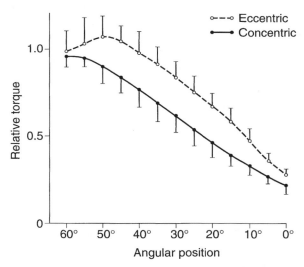

Figure 7.9   Relative knee extension moment as a function of knee position in the unsymptomatic knee. (From Bennett & Stauber 1986.)

exact nature of this error was not elucidated, it was rectified by appropriate training.

Limitations of the patient selection criterion

The use of the 85% Q_{ecc}/Q_{con} criterion has since been criticized (Trudelle-Jackson et al 1989), on

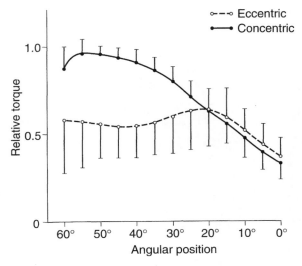

Figure 7.10 Relative knee extension moment as a function of knee position in the symptomatic knee before treatment. (From Bennett & Stauber 1986.)

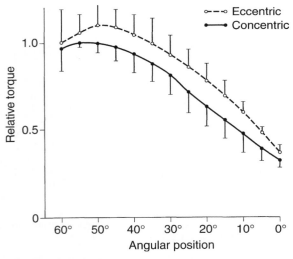

Figure 7.11 Relative knee extension moment as a function of knee position in the symptomatic knee after treatment. (From Bennett & Stauber 1986.)

the grounds that 35–54% of normal subjects demonstrate such deficiency. On the other hand, Conway et al (1992) have claimed that in their experimental group which consisted of 30 patients

with PFPS, the Q_{ecc}/Q_{con} was never less than 0.95. In view of this, it might be concluded that Bennett & Stauber's protocol is particularly suitable for patients with a conspicuous eccentric deficiency.

Support for the eccentric conditioning approach

Although the patient selection process and rehabilitation protocol of the Bennett & Stauber study are still controversial, it is one of the most innovative and intriguing among the many studies which have attempted to incorporate isokinetics as a therapeutic means. Obviously there must be support from research and accumulated experience before this approach can gain acceptance.

A study by Jensen & Di Fabio (1989) has already given some backing. These authors compared patients with patellar tendinitis with control subjects. Each group was divided into a subgroup that performed home muscle stretching exercises only, and one which received additional eccentric isokinetic exercises. The intensity of the isokinetic exercise was enhanced by gradually increasing the velocity of contraction from 30 to 70°/s (a protocol which is not necessarily supported by current knowledge regarding the moment–angular velocity relationship). The isokinetic performance parameter was the QQR of the work done during five consecutive concentric–eccentric contractions at 50°/s. The intensity and occurrence of pain were assessed.

The results indicated that subjects with patellar tendinitis increased their QQR following eccentric input, but that this increase was not significant compared with the matched group which received only stretching input. The authors have attributed this finding to pain inhibition since there was a high negative correlation between pain frequency (−0.80) and occurrence (−0.78) and QQR (work).

Severity of injury and the gender composition of the sample were also implicated. The achievement of optimal strength increases was therefore hampered by pain.

REFERENCES

Arvidsson I, Ericsson E, Haggmark T 1981 Isokinetic thigh muscle strength after ligament reconstruction in the knee joint: results from 5–10 year follow-up after reconstruction of the anterior cruciate ligament of the knee joint. International Journal of Sports Medicine 2: 7–11

Ballmer P M, Jakob R P 1988 The non-operative treatment of isolated complete tears of the medial collateral ligament of the knee. A prospective study. Archives of Orthopaedic and Traumatic Surgery 107: 273–276

Barr A E, Duncan P W 1988 Influence of position on knee flexor peak torque. Journal of Orthopaedic and Sports Physical Therapy 9: 279–283

Bennett J G, Stauber W T 1986 Evaluation and treatment of anterior knee pain using eccentric exercise. Medicine and Science in Sports and Exercise 18: 526–530

Bergfeld J 1979 First, second and third degree sprains. American Journal of Sports Medicine 7: 207–209

Bohannon R W, Gajdosik R L, LeVeau B F 1986 Isokinetic knee flexion and extension torque in the upright sitting and semicircled sitting positions. Physical Therapy 66: 1083–1086

Bonamo J, Colleen F, Firestone T 1990 The conservative treatment of the anterior cruciate deficient knee. American Journal of Sports Medicine 18: 618–623

Borges O 1989 Isometric and isokinetic knee extension and flexion torque in men and women aged 20–70. Scandinavian Journal of Rehabilitation Medicine 21: 45–53

Brown L E, Whitehurst M, Bryant J R 1992 A comparison of the LIDO sliding cuff and the tibial control system in isokinetic strength parameters. Isokinetics and Exercise Science 3: 101–109

Cerullo G, Puddu G, Conteduca F, Ferretti A, Mariani P 1988 Evaluation of the results of extensor mechanism reconstruction. American Journal of Sports Medicine 16: 93–96

Constantin R, Williams A K 1984 Isokinetic quadriceps and hamstring torque level of adolescent female soccer players. Journal of Orthopaedic and Sports Physical Therapy 5: 196–200

Conway A, Malone T R, Conway P 1992 Patellar alignment/tracking: effect on force output and perceived pain. Isokinetics and Exercise Science 2: 9–17

Currier D P 1977 Positioning for knee strengthening exercises. Physical Therapy 57: 148–151

Davies G J, Halbach J W, Carpenter M A 1980 A descriptive muscular strength and power analysis of the US cross-country ski team. Medicine and Science in Sports and Exercise 12: 141

De Carlo M S, Shelbourne K D, McCarroll J R, Rettig A C 1992 Traditional versus accelerated rehabilitation following ACL reconstruction: a one-year follow-up. Journal of Orthopaedic and Sports Physical Therapy 15: 309–316

Dvir Z, Halperin N 1992 Patellofemoral pain syndrome: a preliminary model for analysis and interpretation of isokinetic and pain parameters. Clinical Biomechanics 7: 240–245

Dvir Z, Eger G, Halperin N, Shklar A 1989 Thigh muscle activity and anterior cruciate ligament insufficiency. Clinical Biomechanics 4: 87–91

Dvir Z, Shklar A, Halperin N, Robinson D 1990 Concentric and eccentric torque variations of the quadriceps femoris in patellofemoral pain syndrome. Clinical Biomechanics 5: 68–72

Dvir Z, Halperin N, Shklar A, Robinson D 1991a Quadriceps function and patellofemoral pain syndrome. Part I: pain provocation during concentric and eccentric isokinetic contractions. Isokinetics and Exercise Science 1: 26–30

Dvir Z, Halperin N, Shklar A, Robinson D 1991b Quadriceps function and patellofemoral pain syndrome. Part II: the break phenomenon during eccentric contractions. Isokinetics and Exercise Science 1: 31–35

Elmqvist L-G, Lorentzon R, Langstrom M, Fugl-Meyer A R 1988 Reconstruction of the anterior cruciate ligament: long term effects of different knee angles at primary immobilization and different modes of early training. American Journal of Sports Medicine 16: 455–462

Elmqvist L-G, Lorentzon R, Johansson C, Langstrom M, Fagerlund M, Fugl-Meyer A 1989 Knee extensor muscle function before and after reconstruction of anterior cruciate ligament tear. Scandinavian Journal of Rehabilitation Medicine 21: 131–139

Elton K, McDonough K, Savinar E, Jensen G 1985 A preliminary investigation: history, physical and isokinetic exam results versus arthroscopic diagnosis of chondromalacia patella. Journal of Orthopaedic and Sports Physical Therapy 7: 115–121

Freedson P S, Gilliam T B, Mahoney T, Maliszwewski A F, Kastango K 1993 Industrial torque levels by age group and gender. Isokinetics and Exercise Science 3: 34–42

Ghena D R, Kuth A L, Thomas M, Mayhew J 1991 Torque characteristics of the quadriceps and hamstring muscles during concentric and eccentric loading. Journal of Orthopaedic and Sports Physical Therapy 14: 149–154

Gilliam T B, Sandy S P, Freedson P S 1979 Isokinetic torque levels for high school football players. Archives of Physical Medicine and Rehabilitation 60: 110–114

Goodfellow J, Hungerford D S, Zindel M 1976 Patellofemoral joint mechanics and pathology. Part I: functional anatomy of the patellofemoral joint. Journal of Bone and Joint Surgery 58B: 287–290

Grace T G, Sweetser E R, Nelson M A, Ydens L R, Skipper B J 1984 Isokinetic muscle imbalance and knee joint injury. Journal of Bone and Joint Surgery 66A: 734–740

Gross M T, McGrain P, Demilio P, Plyler L 1989 Relationship between multiple predictor variables and normal knee torque production. Physical Therapy 69: 54–62

Hall P S, Roofner M A 1991 Velocity spectrum study of knee flexion and extension in normal adults: 60 to 500 deg/sec. Isokinetics and Exercise Science 1: 131–137

Halperin N, Dvir Z 1993 Arthroscopic hamstring loop reconstruction combined with ITB strip tenodesis. In: The Ninth International Jerusalem Symposium on Sports Injuries

Hamberg P, Gillquist J, Lysholm J, Oberg B 1983 The effect of diagnostic and operative arthroscopy and open menisectomy on muscle strength in the thigh. American Journal of Sports Medicine 11: 289–292

Hanten W P, Ramberg C L 1988 Effect of stabilization on maximal isokinetic torque of the quadriceps femoris muscle during concentric and eccentric contractions. Physical Therapy 68: 219–222

Hart D L, Stobbe T J, Till C W 1984 Effect of trunk stabilization on quadriceps femoris muscle torque. Physical Therapy 64: 375–380

Hart D L, Miller L C, Stauber W T 1985 Effect of cooling on voluntary eccentric force oscillations during maximal contractions. Experimental Neurology 90: 73–80

Hastings D E 1980 The non-operative management of collateral ligament injuries of the knee joint. Clinical Orthopaedics and Related Research 147: 22–28

Highgenboten C L, Jackson A W, Meske N B 1988 Concentric and eccentric torque comparisons for knee extension and flexion in young adult males and females using the Kinetic Communicator. American Journal of Sports Medicine 16: 234–237

Hoke B, Howell D, Stack M 1983 The relationship between isokinetic testing and dynamic patellofemoral compression. Journal of Orthopaedic and Sports Physical Therapy 4: 150–153

Insall J 1981 Patellar pain. Journal of Bone and Joint Surgery 64A: 147–152

Jensen K, Di Fabio R 1989 Evaluation of eccentric exercise in treatment of patellar tendinitis. Physical Therapy 69: 211–216

Johnson D 1982 Controlling anterior shear during isokinetic knee extension exercise. Journal of Orthopaedic and Sports Physical Therapy 4: 10–15

Kannus P 1988a Ratio of hamstring to quadriceps femoris muscles' strength in the anterior cruciate ligament insufficient knee: relationship to long term recovery. Physical Therapy 68: 961–965

Kannus P 1988b Knee flexor and extensor strength ratios with deficiency of the lateral collateral ligament. Archives of Physical Medicine and Rehabilitation 69: 928–931

Kannus P 1990 Relationship between peak torque, peak angular impulse and average power in the thigh muscles of subjects with knee damage. Research Quarterly 60: 141–145

Kannus P, Jarvinen M 1991 Thigh muscle function after partial tear of the medial ligament compartment of the knee. Medicine and Science in Sports and Exercise 23: 4–9

Kannus P, Jarvinen M, Johnson R et al 1992 Function of the quadriceps and hamstring muscles in knees with chronic partial deficiency of the anterior cruciate ligament. American Journal of Sports Medicine 20: 162–168

Kaufman K R, An K, Litchy W J, Morrey B F, Chao E Y 1991 Dynamic knee joint forces during isokinetic exercise. American Journal of Sports Medicine 19: 305–316

Kirkendall D T, Berfeld I, Calbrese J A 1984 Isokinetic characteristics of ballet dancers and the response to a season of ballet training. Journal of Orthopaedic and Sports Physical Therapy 5: 207–211

Kramer J F, Hill K, Jones I C, Sandrin M, Vyse M 1989 Effect of dynamometer application arm length on concentric and eccentric torques during isokinetic knee extension. Physiotherapy Canada 41: 100–106

Kues J M, Rothstein J M, Lam R L 1992 Obtaining reliable measurements of knee extensor torque produced during maximal voluntary contractions: an experimental investigation. Physical Therapy 72: 492–504

Lopresti C, Kirkendall D T, Street G M, Dudley A W 1988 Quadriceps insufficiency following repair of the anterior cruciate ligament. Journal of Orthopaedic and Sports Physical Therapy 9: 245–249

Lysholm J 1987 The relation between pain and torque in an isokinetic strength test of knee extension. Arthroscopy 3: 182–184

MacIntyre D, Wessel J 1988 Knee muscles torque in patellofemoral pain syndrome. Physiotherapy Canada 40: 20–24

Magnusson P, Geismar R, McHugh M, Gleim G, Nicholas J 1992 The effect of trunk stabilization on knee extension/flexion torque production. Journal of Orthopaedic and Sports Physical Therapy 15: 51–52

Mangine R E, Noyes F R 1992 Rehabilitation of the allograft reconstruction. Journal of Orthopaedic and Sports Physical Therapy 15: 294–302

Mariani P P, Caruso I 1979 An electromyographic investigation of subluxation of the patella. Journal of Bone and Joint Surgery 61B: 169–171

Mariani P P, Ferretti A, Gigli C, Puddu G 1987 Isokinetic evaluation of the knee after arthroscopic meniscectomy: comparison between anterolateral and central approaches. Arthroscopy 3(2): 123–126

Marshall J L, Warren R F, Wickiewicz T L, Reider B 1979 The anterior cruciate ligament: a technique of repair and reconstruction. Clinical Orthopaedics 143: 97–104

Moller R N, Krebs R, Tidemand-Dal C, Aaris K 1986 Isometric contractions in the patellofemoral pain syndrome: an electromyographic study. Archives of Orthopaedic and Traumatic Surgery 105: 24–27

Morris A, Lussier L, Bell G 1983 Hamstring/quadriceps strength ratios in collegiate middle-distance and distance runners. The Physician and Sports Medicine 11: 71–77

Murray P M, Gardner G M, Mollinger L A, Sepic S B 1980 Strength of isometric and isokinetic contractions. Physical Therapy 60: 412–419

Murray S M, Warren R F, Otis J C, Kroll M, Wickiewicz T L 1984 Torque–velocity relationships of the knee extensor and flexor muscles in individuals sustaining injuries of the anterior cruciate ligament. American Journal of Sports Medicine 12: 436–440

Nisell R 1985 Mechanics of the knee: a study of joint load and muscle activity with clinical implications. Acta Orthopaedica Scandinavica, Supplement 216

Nisell R, Ericson M 1992 Patellar forces during isokinetic knee extension. Clinical Biomechanics 7: 104–108

Nisell R, Ericson M O, Nemeth G, Ekholm J 1989 Tibio-femoral joint forces during isokinetic knee extension. American Journal of Sports Medicine 17: 49–54

Nordgren B, Nordesjo L-O, Rausching W 1983 Isokinetic knee extension strength and pain before and after advancement osteotomy of the tibial tuberosity. Archives of Orthopaedic and Traumatic Surgery 102: 95–101

Osternig L R, Hamill J, Sawhill J, Bates B T 1983 Influence of torque and limb speed on power production in isokinetic exercise. American Journal of Physical Medicine 62: 163–171

Paolos L E, Noyes F R, Grood E S 1983 Knee rehabilitation after anterior cruciate ligament reconstruction and repair. American Journal of Sports Medicine 9: 140–149

Patel D, Fahmy N, Sakayan A 1982 Isokinetic and functional evaluation of the knee following arthroscopic surgery. Clinical Orthopaedics and Related Research 167: 84–91

Prietto C A, Caiozzo V J, Prietto P P, McMaster W C 1983 Closed versus open partial meniscectomy: postoperative changes in the force–velocity relationship of muscle. American Journal of Sports Medicine 11: 189–194

Rosenberg T D, Franklin J L, Baldwin G N, Nelson K A 1992 Extensor mechanism function after patellar tendon graft harvest for anterior cruciate ligament reconstruction. American Journal of Sports Medicine 20: 519–526

Sczepanski T L, Gross M T, Duncan W P, Chandler J M 1991 Effect of contraction type angular velocity and arc of motion on VMO:VL EMG ratio. Journal of Orthopaedic and Sports Physical Therapy 14: 256–262

Seto J L, Orofino A S, Morrissey M C, Medeiros J M, Mason W J 1988 Assessment of quadriceps/hamstring strength, knee ligament stability, functional and sports activity levels five years after anterior cruciate ligament reconstruction. American Journal of Sports Medicine 16: 170–180

Shelbourne K D, Nitz P 1990 Accelerated rehabilitation after anterior cruciate ligament reconstruction. American Journal of Sports Medicine 18: 292–299

Shelbourne K D, Porter D A 1992 Anterior cruciate ligament – medial collateral ligament injury: nonoperative management of medial collateral ligament tears with anterior cruciate ligament reconstruction. American Journal of Sports Medicine 20: 283–286

Shelton G L, Thigpen K 1991 Rehabilitation of patellofemoral dysfunction: a review of literature. Journal of Orthopaedic and Sports Physical Therapy 14: 243–249

Sherman O H, Fox J M, Sperling H et al 1987 Patellar instability: treatment by arthroscopic electrosurgical lateral release. Arthroscopy 3: 152–160

Siewert M W, Ariki P W, Davies G J, Rowinski M J 1975 Isokinetic torque changes based upon lever arm pad placement. Physical Therapy 65: 715

Smidt G L 1973 Biomechanical analysis of knee flexion and extension. Journal of Biomechanics 6: 79–92

Smith D J, Quinney H A, Wenger H A 1981 Isokinetic torque output of professional and amateur ice hockey players. Journal of Orthopaedic and Sports Physical Therapy 3: 42–47

Solomonow M, Baratta R, Zhou B H et al 1987 The synergistic action of the anterior cruciate ligament and thigh muscles in maintaining joint stability. American Journal of Sports Medicine 15: 207–213

Souza D R, Gross M T 1991 Comparison of VMO:VL integrated electromyographic ratios between healthy subjects and patients with patellofemoral pain. Physical Therapy 71: 310–320

Taunton J E, Clement D B, Smart C W, McNichol K L 1987 Nonsurgical management of overuse knee injuries in runners. Canadian Journal of Sports Science 12: 11–18

Taylor R L, Casey J J 1986 Quadriceps torque production on the Cybex II dynamometer as related to changes in lever arm length. Journal of Orthopaedic and Sports Physical Therapy 8: 148–152

Tegner Y, Lysholm J, Lysholm M, Gillquist J 1986 Strengthening exercises for old cruciate ligament tears. Acta Orthopaedica Scandinavica 57: 130–134

Timm K 1985 Validation of the Johnson anti-shear accessory as an accurate and effective clinical instrument. Journal of Orthpaedic and Sports Physical Therapy 7: 298–303

Trudelle-Jackson E, Meske N, Highgenboten C, Jackson A 1989 Eccentric/concentric torque deficits in the quadriceps muscle. Journal of Orthopaedic and Sports Physical Therapy 11: 142–145

Walla D J, Albright J P, McAuley E et al 1985 Hamstring control and the unstable anterior cruciate ligament-deficient knee. American Journal of Sports Medicine 13: 34–39

Wild J, Franklin T, Woods G 1982 Patellar pain and quadriceps rehabilitation: an EMG study. American Journal of Sports Medicine 10: 12–15

Wilk K E, Andrews J R 1992 Current concepts in the treatment of anterior cruciate ligament disruption. Journal of Orthopaedic and Sports Physical Therapy 15: 279–293

Worrell T W, Perrin D H, Denrgar C R 1989 The influence of hip position on quadriceps and hamstring peak torque and reciprocal muscle group ratio values. Journal of Orthopaedic and Sports Physical Therapy 11: 104–107

Worrell T W, Denegar C R, Armstrong S L, Perrin D H 1990 Effect of body position on hamstring muscle group average torque. Journal of Orthopaedic and Sports Physical Therapy 11: 449–452

Yasuda K, Ohkoshi Y, Tanabe Y, Kaneda K 1992 Quantitative evaluation of knee instability and muscle thigh strength after anterior cruciate ligament reconstruction using patellar quadriceps tendon. American Journal of Sports Medicine 20: 471–475

Isokinetics of the ankle muscles

Among the major articulations of the lower limb, the talocrural–subtalar joint complex has received moderate attention, more than that accorded the hip, but receiving less interest than the knee, which became the paradigm for isokinetics-related research and clinical practice. With its relatively short, polyarticulated distal 'segment', its variety of movements, and the number of muscles spanning it, the ankle poses difficulties not shared by the hip and knee. These problems are reflected in procedural issues like positioning and alignment of axes, and by substantive issues such as closed versus open kinetic chain testing.

Little work has been done on the clinical applicability of ankle isokinetics. This is indeed surprising, given the high incidence of trauma, particularly ankle sprains which account for 85% of all ankle injuries (Garrick 1977). (A total of 70% of young basketball players have a history of sprain with an 80% recurrence rate (Smith & Reischl 1986).) Some explanation may be found in the already mentioned problems of positioning and stabilization of patients suffering from ankle trauma. In addition, reconstructive surgery, which played a decisive role in the development of knee isokinetics, lags behind with respect to the ankle. It is also true that the muscular machinery of the knee is much simpler than that of the ankle; the difficulty in evaluating the separate contributions of the various muscles operating in the ankle is a substantial practical obstacle.

The topics covered in this chapter are: the procedures for testing the ankle complex; the reproducibility of test findings; representative values, and correlates of ankle instability.

PART 1
ISOKINETIC TESTING OF ANKLE MUSCLES

Measurement of ankle performance involves testing of dorsiflexion and plantarflexion, commonly known as ankle (talocrural) movements, and inversion and eversion, the subtalar movements. The following elements are considered in this section:

1. the tested range of motion (ROM)
2. positioning and stabilization
3. alignment of biological and mechanical axes, and
4. test velocities.

TESTING OF DORSIFLEXION AND PLANTARFLEXION

Test ROM

The ROM for dorsiflexion and plantarflexion is measured relative to the neutral position (0°) of the foot. The values commonly quoted for measurement range from 10 to 30° for dorsiflexion, and from 40 to 65° for plantarflexion. The normative ROM for dorsiflexion is 20°, while for plantarflexion it is 45–50° (Miller 1985). An isokinetic test ROM for dorsiflexion–plantarflexion movements has very seldom been mentioned. In one study (Herlant et al 1992), the full ROM was quoted as being between 55 and 75°, depending on the test velocity and the clinical status of the limb. Clearly the tested ROM in this study coincided with the normal ROM.

Angle of peak moment

Some studies have investigated the angular position of the ankle associated with peak moment, for healthy subjects or patients, and either dorsi- or plantarflexion. As already indicated, this information is essential for decisions regarding the extent of tested ROM.

In a study by Fischer (1982) the isometric strength was measured every 6° from the position of maximal dorsiflexion (here defined as 0°). It was found that the greatest isometric strength of the plantarflexors was achieved at maximal dorsiflexion, where the triceps surae was most lengthened. On the other hand, the dorsiflexors reached maximum strength at 36°, corresponding to approximately 16° of plantarflexion (measured from the neutral position).

Sjostrom et al (1978) indicated that in the unaffected leg of patients who were treated for Achilles tendon rupture, the angle of peak moment shifted towards 30° upon increasing the test velocity from 30 to 180°/s. Gerdle & Fugl-Meyer (1988) applied a similar experimental protocol in a study which involved healthy subjects. The corresponding range was between 24 and 31°, practically identical to the results of Sjostrom et al.

Recommended ROM for testing

Functionally the typical ankle ROM during walking corresponds to 10° dorsiflexion and 20° plantarflexion (McPoil & Knecht 1985), and for running (Soutas-Little et al 1987) it is 20° dorsiflexion and 25° plantarflexion. It is clear that the tested ROM need not correspond to the total ROM. A ROM of 45°, starting from maximal dorsiflexion, is sufficient for strength and endurance testing of both dorsiflexors and plantarflexors. Failure to ensure maximal dorsiflexion will result in a submaximal score for the plantarflexors.

Positioning and stabilization

Positioning and stabilization are cardinal issues whose importance in the reproducibility and validity of ankle isokinetic testing cannot be overstated. Almost the entire repertoire of the plantarflexors consists of coupled eccentric–concentric contractions. These take place during weight-bearing in activities such as the propulsive phases of walking and running, and stair climbing and descending. Additionally, at certain times during these activities, ankle plantarflexors are a component of a chain comprising the knee and hip of the ipsilateral limb as well as all articulations of the contralateral limb.

Kinematic analysis of the lower limb in ambulation reveals that during the propulsive phase the knee is in a near extended position. This may not be equally applicable in stair climbing and descending, where the pitch of the individual step determines the extent of knee flexion, which can reach 60° (Diffrient et al 1974). However it should be borne in mind that even placing the ball of the foot on the stair allows significant dorsiflexion and this helps to offset the loss of gastrocnemius length. Consequently, testing in the position of slight/moderate knee flexion may be logical.

Positioning for plantarflexion

In principle, the plantarflexors could be tested in the upright position, although this would be very awkward and even impractical with most isokinetic systems. For this purpose, the resistance pad would be placed on the shoulders, and the subject would tiptoe (uni- or bilaterally) while the axial skeleton was kept fully erect and stabilized. Assuming minimal spinal arching and/or shoulder sagging, the force developed by the plantarflexors would be easily determinable. However, quite apart from other obstacles, there would be obvious difficulties where the patient could not exert sufficient force in order to tiptoe, or the net force was so small that a reliable measurement could not be obtained.

This means that testing in the prone or supine position is preferred (see also below for testing in the seated position). However, testing in the horizontal position has the conspicuous drawback that it bears no resemblance to the functional position of the plantarflexors: The element of weight-bearing and the closed kinetic chain configuration are missing.

Positioning for dorsiflexion

Positioning for dorsiflexion is more straightforward since the dorsiflexors are not involved in weight-bearing. Moreover, their function, which is to prepare the foot for the initial contact of the stance phase of locomotion is strictly part of an open kinetic chain activity. Thus positioning for dorsiflexor testing is the same as that described for plantarflexors.

Research on positioning

The majority of studies of plantar- and dorsiflexor performance have used horizontal positioning (Fig. 8.1), predominantly supine, with varying hip and knee extension (Fugl-Meyer et al 1980, Fugl-Meyer 1981, Nistor 1981, Karnofel et al 1989, Seymour & Bacharach 1990, Herlant et al 1992). The prone (Gerdle et al 1986, Oberg et al 1987) and seated (Wennerberg 1991, Bobbert & Van Ingen Schenau 1990) positions have also been used. In one study which specifically analyzed dorsiflexor strength, sitting with knees at 90° was the position of choice (Backman & Oberg 1989).

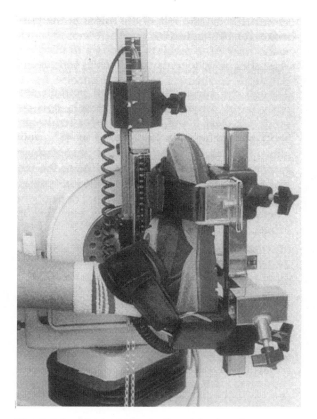

Figure 8.1 Attachment for testing of dorsi- and plantarflexion muscles. Supine test position.

The effect of positioning and test velocity on the strength of plantarflexors was studied by Fugl-Meyer et al (1979) and more recently by Seymour & Bacharach (1990). In the former study it was found that at higher velocities strength was higher by 10–15% when the knee was in extension compared to 90° of flexion.

In the study of Seymour & Bacharach, three test positions were analyzed: (a) supine with knee extended; (b) supine with knee at 90°, and (c) prone with knee extended. Findings indicated that plantarflexion strength scores were highest when subjects were supine with knee in full extension. Strength was less in positions (b) and (c). This observation was valid at all three test velocities. The authors suggested that the low strength scores in supine/knee flexed position resulted from shortening of the gastrocnemius.

However in another study, contrary to these findings, different knee positions did not result in any appreciable variations in plantarflexion strength (Svantesson et al 1991). These authors were not able to offer any explanation of their results but did speculate about the role of the soleus as the prime mover for plantarflexion.

Optimal position for testing plantar- and dorsiflexion

Though the supine/knee extended position obviously favors greater measured strength, it is currently not clear if and how supine (or semi-recumbent) positioning with knee flexed at 45° would affect the results, although some manufacturers recommend this position. In conclusion, the optimal position for plantar- and dorsiflexion testing is supine with the knee in full extension, or nearly full extension for subjects/patients who may find the former inconvenient.

Stabilization

The foot, shank and thigh must all be stabilized, and appropriate foot platforms, bolsters and straps are provided by manufacturers. If stabilization is not carried out properly higher strength scores may be obtained, possibly due to substitutions (Oberg et al 1987).

A recommended position for plantarflexion testing

In the previous edition of this book, the idea of measuring plantarflexion using a *quasi-linear motion pattern* (so-called 'closed kinetic chain') was discussed. In principle the design of the test calls for the subject to be seated with the knee assuming 90° of flexion. For the initial position, the foot is supported by a wedge (Fig. 8.2). Active *concentric* plantarflexion takes place around an axis which generally coincides with the heads of the metatarsal bones. The contracting plantarflexors

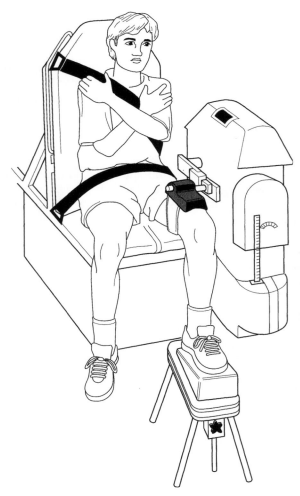

Figure 8.2 Test set-up for ankle plantarflexion strength in 'closed kinetic chain'. (From Möller et al 2000.)

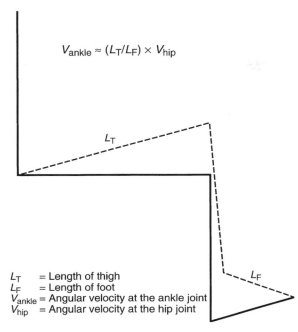

$$V_{ankle} \approx (L_T/L_F) \times V_{hip}$$

L_T

L_F

L_T = Length of thigh
L_F = Length of foot
V_{ankle} = Angular velocity at the ankle joint
V_{hip} = Angular velocity at the hip joint

Figure 8.3 Velocity relationships between hip and ankle joints. (From Möller et al 2000.)

move the shank (tibia + fibula) upwards. The force pad which initially rests on the knee in a substantially collinear configuration with the shank turns around the motor axis via the lever-arm (Fig. 8.2). For eccentric testing the sequence of events is reversed.

It should be borne in mind that the angular velocity of the lever-arm does not apply to that of the ankle. As a result of the differences in lever-arms (Fig. 8.3) the angular velocity of the ankle is approximately 2.5 that of the lever-arm whose axis of rotation is aligned with that of the hip. This test design is significantly more functional than the commonly employed *angular testing* of the ankle plantarflexors and much simpler to apply both in terms of subject and clinician. Its only apparent drawback lies in the fact that the imposed knee flexion results in a shortened gastrocnemius although it does not affect the soleus. However, the results of a dedicated study by Möller et al (2000) indicate that the strength scores are on a par or higher than those derived by other methods besides demonstrating excellent

reproducibility: 0.87–0.97 for the right and left concentric and eccentric exertions.

As the plantarflexion strengths of the right and left sides were similar, the findings were pooled and averaged to yield 177 ± 55 Nm (standard error of measurement, SEM = 14 Nm) and 324 ± 107 Nm (SEM = 26 Nm) for the concentric (Con) and eccentric (Ecc) peak moment, respectively. Worth noting, the Ecc/Con strength would in this case be >1.8, a figure that is generally not typical of comparable 'low' test velocities. Interestingly a similar phenomenon was found with respect to the Ecc/Con ratio applied to combined hip and knee extension (Dvir 1996) strength which was performed at low test velocities, pointing to a variation of this ratio in linear motion pattern.

Alignment of the biological and mechanical axes

The movements of plantar- and dorsiflexion do not pose any difficulties of alignment since the location of the biological axis is well defined. This axis is considered to pass through the malleoli (Inman 1976), forming an angle of approximately 80° with the longitudinal axis of the tibia.

Alignment should therefore be carried out with respect to an imaginary axis which connects the malleoli. A secondary alignment, to take into account the offset angle of 10° from the tibia, is, for all intents and purposes, unnecessary.

Test velocities

A fairly wide variety of velocities has been reported for plantar- and dorsiflexion testing. For instance Bobbert & Van Ingen Schenau (1990) measured plantarflexor strength at 30–300°/s, while Backman & Oberg (1989) used the range 30–240°/s to measure dorsiflexion strength. One reason for using high velocities is to make the testing situation comparable with the functional velocity. For instance, velocities of 150–200°/s have been reported to occur during ankle plantarflexion in terminal stance (Sutherland et al 1980). However, the most commonly used velocities are within the range 30–180°/s.

Whether velocities higher than 30°/s are required depends on the mechanical parameter (e.g. peak moment or mean power) being used as the test criterion.

Peak moment as test criterion

In a study which compared plantarflexion strength at three different velocities, 0, 30 and 180°/s it was found that the moment developed at 30°/s exceeded the isometric moment. There was also a drastic reduction in the strength at 180°/s (Seymour & Bacharach 1990). A parallel observation was made by Karnofel et al (1989), though with respect to a narrower range of velocities. Plantarflexor strength at 60°/s was almost twice that which was recorded at 120°/s. Two possible reasons for these findings are that medium velocities (120–180°/s) may be too high for plantarflexors, and the ROM may be too short.

Stretch–shortening cycle. These arguments cannot fully explain the results obtained in a study by Svantesson et al (1991) which looked into the strength developed by the plantarflexors during a stretch–shortening cycle (SSC). The concentric plantarflexor strength was compared in two experimental situations: first as a result of a single concentric contraction and second, as a result of a concentric contraction which immediately followed (0.03 s) an eccentric contraction. It was found that the moments (near the neutral position of the ankle) in the second case were twice the moments developed by the single concentric contraction, for both angular velocities, 120 and 240°/s. Moreover, plantarflexor moments in SSC-based concentric contractions were minimally affected by test velocity, whereas those developed during a single contraction showed a clear dependence on velocity. It should however be pointed out that, compared with other studies (e.g. Fugl-Meyer 1981) the magnitudes of the SSC moments were very small.

Dorsiflexor strength. When the dorsiflexors are tested concentrically, the moment–angular velocity relationship shows a trend similar to that for the plantarflexors. Backman & Oberg (1989) examined this point in a group of children 6–15 years of age. The decline in concentric strength

with an increase in test velocity was not as dramatic as in plantarflexor testing, but the general impression obtained from this study is of a similar effectiveness of testing using low velocities. It is unfortunate that eccentric testing of the dorsiflexors has not been properly reported, since this contraction mode is of particular importance in the loading response of the stance phase of locomotion.

Mean power as test criterion

However, mean power may be the test criterion, and its maximum is reached at medium/high velocities. In two studies (Fugl-Meyer et al 1982, Gerdle & Fugl-Meyer 1985) the mechanical output of the plantarflexors was examined in relation to the velocities employed and the electrical output (iEMG). It was found that although the strength and total work declined according to the usual moment–velocity relationship, the mean power peaked at 180°/s. It thus appears that the velocity-associated greatest mean power coincides with the velocity for functional demands, namely walking and running.

Conclusion

The above studies lead to the conclusion that a strength-related protocol which does not incorporate SSC activity should consist of low test velocities. Alternatively, if the protocol is power related or if testing is performed in SSC mode the velocities used could be in the medium range. (In the latter case the availability of an active dynamometer is taken for granted.)

It is however clear that the use of very high velocities, i.e. exceeding 300°/s, is of no especial relevance to the ankle complex.

TESTING OF INVERSION AND EVERSION

Test ROM

The movements of inversion and eversion take place in the subtalar joint. In more than one way they are more complex than dorsiflexion and plantarflexion. Inversion results from the combined foot movements of supination, adduction and plantarflexion which occur about the longitudinal, vertical and coronal axes respectively. Eversion is similarly a combination of pronation, abduction and dorsiflexion (Norkin & Levangie 1983). Large individual variations exist in the inclination of the inversion–eversion axis, but a commonly accepted description is that of Manter (1946), according to whom this axis is inclined 42° superioanteriorly and 16° medially, from the transverse and sagittal planes respectively. The ROM about this axis has been described as being between 30 and 50° in inversion, and between 15 and 20° in eversion (Miller 1985). Surprisingly, only one study (Simoneau 1990) has referred explicitly to the tested ROM, quoting an average figure of 82°. Furthermore, there has been no indication regarding the specific angle at which the peak moment was recorded. On the other hand, the use of targets placed at both ends of the active inversion–eversion ROM has been shown to assist subjects in generating a more consistent maximal effort (Leslie et al 1990). In the absence of specific information, it is recommended that the test ROM is the patient's active ROM.

Positioning and stabilization for inversion and eversion

Correct positioning for inversion–eversion testing is as crucial as it is for dorsi- and plantarflexion although some of the difficulties of the latter are absent. In both movement patterns knee position has a significant effect. It has been shown that because of the location of their insertions and line of action, the lateral and medial hamstrings can exert a significant tibial torque component (Osternig et al 1980). This, in turn, may amplify the moment generated by the invertor and evertor muscles. It has been indicated that tibial rotation can be better restrained in the 'close-packed' position of the knee, which takes place near or at full extension (Frankel & Nordin 1980). Consequently, measurement of the moment of the evertors and invertors in this position is likely to be more accurate than testing in a 'loose-packed' position.

Close- or loose-packed positioning

To examine this theory, Lentell et al (1988) studied the moments generated by the invertors and evertors in two different knee angles. In both testing conditions the subject was in the supine position with the hips flexed at 80°. However, whereas for the loose-packed ankle joint position the knee of the tested side was in 70° of flexion, in the close-packed position it was in 10° of flexion. This meant that in the latter case the leg was actually suspended. This was associated with a significant drop in hamstring motor unit activity as shown by EMG. It was suggested that testing in the loose-packed position results in artificially higher invertor–evertor strength because of considerable substitution from the hamstring and other tibial rotators. Hence testing of the invertors and evertors should be conducted in the close-packed position except when it is contraindicated, as in sciatica or tight hamstring.

A survey of studies dealing with isokinetic testing of these muscle groups reveals that the close-packed position was also employed by Karnofel et al (1989), Leslie et al (1990) and Cawthorn et al (1991). Testing in the loose-packed position was used by Wong et al (1984), Simoneau (1990) and Gross & Brugnolotti (1992). Since both methods of positioning offer good to excellent reliability (Simoneau 1990, Cawthorn et al 1991) the decision on which method to employ is based on:

1. clinical contraindications as mentioned above
2. the higher validity of the closed-packed position
3. specific attachments provided by the manufacturer
4. the need to consult representative values and the methods employed in the respective sources.

Angle of plantarflexion

Another issue related to positioning concerns the angle of dorsi- or plantarflexion during the test. Inversion–eversion strength has been measured in three positions: 10° of plantarflexion, 0° (neutral) and 10° of dorsiflexion (Cawthorn et al 1991). In the supine/knee extended position, 10°

of plantarflexion was not only associated with the greatest peak moments but the reproducibility of the test findings was also highest, for both inversion and eversion. On the other hand, Leslie et al (1990) failed to find any significant variation in inversion–eversion strength between the positions of 0 and 20° of plantarflexion. The latter position probably produced an overlengthened configuration of the plantarflexors. Therefore, the question of ankle position in terms of the plantarflexion angle cannot be currently resolved, although it seems that slight plantarflexion would benefit strength production by these muscles.

Recommended positioning

To summarize, in the absence of limitations or contraindications a single evaluation of inversion–eversion performance should preferably be performed in the close-packed position. If follow-up is intended or other structures are involved, the position – close or loose packed – should be determined according to the patient's safety and comfort. The ankle should be maintained at an angle of 10° of plantarflexion.

Stabilization

Stabilization of the subject, in both the supine or semirecumbent/seated position, involves positioning the foot in the attachment with the use of Velcro straps to ensure minimal movement of the foot. The lower leg and the pelvis should be stabilized, using similar means.

Alignment of the biological and mechanical axes

Because of the particular inclination of the inversion–eversion axis, it is debatable whether there is any possibility of proper alignment with current dynamometer designs. Hence, available attachments are based on approximations. One such attachment is shown in Figure 8.4.

To align the axes the dynamometer head is tilted away from the table/bench at an angle which corresponds to the offset of the biological axis. For instance, Lentell et al (1988), who used

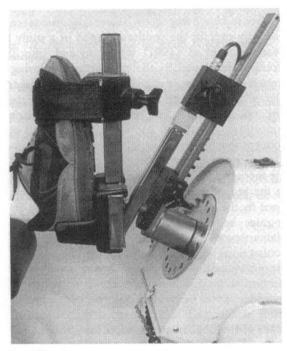

Figure 8.4 Attachment for testing of inversion and eversion muscles. Supine test position.

the Cybex UBXT-Iv/Ev attachment–dynamometer combination, set this angle at 55°. The mechanical axis was made to extend through the superior edge of the lateral malleolus. The same basic configuration has been used by others, sometimes using other dynamometers (Simoneau 1990, Cawthorn et al 1991). No account was taken for the inclination of the other axis of the joint.

Test velocities for inversion–eversion

The range of test velocities for inversion–eversion testing has typically been 30–120°/s. There is only one reported exception, the study by Cawthorn et al (1991), where the test velocity was 160°/s. This was used in an attempt to stimulate subtalar motion during normal walking. In some respects, the arguments for the use of lower velocities in dorsi- and plantarflexor testing apply similarly for inversion–eversion testing. Moreover, for the purpose of normal walking/running, the mean power (which is an important parameter in ankle motion) may not be of parallel significance in subtalar motion.

However, if the main clinical problem is recovery of mechanical output after ankle complex sprain, medium velocity testing may be very relevant. If the concept of primary and secondary restraints as used in the knee, namely the ligamentous and muscular protection of the joint, is applied to the ankle, the speed with which the neuromuscular system reacts to a sudden external inverting force may affect the end result of that force. One might therefore speculate that if the evertors come into play rapidly enough, and their eccentric performance is preserved, the chance for recurrence of injury is likely to be lower.

Admittedly isometric testing, using software routines provided with modern isokinetic systems, can yield valuable information regarding rapidity of mobilization. On the other hand such a test cannot demonstrate strength variations throughout the ROM, which may be vital. Consequently, the present author suggests that medium velocity inversion–eversion testing of patients with sprained ankle is advisable once all symptoms have subsided and normal activity has been resumed. The strength and the time within which the preset speed is reached are the parameters to observe.

PART 2
REPRODUCIBILITY OF ANKLE TESTING

DORSI- AND PLANTARFLEXION

Ostensibly, there is a lack of unanimity regarding this issue. Findings from four studies, with differing test-retest periods are discussed here.

Test-retest gap of at least 24 hours

Karnofel et al (1989) examined the reproducibility of strength findings in a group of 41 subjects. The protocol consisted of three different testing sessions, with at least 24 hours between each one

using 60 and 120°/s as the test velocities (supine position). Intrarater and inter-rater reproducibility, using the correlation coefficient Pearson's r, were in the ranges 0.86–0.94 and 0.87–0.94, respectively. No significant differences in strength values across the three test sessions were evident.

Test-retest period of 3 weeks

Reinking (1992) tested and retested strength and work, at the velocities of 30 and 90°/s in a group of healthy subjects, a period of 3 weeks apart. The intraclass correlation coefficients (ICCs) ranged from 0.87, for peak concentric moment at 90°/s, to 0.96 for peak eccentric moment at 30°/s.

Retesting within 10 minutes

In another study, using the same dynamometer as Reinking, 32 subjects took part in what might be described as an intrasession reproducibility assessment (Wennerberg 1991). Retesting followed testing within 10 minutes. The test velocities were 30 and 120°/s and the seated position was used.

Reproducibility as assessed by Pearson's r was below 0.8 for both dorsi- and plantarflexion and for both velocities. These are of course unacceptable values, especially given the very short retest period. The author suggested that the low correlations could derive from improper positioning, testing in bare feet, and possibly from fatigue because of the short pause between trials.

The points mentioned by Wennerberg raise doubts about the procedural rigor of his study, and stimultaneously help to validate the findings of the other two studies. It is indicated that a well defined protocol ensures acceptable reproducibility of dorsi- and plantarflexion strength scores.

Retesting after 2 years

Fugl-Meyer et al (1985) studied the reproducibility of strength and work in the context of plantarflexor endurance, using a Cybex II system. A group of 13 subjects were tested twice, years apart. Although no correlational analysis was presented, the shape of the endurance curves, peak moment and work versus repetition number were similar in both tests. Moreover, the differences between the two tests were consistently not significant, and less than 10 Nm throughout the test, except for the last 20 of the 200 repetitions.

It was therefore concluded that 'in randomly selected middle-aged males with stabilized levels of physical activities, maximum supine isokinetic plantarflexor output varies only slightly'. Thus plantarflexion endurance, as well as strength, is a reproducible factor.

INVERSION AND EVERSION

In view of their complexity and their involvement in ankle sprain, the reproducibility of performance of the invertors and evertors is of obvious interest. However it was not until the late 1980s that studies were undertaken with contradictory results.

Karnofel et al (1989)

Alongside their analysis of dorsi- and plantarflexion, Karnofel et al (1989) examined the reproducibility of inversion–eversion, using the same protocol with velocities of 60 and 120°/s with the exception that the subjects were seated. Intrarater and inter-rater correlation coefficients (Pearson's r) ranged from 0.85 to 0.93 for inversion, and from 0.78 to 0.89 for eversion. Although the correlation coefficients varied only slightly with test velocity, where there was a difference, correlation was better at 120°/s. Clearly the reproducibility level of invertor testing was on a par with that of dorsi- and plantarflexion, but eversion scores were more variable. The authors suggested that the difference derives from two sources: dorsi- and plantarflexion is a more commonly performed and a more functional activity, and inversion– eversion testing is more complicated. Nevertheless, the reproducibility of inversion testing is definitely acceptable, according to this study.

Simoneau (1990)

Quite opposite results were obtained by Simoneau (1990), who examined reproducibility based on

three testing sessions, 1 week apart. Two velocities were used – 60 and 120°/s – and the test was conducted in the sitting position. The ICCs were consistently higher at the velocity of 60°/s and greater in eversion. Reproducibility improved with additional test sessions. For eversion the ICCs were 0.82–0.93 for strength and 0.83–0.94 for total work. For inversion, the corresponding figures were 0.80–0.86 and 0.72–0.88. These findings indicate acceptability of eversion test findings. Two possible sources for the discrepancy between these studies are the use of different dynamometers, and different positioning and stabilization.

Cawthorn et al (1991)

These authors used a retesting period similar to Wennerberg's to examine inversion–eversion reproducibility. Only a few minutes were allowed until retesting was carried out. Apparently, reproducibility was not affected by the test velocity. The correlation coefficients were acceptable (0.87–0.94) but consistently higher for inversion.

Leslie et al (1990)

In another study, Leslie et al (1990) used a Cybex II system to examine the effect of ROM targets and ankle position of inversion–eversion reproducibility, using two sessions at least 24 hours apart. Tests were performed at 30 and 120°/s. With the use of these targets, 88% of the values of r were significant, compared to only 56% without ROM targets. In addition, a 50% increase in reproducibility, as judged by the number of significant r values, was observed in the test position of 20° plantarflexion. These correlation coefficients were greater than 0.8. No velocity effect on reproducibility was mentioned.

Conclusion

The studies of Leslie et al (1990) and Cawthorn et al (1991) do not help to resolve the contradictions, although it does seem that the reproducibility of inversion test findings is better than that of eversion testing. Moreover, testing in the close-packed position should yield more consistent results. Hence if the aim of the test is to reflect variations over time, the protocol of Karnofel et al (1989), at low angular velocities, is recommended.

PART 3
REPRESENTATIVE VALUES

There is a wide variation among different sources regarding the performance of ankle complex muscles. This is sometimes evident even between studies performed by the same group (see below). As with other joints, side dominance has not been proven to be a significant factor, at least with regard to strength (Fugl-Meyer et al 1980, Wong et al 1984, Leslie et al 1990, Simoneau 1990). Consequently the values refer, where applicable, to the dominant side.

DORSI- AND PLANTARFLEXOR REPRESENTATIVE VALUES
Strength and angular velocity

Performance norms in terms of strength, as a function of the test angular velocity, are shown in Table 8.1. The entries are based on a series of studies by Fugl-Meyer and his colleagues. It should

be noted that whereas considerable differences in plantarflexor strength were recorded between sedentary and trained subjects, the scores for dorsiflexors were very similar and hence quoted only for the former group.

The findings by Karnofel et al (1989) were not incorporated since they did not distinguish between women and men, and the findings of all subjects, who covered a wide range of ages, were pooled together. The findings by Oberg et al (1987) were based, in the case of plantarflexion, on the uncommon prone position and consisted of a relatively small sample, and hence are not outlined here.

Variation of plantarflexion strength with age

Variations in plantarflexor strength as a function of age form an important component of any normative database. Thus although the size of each age category is small ($n = 15$), Table 8.2 which is based on the performance of sedentary Swedish subjects (Fugl-Meyer et al 1985) is of specific significance.

Prediction of peak moment and work

Using the above database, Fugl-Meyer et al (1985) derived the coefficients which appear in Table 8.3. These enable the prediction of plantarflexion peak moment and work from gender (male = 1, female = 0), age and crural circumference. It is of interest to note that weight was not incorporated

Table 8.1 Dorsiflexor and plantarflexor concentric strength. Subjects were tested supine, with full knee extension

Velocity (°/s)	Gender	Peak moment (SD), Nm		
		Dorsiflexors*	Plantarflexors	
			Sedentary*	Trained[†]
30	F	26 (8)	84 (13)	140 (19)
	M	33 (6)	126 (17)	183 (24)
60	F	20 (6)	64 (12)	113 (15)
	M	26 (6)	96 (19)	145 (21)
120	F	15 (5)	39 (7)	75 (13)
	M	18 (5)	60 (14)	95 (26)
180	F	12 (6)	27 (5)	52 (9)
	M	12 (5)	41 (10)	64 (9)

* Fugl-Meyer et al (1980); [†] Fugl-Meyer (1981).

Table 8.2 Age variations of plantarflexor strength at three angular velocities*

Age group (years)	Gender	Plantarflexor strength, mean (SD), Nm		
		30°/s	60°/s	180°/s
40–44	F	108 (13)	87 (12)	41 (8)
50–54	F	101 (19)	78 (14)	35 (7)
60–64	F	78 (15)	64 (13)	30 (5)
40–44	M	171 (27)	133 (22)	62 (13)
50–54	M	154 (21)	119 (16)	57 (11)
60–64	M	139 (16)	106 (14)	46 (9)

* Based on Fugl-Meyer et al (1985).

into the optimal formulae. In the following example the plantarflexor strength of a woman 41 years of age, with a crural circumference of 36 cm, is calculated:

Plantarflexor strength
= gender coefficient + age group coefficient
+ (crural circumference × crural circumference coefficient)
= (39.2 × 0) − 24.4 + (36 × 3.1) = 87.2 Nm

EVERSION AND INVERSION REPRESENTATIVE VALUES

In this instance the sources of representative values are more versatile and up-to-date. As is evident from Table 8.4, there is a surprising compatibility among the three different sources even though the experimental conditions were dissimilar.

Table 8.5 stratifies the representative values in terms of age groups. The data are based on Gross & Brugnolotti (1992). It should be noted that these findings are somewhat higher than those quoted in Table 8.4. It is seen from Table 8.5 that:

1. invertor–evertor strength in women is generally maintained at the same level throughout from 19 to 50 years, and only then declines
2. invertor–evertor strength in men is maximal at the third decade and then declines, thereafter staying generally at the same level throughout the tested age spectrum.

Table 8.3 Coefficients for prediction formulae for plantarflexor performance. Based on Fugl-Meyer 1981 copyright © Springer-Verlag

	Peak moment	Work (joules)
Gender coefficient (× 1 for men, × 0 for women)	39.2	23.4
Age group		
40–44	−24.4	−6.2
50–54	−35.2	−17.9
60–64	−45.4	−24.8
Crural circumference coefficient	3.1	1.8
r^2	0.79	0.63
SD	13.4	12.7

Table 8.5 Age variations of invertor and evertor strength*, in Nm to the nearest integer

	Age group (years)			
	19–30	30–40	40–50	50–62
Women				
Invertors				
60°/s	23 (4)	25 (6)	23 (4)	20 (3)
120°/s	20 (3)	21 (6)	18 (4)	17 (3)
Evertors				
60°/s	20 (3)	18 (4)	20 (5)	16 (4)
120°/s	16 (4)	14 (3)	13 (4)	13 (2)
Men				
Invertors				
60°/s	36 (5)	31 (6)	29 (10)	30 (5)
120°/s	32 (7)	26 (7)	25 (7)	23 (4)
Evertors				
60°/s	29 (3)	25 (5)	25 (7)	24 (4)
120°/s	23 (5)	19 (6)	18 (5)	18 (4)

* Based on Gross & Brugnolotti (1992).

Table 8.4 Invertor and evertor concentric strength (SD*, in Nm)

Source	Velocity (°/s)	Women		Men	
		Invertors	Evertors	Invertors	Evertors
Wong et al (1984)	30	24 (5)	20 (3)	32 (6)	28 (6)
Leslie et al (1990)	30	25 (3)	23 (4)		
Wong et al (1984)	60	20 (4)	16 (2)	26 (5)	24 (6)
Simoneau (1990)	60	19 (5)	17 (4)		
Wong et al (1984)	120	16 (3)	13 (2)	22 (4)	19 (3)
Leslie et al (1990)	120	17 (3)	13 (3)		
Simoneau (1990)	120	14 (4)	12 (3)		

* To nearest integer.

Box 8.1   **Prediction formulae for invertor and evertor strength at 60°/s, based on Gross & Brugnolotti (1992)**

Women
Invertors = 14.312 + (0.057 × weight) − (0.371 × % body fat) + (0.504 × shoe size)
Evertors = −15.726 − (0.061 × age) + (0.977 × leg dominance) + (0.468 × height)

Men
Invertors = 9.188 − (0.114 × age) + (0.83 × weight)
Evertors = −14.433 + (0.086 × weight) + (0.495 × leg girth) − (0.416 × % body fat) + (1.162 × shoe size)

Units: strength (peak moment), ft-lb; weight, kg; shoe size system, American; age, years; height, inches; leg girth, inches, measured at a point one-third of the distance between the fibular head and the lateral malleolus distal to the former; leg dominance factor: dominant leg = 1, non-dominant leg = 2.

Prediction formulae, derived from these findings, for the strength of the invertors and evertors, at 60°/s only are shown in Box 8.1.

STRENGTH RATIOS

The strength ratios – dorsiflexors, plantarflexors and evertors/invertors – have been investigated and are tools for interpretation of isokinetic test data.

Ratio of dorsiflexor to plantarflexor strength

Fugl-Meyer (1981) studied the dorsiflexor/plantarflexor strength ratio in relation to activity level, using sedentary and trained subjects. The value of this ratio appears to be inversely proportional to the test velocity, for both activity groups and for women and men alike. The reason for this decline is a sharper reduction in plantarflexor strength compared with that of the dorsiflexors. This decline should not however be confused with the ability of the muscle to function at higher velocities, as indicated earlier. The variations in this ratio are outlined in Table 8.6.

Ratio of evertor to invertor strength

The particular ratio of evertor/invertor strength was studied by Wong et al (1984), Nickson (1987) and Leslie et al (1990). The findings appear in Table 8.6. Whereas no velocity dependence is apparent from the study of Wong et al, there seems to be a certain decline in this ratio as indicated by that of Leslie et al.

Table 8.6   Ankle muscles strength ratios, as percentages

	30°/s	60°/s	120°/s	180°/s
Dorsiflexor/plantarflexor				
Fugl-Meyer (1981)				
Sedentary				
Women	30	32	38	45
Men	26	27	29	30
Trained				
Women	19	19	20	24
Men	19	19	21	28
Evertors/invertors				
Wong et al (1984)				
Women	81	80	82	
Men	87	90	86	
Nickson (1987)				
Women	79	80	80	
Men	79	76	74	
Leslie et al (1990)	80		63	

PART 4
ISOKINETIC CORRELATES OF CHRONIC ANKLE INSTABILITY

The issue of chronic ankle instability (CAI), which refers to repetitive incidences of lateral ankle instability resulting in numerous ankle sprains (Hertel 2002), occupies, justifiably, a specific niche in the isokinetic literature. CAI engulfs two well established concepts, that of mechanical and functional ankle insufficiency (MAI and FAI, respectively). Rather than two distinct entities MAI and FAI are probably complementary in nature (Kaminski & Hartsell 2002). Hertel (2002) suggests that MAI, which relates to structural changes following an initial ankle sprain that predispose the ankle to CAI, consists of four elements: pathologic laxity, arthrokinematic restrictions, degenerative changes and synovial changes. On the other hand, FAI, which relates to a compromised neuromuscular apparatus, comprises impaired proprioception, postural and neuromuscular control and strength deficits. It is the latter element that has been the focus of a number of studies which have largely applied isokinetic dynamometry.

The reason for attaching specific importance to the ankle muscle complex and its level of performance is the critical dependence of ankle stability on dynamic muscular control. Although its ligamentous protection is far more robust compared to other joints that suffer from inherent instability (e.g. the glenohumeral), the mechanical demands put on this joint system are immense. The combination of a high center of gravity and hence a relatively large gravitational lever-arm, uneven surfaces and speed of motion as well as sudden high velocity impacts may result in a biomechanical combination that exceeds the physiological tolerance of the lateral aspect. This in turn leads to various degrees of collapse of the passive defense provided by the lateral ligaments of the ankle.

Together with the lateral ankle ligaments – the anterior talofibular, calcaneofibular, posterior talofibular, talocalcaneal and cervical – the peronei muscles act to counteract the external inversion–supination moment. As the peronei contract they also elongate and given the fast nature of this contraction it is feasible that the force generated within these muscles is near or at its maximum. Hence the pivotal role that eccentric testing has in the muscular assessment of the ankle in general and cases of instability in particular.

STRENGTH VARIATIONS IN CAI

There is a controversy regarding weakness of the peronei in CAI. In one of the first studies of its kind Tropp (1986) compared eversion strength in subjects with FAI. Significant reduction in peak moment was revealed and attributed to inadequate

rehabilitation and atrophy. Using concentric tests, Lentell et al (1990), Ryan (1994), Lentell et al (1995), Wilkerson et al (1997), McKnight & Armstrong (1997) and Porter et al (2002) reported no selective weakness in the *evertors* of the involved side in patients presenting with CAI although tests covered substantially the full spectrum of test velocities (30–210°/s). In variance with the findings associated with eversion strength Ryan (1994) and Wilkerson et al (1997) reported a seemingly unexpected weakness in inversion strength among CAI patients. This weakness was explained by compression of the deep peroneal nerve, an outcome of lateral sprain, and reduced ability to control the lateral displacement of the foot due to compromised lateral ligaments. As a result, eccentric conditioning of the invertor group was suggested (Wilkerson et al 1997). Eccentric testing in patients with CAI was conducted by Bernier et al (1997) and Kaminski et al (1999). In the former study no differences in either the invertor or evertor muscles was noted. The latter study returned similar findings with respect to eversion strength.

On balance, these studies deny a specific weakness of the evertors but point to a possible compromise to the invertors. Though the absence of expected eversion insufficiency may reflect a genuine situation, it is possible that a number of factors conceal a real problem. First, the possible misalignment of axes (biological versus motor) as well as the test position for eversion–inversion may not impose a pure external inversion–eversion countermoment in the same way it does, for instance, during testing of the other major ankle muscle groups: the plantar- and dorsiflexors. This misalignment, which due to their design and construction takes place in all dynamometers, could put the force vectors of the evertors and invertors in an off-plane position and consequently enable recording of only a fraction of their true potential. In much the same way testing in the seated position is quite at variance with the functional demand and the static effect of gravity. In other words, the operating muscles may already be under a 'bias level' of tension. It is not at all clear whether the test protocols employed have incorporated a sufficient isometric preactivation bias. In addition to these and as pointed out previously, lateral ankle sprain may occur within a very short duration, typically shorter than what is needed for a reflex arch to activate the muscle. Thus, enhanced strength may not offer enough protection in such situations, anyway. On the other hand, lower velocity threats may be averted by higher performance muscles and a better tuned proprioceptive apparatus. These indeed are the major objective of CAI rehabilitation.

STRENGTH RATIOS

The limited value of 'reference' scores as reflected by the sizeable range they span, results mainly from the application of different dynamometers and test protocols. An alternative approach, albeit inherently limited, is provided by using within subject-based strength ratios. The limitation stems from the fact that although the ipsilateral antagonist muscles (e.g. invertors and evertors) may be weaker than their contralateral counterparts, their strength ratio can still be equivalent to the uninvolved side as long as the weakness is fairly uniform.

Strength ratios may generally be divided into two variants: one relates to the more traditional concentric agonist versus concentric antagonist ratios (or their eccentric counterparts), reminiscent of the knee-based H/Q ratio; the other embodies the concept of dynamic control ratio (DCR) as originally proposed by Dvir et al (1989). This ratio is obtained by dividing the eccentric strength of the antagonist by the concentric strength of the agonist or vice versa. It was later adopted and renamed the functional ratio by Bak & Magnusson (1997) to differentiate between painful shoulders and their contralateral uninvolved side as well as by Aagard et al (1998).

Whereas the same mode strength ratios were largely unremarkable with respect to CAI, there was some hope that DCR-type ratios would allow a clear differentiation between involved and uninvolved sides. Specifically targeted was the EV_{ecc}/INV_{con} which relates to the effect the peronei exert while attempting to control the turning (inversion) moment produced by the invertors (Buckley et al 2001, Kaminski et al 2001) upon performance of an angular ('open chain') isokinetic test. However, both studies failed to establish a specific role for either the EV_{ecc}/INV_{con} or the EV_{con}/INV_{ecc} ratios. Thus whether DCR-type ratios have a parallel place to the one they serve for the shoulder and knee is questionable but certainly deserves further research.

REFERENCES

Aagard P, Simonsen E B, Magnusson S P, Larsson B, Dyhre-Poulsen P 1998 A new concept for isokinetic hamstring:quadriceps muscle strength ratio. American Journal of Sports Medicine 26: 231–237

Backman E, Oberg B 1989 Isokinetic muscle torque in the dorsiflexors of the ankle in children 6–15 years of age. Scandinavian Journal of Rehabilitation Medicine 21: 97–103

Bak K, Magnusson S P 1997 Shoulder strength and range of motion in symptomatic and pain-free elite swimmers. American Journal of Sports Medicine 24: 454–459

Bernier J N, Perrin D H, Rijke A M 1997 Effect of unilateral functional instability of the ankle on postural sway and inversion and eversion strength. Journal of Athletic Training 32: 226–232

Bobbert M F, Van Ingen Schenau G 1990 Mechanical output about the ankle joint in isokinetic plantar flexion and jumping. Medicine and Science in Sports and Exercise 22: 660–668

Buckley Bd, Kaminski T W, Powers M E, Ortiz C, Hubbard T J 2001 Using reciprocal muscle group ratios to examine isokinetic strength in the ankle: a new concept. Journal of Athletic Training 36: S93

Cawthorn M, Cummings G, Walker J R, Donatelli R 1991 Isokinetic measurement of foot invertor and evertor force in three positions of plantarflexion and dorsiflexion. Journal of Orthopaedic and Sports Physical Therapy 14: 75–81

Diffrient N, Tiley A R, Bardagjy J C 1974 Humanscale 7/8/9. The MIT Press, Cambridge, Massachusetts

Dvir Z 1996 An isokinetic study of combined activity of the hip and knee extensors. Clinical Biomechanics 11: 135–138

Dvir Z, Eger G, Halperin N, Shklar A 1989 Thigh muscles activity and ACL insufficiency. Clinical Biomechanics 4: 87–91

Fischer R D 1982 The measured effect of taping, joint ROM and their interaction upon the production of isometric ankle torques. Athletic Training 17: 218–223

Frankel V, Nordin M 1980 Basic biomechanics of the skeletal system. Lea & Febiger, Philadelphia

Fugl-Meyer A R 1981 Maximum isokinetic ankle plantar and dorsiflexion torque in trained subjects. European Journal of Applied Physiology 47: 393–404

Fugl-Meyer A R, Sjostrom M, Wahlby L 1979 Human plantarflexion strength and structure. Acta Physiologica Scandinavica 107: 47–56

Fugl-Meyer A R, Gustavsson L, Burstedt Y 1980 Isokinetic and static plantarflexion characteristics. European Journal of Applied Physiology 45: 221–234

Fugl-Meyer A R, Mild K H, Hornsten J 1982 Output of skeletal muscle contraction: a study of isokinetic plantarflexion in athletes. Acta Physiologica Scandinavica 115: 193–199

Fugl-Meyer A R, Gerdle B, Eriksson E, Jonsson B 1985 Isokinetic plantarflexion endurance. Scandinavian Journal of Rehabilitation Medicine 17: 47–52

Garrick J G 1977 The frequency of injury, mechanism of injury and epidemiology of ankle sprains. American Journal of Sports Medicine 5: 241–242

Gerdle B, Fugl-Meyer A R 1985 Mechanical output and iEMG of isokinetic plantar flexion in 40–64-year-old subjects. Acta Physiologica Scandinavica 124: 201–211

Gerdle B, Fugl-Meyer A R 1988 Rank order of peak amplitude of EMG between the three muscles of triceps surae during maximum isokinetic contractions. Scandinavian Journal of Rehabilitation Medicine 20: 89–92

Gerdle B, Hedberg B, Angquist K, Fugl-Meyer A R 1986 Isokinetic strength and endurance in peripheral arterial insufficiency with intermittent claudication. Scandinavian Journal of Rehabilitation Medicine 18: 9–15

Gross M T, Brugnolotti J C 1992 Relationship between multiple predictor variables and normal Biodex eversion–inversion peak torque and angular work. Journal of Orthopaedic and Sports Physical Therapy 15: 24–31

Herlant M, Delahaye H, Voisin Ph, Bibre Ph, Adele M F 1992 The effect of anterior cruciate ligament surgery on the ankle plantar flexors. Isokinetics and Exercise Science 2: 140–144

Hertel J 2002 Functional anatomy, pathomechanics and pathophysiology of lateral ankle instability. Journal of Athletic Training 37: 364–373

Inman V T 1976 The joints of the ankle. Williams & Wilkins, Baltimore

Kaminski T W, Perrin D H, Gansneder B M 1999 Eversion strength analysis of uninjured and functionally unstable ankles. Journal of Athletic Training 34: 239–245

Kaminski T W, Buckley Bd, Powers M E et al 2001 Eversion and inversion strength ratios in subjects with unilateral ankle instability. Medicine and Science in Sports and Exercise 33S: 135

Kaminski T W, Hartsell H D 2002 Factors contributing to chronic ankle instability: a strength perspective. Journal of Athletic Training 37: 394–405

Karnofel H, Wilkinson K, Lentell G 1989 Reliability of isokinetic muscle testing at the ankle. Journal of Orthopaedic and Sports Physical Therapy 11: 150–154

Lentell G, Cashmnan P A, Shiomoto K J, Spry J T 1988 The effect of knee position on torque output during inversion and eversion movements at the ankle. Journal of Orthopaedic and Sports Physical Therapy 10: 177–183

Lentell G, Katzman L, Walters M 1990 The relationship between muscle function and ankle stability. Journal of Orthopaedic and Sports Physical Therapy 11: 605–611

Lentell G, Baas B, Lopez D et al 1995 The contribution of proprioceptive deficits, muscle function and anatomic laxity to functional instability of the ankle. Journal of Orthopaedic and Sports Physical Therapy 21: 206–215

Leslie M, Zachazewski J, Browne P 1990 Reliability of isokinetic torque values for ankle invertors and evertors. Journal of Orthopaedic and Sports Physical Therapy 12: 612–616

Manter J T 1946 Distribution of compression forces in joints of the human foot. Anatomical Record 96: 313–324

McKnight C M, Armstrong C W 1997 The role of ankle strength in functional ankle instability. Journal of Sport Rehabilitation 6: 21–29

McPoil T G, Knecht H G 1985 Biomechanics of foot in walking: a functional approach. Journal of Orthopaedic and Sports Physical Therapy 7: 69–72

Miller P J 1985 Assessment of joint motion. In: Rothstein J M (ed) Measurement in physical therapy. Churchill Livingstone, New York, pp 104–109

Möller M, Lind K, Styf N, Karlsson J 2000 The test-retest reliability of concentric and eccentric muscle action during plantar flexion of the ankle in a closed kinetic chain. Isokinetics and Exercise Science 8: 223–228

Nickson W 1987 Normative isokinetic data on the ankle invertors and evertors. Australian Journal of Physiotherapy 33: 85–90

Nistor L 1981 Surgical and non-surgical treatment of Achilles tendon rupture. Journal of Bone and Joint Surgery 63A: 394–399

Norkin C C, Levangie P K 1983 Joint structure and function: a comprehensive analysis. F A Davis, Philadelphia, pp 341–346

Oberg B, Bergman T, Tropp H 1987 Testing of isokinetic muscles strength in the ankle. Medicine and Science in Sports and Exercise 19: 328–332

Osternig L, Bates B, James S 1980 Patterns of tibial rotatory torque in knees of healthy subjects. Medicine and Science in Sports and Exercise 12: 195–199

Porter G K, Kaminski T W, Hatzel B, Powers M E, Horodyski M 2002 An examination of the stretch-shortening cycle of the dorsiflexors and evertors in uninjured and functionally unstable ankles. Journal of Athletic Training 37: 494–500

Reinking M F 1992 The effect of concentric and eccentric training on the strengthening of tibialis anterior. Isokinetics and Exercise Science 2: 193–201

Ryan L 1994 Mechanical stability, muscle strength and proprioception in the functional unstable ankle. Australian Journal of Physiotherapy 40: 41–47

Seymour R J, Bacharach D W 1990 The effect of position and speed on ankle plantarflexion in females. Journal of Orthopaedic and Sports Physical Therapy 12: 153–156

Simoneau G G 1990 Isokinetic characteristics of ankle evertors and invertors in female control subjects using the Biodex dynamometer. Physiotherapy Canada 42: 182–187

Sjostrom M, Fugl-Meyer A R, Wahlby L 1978 Achilles tendon injury: plantar flexion strength and structure of the soleus muscle after surgical repair. Acta Chirurgica Scandinavica 144: 219–226

Smith R W, Reischl S F 1986 Treatment of ankle sprains in young athletes. American Journal of Sports Medicine 14: 465–471

Soutas-Little R W, Beavis G C, Verstraete M C, Markus T L 1987 Analysis of foot motion during running using a joint coordinate system. Medicine and Science in Sports and Exercise 19: 285–293

Sutherland D H, Cooper L, Daniel D 1980 The role of the ankle plantar flexors in normal walking. Journal of Bone and Joint Surgery 62A: 354–363

Svantesson U, Ernstoff B, Bergh P, Grimby G 1991 Use of a Kin-Com dynamometer to study the stretch-shortening cycle during plantar flexion. European Journal of Applied Physiology 62: 415–419

Tropp H 1986 Pronator muscle weakness in functional instability of the ankle joint. International Journal of Sports Medicine 7: 291–294

Wennerberg D 1991 Reliability of an isokinetic dorsiflexion and plantar flexion apparatus. American Journal of Sports Medicine 19: 519–522

Wilkerson G B, Pinerola J J, Caturano R W 1997 Invertor vs evertor peak torque and power deficiencies associated with lateral ankle ligament injury. Journal of Orthopaedic and Sports Physical Therapy 26: 78–86

Wong D L, Glasheen-Wray M, Andrews L F 1984 Isokinetic evaluation of the ankle invertors and evertors. Journal of Orthopaedic and Sports Physical Therapy 5: 246–252

Isokinetics of the trunk muscles

The literature relating to isokinetic testing of the trunk has continued to flourish during the 1990s reflecting the great clinical interest in various muscle performance characteristics of low-back dysfunction (LBD) patients, the relationship between these and other characteristics belonging to different context structures (e.g. neurophysiological and psychological), the possibility of using this tool in screening of employees and the verification of effort in LBD patients. Other than in the latter application, the scientific evidence emerging from a large number of studies is in some instances confusing and even contradictory. This situation is a direct outcome of the diversity of instruments, protocols, normalization factors, the specific diagnoses and the study samples (gender, age, activity levels) on one hand and the multimodal nature of LBD on the other. Specifically, each of the above five factors contributes significantly to the *error* associated with isokinetic measurements of trunk muscle performance. Thus so-called 'normative' values may only serve as general guidelines and extreme care should be exercised upon their application to individual patients or groups of patients. In this chapter new information on trunk testing has been incorporated and a more critical interpretative approach assumed, particularly in view of the above complexities.

PART 1
GENERAL ISSUES

IMPORTANCE OF SAGITTAL MOTION

The trunk is capable of performing three major rotations: in the sagittal (flexion and extension), frontal (lateral flexion) and transverse (axial rotation) planes. By far the most important among these is the sagittal. Lateral flexion and axial rotation have attracted limited attention partly because of the serious technical difficulty of effectively isolating and accurately aligning the relevant segments. Furthermore, research, not exclusively isokinetic, has found that performance, as shown in the strength curves, of antagonistic lateral flexion and axial rotation muscle groups is basically symmetrical (Thorstensson & Nilsson 1982), and this symmetry is preserved in LBD patients (Thorstensson & Arvidson 1982, Mayer & Gatchel 1988). Although there may be a reduction of up to 25% in rotatory strength in LBD, compared with controls, this is less dramatic than the deficit in sagittal flexion–extension strength (Mayer et al 1985a). The clinical benefit of axial rotation testing may thus be questionable.

Finally, isokinetic test-lift instruments have been used so far to test sagittal plane motions, only. However by creative use of these instruments, lifts in a plane which is not strictly sagittal could be devised, and here lateral extension and axial rotation would also be tested. Nevertheless, this chapter is generally dedicated to the testing, interpretation and clinical applications of sagittal isokinetic motions of the trunk.

CONCENTRIC AND ECCENTRIC ACTIVITY

The mode of contraction under evaluation is of paramount importance in the trunk region. Until the mid-1980s isokinetic studies of trunk performance were almost exclusively limited to concentric contractions. These studies emphasized the 'active' component of extensor performance, namely extension of the trunk from a flexed position. Additionally, based on the controversial

'abdominal balloon' theory, the abdominal muscles were considered a key factor in extending the spine, so measuring their concentric activity was as integral to comprehensive trunk testing as measuring that of the extensors.

However, simple kinesiological analysis shows that except when trunk flexion is performed against gravity (e.g. in a forward rise from a supine position), it is generally assisted by it. Therefore, as soon as the trunk moves anteriorly from an upright position, possibly due to a brief, low-level contraction of the abdominals and hip flexors, eccentric contraction of the extensors is required to control the otherwise 'free fall' of the trunk. This activity becomes even more crucial where handling a load is concerned, particularly when it has to be carefully lowered onto a platform.

It is for this reason that, for a comprehensive trunk evaluation, it is equally important to test the eccentric performance of the extensor mechanism as it is to test its concentric performance. Comparison of concentric and eccentric performance may yield significant information, particularly in the clinical setting and therefore excluding the eccentric component may limit the scope of the assessment, and any conclusions drawn from it. Eccentric trunk muscle activity has been studied in normal subjects and chronic LBD (CLBD) patients in the sagittal plane (Shirado et al 1992, 1995), in the coronal plane (Huang & Thorstensson 2000) and in maximal as well as submaximal levels in normal individuals (Dvir 1997, Dvir & Keating 2001a,b) as well as in CLBD patients (Dvir & Keating 2003). These studies shed new light on the mechanical behavior of the trunk extensors in particular and their differential capacity compared to their concentric counterparts in healthy subjects and especially in CLBD patients.

HARDWARE IN TRUNK ISOKINETICS
ANGULAR MOTION TESTING

Angular motion (AM) isokinetic dynamometers for trunk testing developed along two lines. One used slight modifications to the basic system, fitting special attachments or even incorporating the dynamometer within a totally reconstructed frame. The other approach was to use entirely originally designs, culminating in special purpose dynamometers.

Special attachments

Special attachments/frames, normally used in conjunction with a Cybex dynamometer, were reported in a number of studies. Hause et al (1980), Smidt et al (1980, 1983), Thorstensson & Nilsson (1982), Thorstensson & Arvidson (1982) and Huang & Thorstensson (2000) tested subjects, both with and without LBD in the supine, side-lying and supine and side-lying positions. Langrana & Lee (1984) and Marras & Mirka (1989) tested subjects in the seated and upright positions. The systems used in these studies generally required a great deal of mechanical design work and ingenuity.

There are a number of special attachment designs which lock onto the mainframe and allow testing in the seated position. One such design, the Biodex Back Attachment (Fig. 9.1), consists of a reclined seat, in which the subject is partially reclined but otherwise in almost full body extension, and stabilized. This attachment does not seem to offer accurate alignment since the actuator is connected directly to the seat hinge, which is fixed at the lumbar region. It does however afford

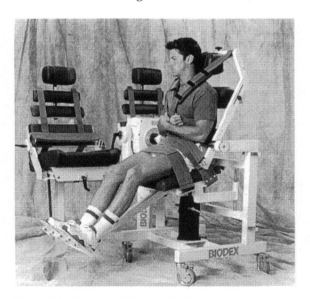

Figure 9.1   The Biodex back attachment.

a full range of trunk flexion and hyperextension. Another advantage is that Biodex is an active system and hence enables eccentric testing or conditioning, in addition to all other modes. The trunk attachment by KinCom also operates on the stand-alone principle. However, there is a striking difference in alignment procedure between this and the Biodex attachment. In the KinCom design, the positions of both the force pad and the mechanical axis are adjustable, using a fairly elaborate assembly of sliding blocks for the pad. The initial position of the subject is sitting, with hips semi-flexed. The KimCom is also an active system, enabling eccentric testing/conditioning.

Special purpose dynamometers

Two manufacturers have produced special purpose AM dynamometers. The Cybex trunk extension and flexion (TEF) unit was the first special purpose trunk machine. The subject is tested in a standing position, and concentric performance may be measured.

This company also produced another special purpose trunk dynamometer, the Torso Rotation Device, which tested torsional trunk muscle performance in the seated position. This machine has not acquired popularity, probably because of the studies of Mayer et al (1985b), as well as its bulk and price. The indications concerning the limited value of trunk rotation testing have recently been significantly reinforced by Newton et al (1993). The authors claimed that rotational testing did not add any useful clinical information to findings based on sagittal measurements. However for the sake of comprehensiveness, data relating to both axial rotation and lateral flexion are presented later in the text.

The Lido isokinetic sagittal tester is a passive special purpose dynamometer system, which allows testing in the standing as well as the sitting position, an option which is exclusive to this design.

LINEAR MOTION TESTING

Alongside the AM devices conventionally used for analysis of trunk isokinetic performance, linear motion (LM) dynamometers enable the measurement of forces developed during combined motion of the trunk and the lower extremities with a possible contribution from the upper extremity. This motion is typically exemplified by lifting tasks. The operation of a typical LM isokinetic dynamometer is based on either a cable which unwinds at a preset linear velocity or a sliding block. The adjustments of the displacement of the handle, by which the cable is pulled, and its linear speed is carried out in a fashion similar to that of conventional testing. Subjects may assume any of the accepted test positions, for example straight knees and bent back, or alternatively bent knees and a slightly flexed back. Figure 9.2 illustrates an LM system (Lift simulator) manufactured by Biodex.

The test consists of pulling up the handle, exerting a submaximal or maximal effort. The test findings show the total force and cannot discriminate trunk muscle output from that of other segments. Hence, although this isokinetic testing method is more nearly functional, its inability to locate deficiencies at the individual joint level is a weakness. Moreover, unlike the situation in AM flexion–extension testing, the subject cannot be accurately positioned, and proven testing practices cannot be followed.

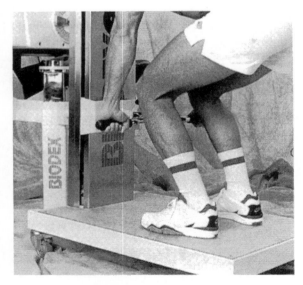

Figure 9.2   The Biodex lift simulator.

In the following sections, isokinetics of the trunk will be discussed in terms of general testing procedures, reference values, interpretation of findings and clinical applications. Where relevant, these sections will separately consider AM versus LM testing.

PART 2
TESTING PROCEDURES FOR THE TRUNK

Trunk evaluation poses particular problems, particularly with respect to LBD patients. Since LBD may be directly or indirectly associated with muscle dysfunction, patients suffering from this syndrome must be tested with extreme care. It should however be emphasized that all studies of trunk extension strength in CLBD reported excellent compliance even in the presence of pain. Notably in a study of the effect of facet joint anesthesia on isokinetic performance of patients with chronic degenerative low back disorders, it was reported that all 87 patients could perform the concentric isokinetic tests despite the presence of pain (Holm et al 2000). In another study CLBD patients performed maximal concentric and eccentric tests and all but one did not complain of pain provocation following the test (Dvir & Keating 2003). Thus trunk testing may be conducted reasonably safely while maintaining the necessary precautions, particularly the general and specific warm-up. Furthermore, it has been pointed out (Mayer et al 1985a) that patients may not produce their maximal force output for fear of injury or pain. It is therefore advisable to extensively use the feedback force/moment signals, available in most systems, as a means of both motivation and instruction. The present author would also suggest that pain scales be used during the tests, so that the examiner is fully aware of any ominous sign.

The issues dealt with in this section are:

1. Alignment of the biological and mechanical axes
2. Positioning and stabilization
3. Range of motion

4. Test velocities
5. Gravity correction
6. Strength normalization for bodyweight
7. Isometric preactivation.

ALIGNMENT OF THE BIOLOGICAL AND MECHANICAL AXES

Trunk motion during isokinetic testing involves a large number of joints including the lumbosacral, the intervertebral (up to the thoracic articulations) and potentially the hip. Consequently, the optimal alignment of the biological and mechanical axes is not as straightforward as is the case with, for example, the knee joint. Consistent alignment is of course a normal prerequisite for repeatability; in the trunk, inconsistency is also liable to lead to differing contributions from the various muscle groups.

Hip joint versus midlumbar alignment

In an early attempt to define the extent of the problem, Thorstensson & Nilsson (1982) compared the effect of aligning the force actuator of the dynamometer with the greater trochanter (hip joint) level, with alignment with an imaginary axis passing through the L2–L3 intervertebral junction. It was indicated that the peak moment, in both flexion and extension, was significantly higher when the axis was aligned with the L2–L3 level compared to the trochanteric level. Furthermore, the difference was greater for flexion than for extension, and resulted in significantly lower extension/flexion ratios, when alignment was made with respect to L2–L3. The authors suggested that these differences could be attributed to hip flexor function and hence use of the term 'abdominal' strength was inappropriate.

LBD patients and controls

In another study (Thorstensson & Arvidson 1982) it was found that the strength of trunk flexion, when the axes were aligned at the hip joint level, was significantly lower in LBD patients compared with control subjects. No significant differences were noted at the L2–L3 level alignment, suggesting a selective hip flexor deficiency in the former group.

Anterior and posterior superior iliac spine, and hip joint alignments

The effect of axis alignment on measured trunk strength was assessed in the seated position, at three velocities, using the Biodex dynamometer (Grabiner et al 1990). Alignment was made with respect to the anterior superior iliac spine, the posterior superior iliac spine and the greater trochanter.

While the statistical analysis did not demonstrate the superiority of any alignment, the data based on the anterior superior iliac spine were associated with the smallest variability overall. Because of the test position and lack of stable pelvic restraint, these findings may be applicable to the Biodex back attachment only.

Lumbosacral versus mid-lumbar alignment

It should be emphasized that in most studies alignment has been made with respect to the lumbosacral joint, L5–S1 (Langrana & Lee 1984, Langrana et al 1984, Marras et al 1984, Smith et al 1985, Mayer et al 1985a,b, Marras & Mirka 1989, Jerome et al 1991), possibly due to ease of location.

This practice was challenged by Stokes (1987) using a simulation of the movement of T12 about a fixed pelvis. It was demonstrated that under normal conditions, the motion of the instantaneous center of rotation of T12 was similar to that of L3 along the total simulated range of motion (ROM) in both flexion and extension. It was therefore suggested that the mechanical axis should be aligned with the L3 vertebra, and pelvic as well as thoracic motion should be maximally controlled. It was also argued that: 'failure to observe these precautions would tend to make the motion of the lumbar spine nonisokinetic and, thus, interfere with angular measurement of spinal motion'. Unfortunately no error analysis was performed, and hence the significance of misaligning the axes at the level of L5–S1 rather than L2–L3 was not determined.

A more recent study sheds additional light on the issue of axes alignment. Amell et al (2000) tested concentric isokinetic flexion and extension in a group of 30 healthy subjects in the standing and seated position where alignment was made relative to five distinct anatomical landmarks (Fig. 9.3) displaced from the reference marker by 25 and 50 mm in the anterior–posterior and superior–inferior directions, respectively. No significant differences were indicated between the two test positions. However, all measurement axes yielded significantly different strength scores (although not between the two superior and two inferior axes) with the inferior axes providing the largest scores, as expected.

Since axis alignment is a significant source of error, its relevance could be diminished if instead of expressing strength in moment (Nm) units, force units (N) were used. That force was a more stable parameter compared to moment was first shown in a study of *isometric* strength of the trunk flexors

and extensors (Rantanen et al 1994). In this study the force sensor was kept constantly at shoulder level while the fulcrum was gradually moved down from the posterior superior iliac spine to the gluteal fold (Fig. 9.4). As clearly evident from Figure 9.5 the flexion and extension average moments increased significantly ($p < 0.0001$) by about 77 and 60%, respectively. On the other hand, the flexion force remained stable while the extension force decreased by about 15%.

The incorporation of force in addition to moment units was applied by Dvir & Keating (2001a) in a study of trunk extension strength in

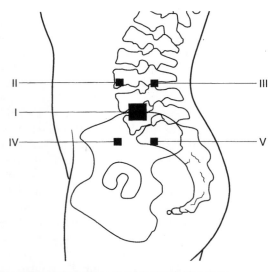

Figure 9.3   Test axis locations for trunk alignment. Measurement axis I (reference axis), the most superior aspect of the iliac crest, was aligned with the axis of rotation of the dynamometer. Measurement axis II was located at a point 25 mm anterior to and 50 mm superior to reference axis I. Measurement axis III was located at a point 25 mm posterior to and 50 mm superior to reference axis I. Measurement axis IV was located at a point 25 mm anterior to and 50 mm inferior to reference axis I, while measurement axis V was located at a point 25 mm posterior to and 50 mm inferior to reference axis I. (From Amell et al 2000.)

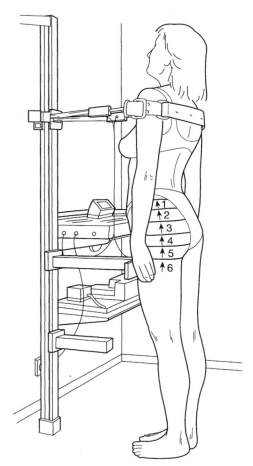

Figure 9.4   Trunk extension strength measurement. The fulcrum is at the lowest level (6) and the black marks drawn on the skin show the other levels. Trunk flexion measurement was similarly measured with the subject's back against the board. (From Rantanen et al 1994.)

which a short ROM of 20° was divided into 10° of hyperextension and 10° of flexion relative to the trunk upright position of the seated subjects. The force sensor was aligned with the vertebral angles of the scapulae while the location of the mechanical axis which was dictated by the structure of the seat and its connection to the mainframe of the dynamometer was above the greater trochanter.

This configuration and the relative length of the lever-arm meant that the thrust against the force pad could be interpreted in terms of quasi-linear motion. The test protocol consisted of concentric (Con) and eccentric (Ecc) contractions performed at 10 and 40°/s. The strength scores which are expressed in both N and Nm were compatible with other studies, conformed with the M–ω

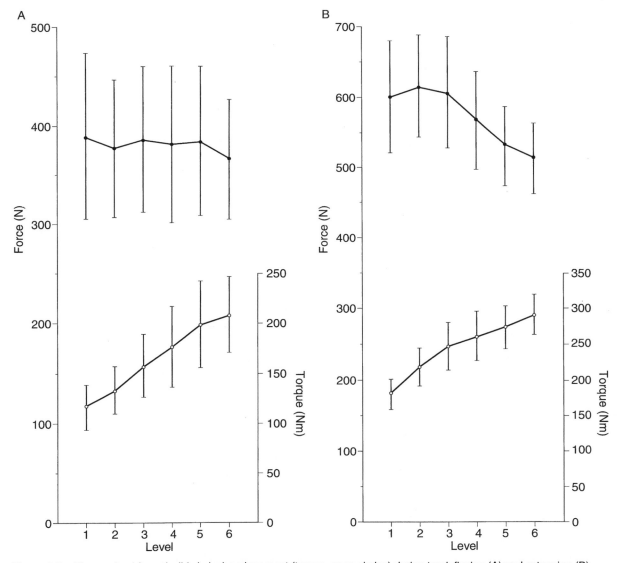

Figure 9.5 The maximal force (solid circles) and moment (torque, open circles) during trunk flexion (A) and extension (B) using different levels of fulcrum. Error bars indicate 99% confidence intervals. 1 and 6 indicate fulcrum at highest and lowest position, respectively. (From Rantanen et al 1994.)

(moment–angular velocity) curve and exhibited Ecc/Con ratios that were well within the expected range. The additional benefit of this protocol is the fact that subjects but especially patients do not have to bend over substantially thus eliminating a significant risk factor. Moreover, bearing in mind the fact that joint motion involves significant non-axial components, the larger the ROMs, the larger is the error. This rule is very much applicable in the case of the trunk as it also involves movement at several intervertebral levels. Consequently, clinicians who insist on testing along large ROMs (e.g. 60° or more) and are also comfortable in locating spinal landmarks are advised to align the axes at the L3 level. Otherwise and where possible, emphasis should be given to the location of the force sensor (pad) and the application of a short ROM.

POSITIONING AND STABILIZATION

Positioning for angular motion

Among procedural parameters, the positioning and stabilization of subjects for trunk sagittal evaluation occupy a central role. Different methods of positioning have been studied over the years and the experience gathered has been incorporated in a number of commercial trunk systems. Early studies used side-lying positions, thus cancelling the effect of gravity (Smidt et al 1980, 1983, Thorstensson & Nilsson 1982). However, this position was not only non-functional, but complex methods were needed to interface the dynamometer with the frame which supported the subject. Other solutions concentrated on standing or sitting test positions but these meant that the gravitational effect had to be accounted for (see below).

To examine the effect of test position on flexion and extension strength, Langrana & Lee (1984) designed a special isokinetic system which permitted tests both standing and sitting. In a group of 25 men, the average extension strengths were 253 and 313 Nm, for sitting and standing, respectively with an extension/flexion ratio of 1.18. (These data were probably not corrected for gravitational effect.) On the other hand the

corresponding figures for flexor strengths were 125 and 220 Nm respectively with an extension/flexion ratio of 1.97.

These results showed that both the extensors and flexors exert greater effort in standing compared to sitting; the sitting position had however a greater effect on flexor strength, reducing this to some 50% of its capacity in standing. This effect was attributed to the involvement of the iliopsoas in the standing position. The authors also mentioned that testing in the sitting position was tolerated better than in the standing position. This finding echoed those of an earlier study (Smidt et al 1983), in which it was noted that the sitting position, compared to standing, allowed greater ROM, both in flexion and extension, and hence was the preferred testing position.

In an attempt to isolate the factors responsible a more recent study (Gallagher 1997) looked into the differences in trunk extension strength as a result of testing in the kneeling versus standing position using a specially fabricated frame. EMG records were collected from eight trunk muscles in order to assess recruitment patterns under each condition. It was revealed that testing in the kneeling posture was associated with a decrease of some 15% in extension strength despite equivalent muscular activity. As a result the altered capacity was attributed to a reduced capability of pelvic rotation in kneeling compared to standing due to disruption of the biomechanical linkage of the leg structures.

In conclusion, testing in the seated position seems preferable as it isolates more efficiently the pelvic–lower extremity component and thus portrays in a better way the singular capacity of the spinal musculature.

Positioning for linear motion

Isokinetic linear motion testing of the trunk is carried out basically in one position, i.e. standing. However, even within this position the initial configuration of the joints may differ as mentioned earlier. Furthermore, the distance between the feet and the external force vector is another factor which ought to be taken into account when setting the test parameters.

Porterfield et al (1987) studied the effect of these parameters on the total work, in two age groups of LBD-free male subjects. The two initial positions were:

1. squatting with arms as straight as possible and head looking forward
2. knees locked and trunk fully curled forward.

The foot positions were toes in a line with the exit point of the cable, or toes 10 cm behind this point. It was indicated that the amount of work generated from the squatting position was greater than that from the straight leg position, and the same applied for the toe-forward compared with toe-backward position. These findings may serve as general guidelines for multijoint isokinetic trunk testing.

Because of the high stresses that are likely to be exerted by the lumbar extensors, lifting activity has to be closely monitored and controlled. For this purpose, and particularly in the case of subjects with or prone to LBD, the test must be preceded by a warm-up session consisting of stretch maneuvers and then submaximal lifts.

Stabilization in trunk testing

Stabilization of body segments, particularly the pelvis, is the next essential step after the selection of test position. Failure to adequately stabilize the segments below the force application point may result in substitution with variations in moment output.

Effect of level of stabilization

Smidt et al (1983) compared the effect of three levels of stabilization on the spatial movement of the spinous process of L5, during testing in the sitting position. Rigorous stabilization was ensured by placing rigid pads in firm contact with the anterior shank (pointing against the tibial tuberosity), anterior thigh, anterior superior iliac spine and immediately below the level of L5–S1. For medium stabilization, the thighs and feet were strapped and for minimal stabilization only the feet were strapped leaving the pelvis, in both cases, unstabilized. It was indicated that although all modes of stabilization were effective in preventing side (lateral) movements, anteroposterior and vertical movements increased with relaxation of strapping.

Another systematic study which examined the effect of several levels of stabilization on trunk flexion and extension strength, was conducted by Timm (1991) using a Cybex TEF system. The ankle, knee, and hip/pelvis regions were independently stabilized. Blocking motion in all of these regions resulted in a configuration of 'maximal stabilization'. The footplate which served to stabilize the ankle could be removed, resulting in 'no ankle stabilization', or the anterior knee pads could be removed resulting in 'no knee stabilization'. Finally, the lowest level of stabilization (minimal) consisted of blocking of hip/pelvic motion only.

The results demonstrated highly significant differences between the above configurations. Analysis revealed significant differences between maximal stabilization and all the others; between minimal stabilization and no ankle stabilization; between minimal stabilization and no knee stabilization, but not between no ankle and no knee stabilization.

The importance of these findings is that they indicate not only that the level of stabilization has a direct bearing on trunk muscle strength, but also that this effect is not necessarily 'linear'. In other words, a more distal stabilization is not directly correlated with a higher force input and vice versa. Therefore, in order to maximize trunk muscle strength in normal subjects, stabilization should be applied to all major joint systems distal to the axis of alignment.

RANGE OF MOTION
ROM in angular motion testing

The literature concerning this topic is not particularly extensive and some studies even fail to specify the ROM. However, in most cases an angular range of some 80–100° is quoted as relevant for trunk testing. For pain-free subjects, the following ROMs were typically used: −10° of 'hyperextension' to 90° of flexion (Delitto et al 1989), or 0–80° of flexion (Smidt et al 1983, Hazard et al 1988, Jerome et al 1991). Langrana & Lee (1984) used a range of 110°

in standing and 50° in sitting, even though Smidt et al (1983) noted that a greater ROM in sitting could be better tolerated, particularly by patients. The isokinetic testing ROM for LBD patients is obviously more limited. Mayer et al (1985a) used 45° for pain-free LBD patients and reduced this range to 30° when clear limitations of motion were noted.

A different approach to trunk strength testing in both healthy subjects and patients has been proposed by Dvir & Keating (2001a,b, 2003). Termed 'short ROM testing' (SRT) it is based on observations indicating that when the angular velocities were adjusted to the ROM in such a way that the nominal lever-arm movement times were compatible with those applied in common protocols (between 0.5 and 2 s) the strength values were compatible with those reported in previous studies. Specifically this protocol was applied for measuring concentric and eccentric trunk extension. The range was 20°, 10° each of flexion and extension about the upright position. The derived M–ω curve exhibited the typical characteristics in both subjects and patients. Research is still to be done on SRT with respect to the trunk flexors in order to generalize and standardize this protocol.

ROM in linear motion testing

The available information regarding LM testing is very limited as this is a rather novel technology. Moreover, since the motion of the end segment is linear, the normalizing effect of angular motion is no longer relevant. The 'ROM' in LM tests depends on the linear dimensions of the subject; given the same angular joint displacements, a tall subject would obviously have to pull the handle a proportionally greater distance than a shorter one. Hence, even if the peak moment is the same for both subjects, the work output may not be comparable.

Since the starting position assumed by the subject depends on personal preference to a great extent, care should be taken to record knee angle, handle height and feet position relative to the handle, in order to ensure ROM repeatability if retesting is envisaged.

TEST VELOCITIES

Angular motion testing

The issue of test angular velocities is more complex and the variations in this case are wider. Goniometry-based measurements of trunk velocities have indicated that these could reach a maximum of 200–300°/s (Thorstensson & Nilsson 1982) while in walking and running the range was 15–75°/s. This observation also fits well with another study (Parnianpour et al 1988) which indicated that the velocity of 60°/s closely approximated the flexion and extension velocities in a number of activities of daily living.

The kinematic behavior of the trunk in LBD and control groups was studied by Marras & Wongsam (1986) using a lumbar motion monitor. It was found that LBD patients differed significantly from controls, presenting with dramatically reduced velocities in flexion and extension. These differences were particularly marked in hyperextension, where patients did not exceed 10°/s in both normal and maximal velocity, versus averages of 35 and 65°/s in the control group. In flexion and extension from flexion, the velocities in the LBD group were within the 30°/s range, whereas the figures for control subjects were roughly between 50 and 100°/s for flexion and 30–75°/s for flexion from re-extension.

In a later study, ROMs, velocities and accelerations in the sagittal as well as off-sagittal planes were measured in 85 subjects (Marras et al 1990). It was indicated that the average velocity in both flexion and extension was 100°/s, and that there was a significant reduction in flexion and extension velocities for motion in the off-sagittal planes.

In the most recent variation of protocol, angular velocities of 10 and 40°/s were employed by Dvir & Keating (2001a,b, 2003) for measuring trunk extension in the seated position. Dividing the ROM (20°) by these velocities and assuming ideal isokinetic conditions would have resulted in segmental movement times of 2 and 0.5 s while testing at 10 and 40°/s, respectively.

Broader performance indices

Alongside the measurement of the strength of the different muscle groups involved in trunk function, there is a growing school of researchers who are looking into broader aspects of trunk muscle performance (see the section on Interpretation for a more detailed analysis). Parameters such as average power and total work at the medium velocities of 120 and 150°/s have been used, in order to arrive at a single performance parameter: the muscle performance index (MPI) devised by Jerome et al (1991), or the average performance deficit (APD) suggested by Timm (1992). Using an alternative approach, Grabiner & Jeziorowski (1992) tested LBD and control subjects at 60, 120 and 180°/s and demonstrated the crucial value of adding the latter velocity to the test protocol. It should be emphasized, however, that the testing of patients in this study took place 8 years, on average, after the initial injury, permitting the incorporation of this relatively high velocity.

Velocities in linear motion testing

The velocities employed in LM testing have normally been quoted in inches per second (ips). Since the metric system is adopted throughout this book, metric units will be used for this parameter also. For some reason, the 'quantal speed unit' reported in most studies has been 15 cm/sec (6 ips). Thus for instance Mayer et al (1985a) tested subjects at 45, 75 and 90 cm/s, speeds which have also been used by Hazard et al (1988). A wide spectrum of testing velocities was reported by Timm (1988): 15, 30, 45, 60, 75 and 90 cm/s.

Prescribing an LM testing velocity in this case is a more difficult undertaking, not only because of the paucity of data, but also on account of individual differences. For instance, given the same angular excursion, a velocity of 15 cm/s may be reasonable for a short subject but unsafe for a very tall one. Subject comfort as well as pain levels should therefore be carefully checked and recorded before initiating a maximal effort test of this kind.

GRAVITY CORRECTION

Due to the mass of the trunk – 63 and 67% of bodyweight in women and men respectively (Diffrient et al 1978) – its gravitational moment can be quite considerable. The magnitude of this moment depends on the location of the trunk's center of mass which is a function of individual anthropometry and the extent of flexion. Clearly, the deeper the bending, the greater is the gravitational moment. Moreover, while in extremity testing the contralateral segment serves as the criterion, the trunk has no such basis of comparison other than in lateral flexion when it is performed in the upright position. In any case the fact that isokinetic trunk testing is regularly performed either in the standing or sitting position necessitates consideration of the gravitational effect.

For a rough estimate of the significance of the gravity factor consider the following example which uses data from different sources. Calculations based on the anthropometric tables of Diffrient et al (1978) indicate that for an adult male, with an 'average' build whose height and weight are 180 cm and 80 kg respectively, the gravitational moment at 30° of trunk flexion is approximately 90 Nm. At this flexion angle, the peak moment-based extension/flexion ratio, for subjects in a side-lying position with L2–L3 alignment and at a velocity of 30°/s, was 2.93 (Thorstensson & Nilsson 1982). Consider now the corresponding extension/flexion ratio of Delitto et al (1991), calculated without incorporating a gravity correction. Measured at a velocity of 60°/s, the average male trunk strength was 223 and 305 Nm for flexion and extension respectively, giving an extension/flexion ratio of 1.36. The average weight of the participants in the study of Delitto et al was 80 kg and therefore as a post hoc 'gravity correction', one should add and subtract 90 Nm to the peak extension and flexion moments respectively. The ratio then becomes (305 + 90)/(223 − 90), i.e. 2.96 which is almost identical to the 'zero gravity' ratio of 2.93 obtained by Thorstensson & Nilsson (1982). This is drastically different, by a factor of more than 100%, from the ratio of 1.36.

Bygott et al (2001a,b)

The most comprehensive and systematic study of gravity correction in trunk testing was carried out by Bygott et al (2001a,b). In the first part, the reproducibility of three methods of gravity correction was analyzed with respect to a KinCom dynamometer. Subjects were tested twice, one week apart. In method I, the dedicated software of the system had been applied over a *randomized* series of test angles at 5° increments spanning 5–40° of flexion and extension. For each angle (and in all methods) subjects were asked to lean on the force pad and relax. In method II, measurements were performed using a *sequential* order which spanned the same angular sectors as in method I. Method III, the dynamic approach, was based on measuring the gravitational effect while moving the lever-arm at 10 and 30°/s. During performance of the tests subjects were asked to close their eyes. Analysis of the findings highlighted the following major trends:

1. the retest was characterized by a lesser variability compared to the test
2. error was greater at angles closer to the vertical
3. trunk extension showed greater variability than trunk flexion
4. method I yielded the most variable findings
5. the most reliable tests were performed at angles of 25–40°.

It was suggested that these results reflected various factors and mechanisms. First, decreased somatosensory input (pressure feedback) was probably responsible for the higher variability in positions nearer to the upright. Second, absence of visual feedback, particularly when the lever-arm was pushing them back may have been disconcerting for some of the subjects. It was also indicated that eccentric test direction probably enhanced relaxation. The authors have therefore recommended that if a single measure was to be used it should be taken from 20–35° of trunk flexion range and 20–30° of trunk extension range as this seems to be the least variable range irrespective of the method.

In the second part of the study the validity of gravity correction procedures was analyzed using estimates of the weight of the HAT (head, arms, trunk) segment and its effect at 25° of flexion and extension. Actual findings were approximated by polynomial regression and compared to the cosine curve yielded by the dedicated software.

Analysis has indicated that none of the procedures closely matched the anthropometry-based estimates. Furthermore, based on all procedures, trunk extension curves were lower than their flexion counterparts. The authors have offered a list of possible factors, some of which accounted for the compromised reproducibility, that could take part in producing the error:

1. inclusion of the pelvic mass in bodyweight estimates
2. difficulty with relaxation
3. attenuation of forces by spinal structures
4. absorption of force by the pad
5. inadequate match between lever-arm angle and trunk angle
6. non-attachment of the subject to the force pad.

As a result caution was recommended when applying these procedures in trunk testing.

Conclusion

The above studies as well as the calculations presented serve to underline the importance of introducing gravity corrections to trunk muscle performance analysis on one hand, and the error incurred when attempting one on the other. Clearly, those studies where the contribution of gravity was ignored, have seriously under-rated extensor strength and conversely over-rated that of the flexors. This has obvious clinical implications besides rendering difficult or even irrelevant any comparison between data which do or do not include a correction. One possible way of dealing with problem of gravity correction in trunk testing is to eliminate its effect as much as possible. Since side-lying testing is non-functional, necessitates complex set-ups and is problematic in higher velocities (see later in this chapter under Lateral flexion), the alternative approach is by limiting the tested ROM to a very short sector in flexion and in extension, both with respect to the upright position. In this way the effect of the gravitational component is considerably limited. Such an approach has indeed been taken by Dvir & Keating (see under ROM in angular motion testing).

STRENGTH NORMALIZATION FOR BODYWEIGHT

In a growing number of studies strength, hitherto expressed in newton-meters (Nm) or foot-pounds (ft-lb), is quoted relative to the subject's bodyweight. The unit of measurement is therefore newton-meters per kilogram (Nm/kg) of bodyweight or ft-lb/lb. Often, as quoted in Mayer's series of studies on trunk function the latter unit was multiplied by 100 to yield a percentage expression. This practice is based on the assumption that individual weight differences partly account for variance in isokinetic measurements.

This assumption is controversial. In a study by Delitto et al (1989), it was indicated that although weight and strength were positively related, the correlation was not significant in women, and in men it accounted for less than 20% of the peak moment variance. It was therefore concluded that normalizing strength by bodyweight cannot be justified in women, and that in men, the range of expected values is quite wide. For instance, based on the findings collected in this study, trunk extensor strength could be regarded deficient if 64% or less of the subject's bodyweight was developed. It was suggested that if factors other than weight (i.e. age and activity level) were added, the variance could be reduced.

These observations were supported by a later study (Jerome et al 1991) which indicated that bodyweight indeed exerted a major effect, greater than that of age or height, on the variance, but increased weight was not necessarily correlated with an increase in strength. The findings of Newton et al (1993) are much the same as those of Delitto et al (1989). In this study of patients with low back dysfunction and normal subjects, gender-based analysis indicated that consistent correlations between bodyweight and isokinetic measurements associated with trunk flexion, extension and rotation were apparent only in normal men. However, even in this individual group, there was no significant correlation between bodyweight and the moment developed during multijoint motion (linear lift). No correlations between bodyweight and any of the isokinetic measurements were found in the male and female patient groups. The authors have therefore concluded that there are no grounds for presenting trunk isokinetic measurements in terms of bodyweight.

The study by Mayer et al (1993) reintroduced the concept of strength normalization. This study included male workers only and is therefore not suitable for estimating normalization to bodyweight in women. Three normalization variables were explored: actual bodyweight, 'ideal' bodyweight (a height/weight estimate based on weight control charts) and 'adjusted' bodyweight which represented the lesser of the other two. The applicability of these variables was tested with respect to isokinetic angular (flexion/extension) and linear ('floor to knuckle' lifting) exertions. It was indicated that the best correlation was achieved using actual bodyweight, with significant r values ranging from 0.49 to 0.67. Two points should however be emphasized:

1. Even though the r score in some instances would seem impressive, it is really R^2 that explains the variability and in this respect the values quoted will account for only between 20 and 40% of the variation.
2. Pearson's r is very vulnerable to the actual range of the base scores and hence outliers would tend to significantly increase its values.

Therefore, the conclusion reached by the authors – namely that bodyweight is the best normalizing factor for isokinetic angular and linear exertions – is questionable. Consequently it is recommended that in all instances, the absolute moment or force (linear lift) values should be quoted, leaving normalization to bodyweight an option.

ISOMETRIC PREACTIVATION

Isometric preactivation (IP) refers to the exertion of static tension immediately prior to the initiation of motion. When IP is employed, the concentric strength curve does not demonstrate the typical inverted U shape. IP therefore has a decisive influence on the average moment but less so in terms of the peak moment. The extent of this influence depends on the magnitude of the IP. The significance of IP in the context of trunk testing has been studied by Grabiner & Kasprisin (1994). Trunk extension was tested concentrically and eccentrically with an IP equal to 0, 25 and 50% of their bodyweight. Results have indicated a trend towards enhancement of performance but this trend was not statistically significant. It is therefore concluded that incorporation of some level of IP may be beneficial but is not strictly necessary in the context of trunk testing.

PART 3
REPRODUCIBILITY OF TRUNK TESTING

Chapter 3 presents a detailed analysis of various reproducibility indices in the context of isokinetic dynamometery, including reference to a study by Madsen (1996) which was dedicated to concentric trunk extension strength using an absolute index, the CVp. Furthermore, given the low significance given in recent years to studies that were solely dependent on the use of Pearson's r, reference to such studies has generally been omitted in this edition.

ANGULAR MOTION AND REPRODUCIBILITY

This issue was studied for the first time by Smidt et al (1980) with respect to the side-lying position. In a later study by this group (Smidt et al 1983) consistency and reproducibility of strength scores were investigated for the sitting position. Scores from 24 subjects were used in the consistency analysis. It was indicated that the intraclass correlation coefficients (ICCs) for concentric flexion and extension were good to excellent ranging from 0.88 to 0.99. Four subjects were retested a week later and the average reproducibility variations in concentric flexion and extension were 13 and 21% respectively. These figures could be partly attributed to the very small sample size.

Study of Smidt et al (1989)

Using the KinCom back attachment, Smidt et al (1989) calculated the reproducibility of a very

large number of variables which they divided into kinetic, electromyographic and trunk angle categories. Using a small group ($n = 7$) and a retesting period of 3 days, it was discovered that:

1. none of the measured variables demonstrated significant variations on retesting
2. the kinetic parameters, peak moment, range of moment rise and decay (between 25 and 75% of maximum), impulse and work were highly reproducible
3. reproducibility of extension/flexion ratios for the concentric and eccentric peak moment and work were clinically agreeable
4. there was good reproducibility of the eccentric/concentric ratio in extension but it was poor in flexion.

It should be mentioned that in this outstanding study, tight control of stabilization and axis alignment, as well as the position of testing (sitting), probably played a decisive role in reducing intertest variations to a minimum.

Delitto et al (1991)

Delitto et al (1991) used another dynamometer, the Lidoback, to test the reproducibility of the normalized peak moment, extension/flexion ratio and average work/repetition, using velocities of 60, 120 and 180°/s. A total of 62 asymptomatic subjects were tested three times with intervals of 1 week and 2 weeks between the initial and retesting sessions respectively. The tests were performed standing and did not include gravity corrections. Intraclass correlation coefficients (ICCs) varied from 0.74 to 0.88, and 0.88 to 0.93, for the peak moment measures and work respectively. However, the standard error of the mean increased with the increase in test velocity. The authors concluded that: 'isokinetic measurements of muscle function offer … sensitive and reliable measurements of trunk muscle performance'.

Newton et al (1993)

In one of the most comprehensive studies so far, Newton et al (1993) tested trunk muscle performance in a group of 70 normal subjects and 120 low back pain (LBP) patients using sagittal and rotational movements. For the reproducibility and learning effect study, a subgroup of 21 subjects and 20 patients was selected and tested on four consecutive occasions, 2–3 days apart. Reproducibility was assessed using intraclass correlation coefficients (ICCs) which, in view of an apparent learning effect, referred to the tests carried out on days 2–4. (The learning effect refers to the variation in the strength scores which cannot be attributed to changes in the actual performance of the muscle(s) but to the acquisition of skill or familiarity with the testing procedures. Thus the first testing day was dropped from the analysis.) The spectrum of velocities for testing extension and flexion consisted of 60, 90 and 120°/s, and for rotations the velocities were 60, 120 and 150°/s.

The peak moments in all test conditions proved to be highly reliable, with ICCs ranging from 0.93 to 0.98 for the 'interobserver' situation and 0.84 to 0.96 and 0.85 to 0.98 for the two intraobserver situations respectively. On the other hand, isokinetic ratios such as flexion/extension, left/right rotations, endurance or recovery, were shown to be unreproducible. It was therefore claimed that these ratios could not be used for clinical purposes. Additionally, the average points variance (APV), which was used in the context of identifying consistency of effort, was not a reproducible parameter. There was a considerable learning effect expressed in increments in the measured variables, ranging from 2 to 16% between day 1 and day 2. The authors recommended therefore that isokinetic performance should be assessed on the second test session, on a different day. Though this is an important reflection, it is doubtful whether such advice can be effectively carried out. It should also be mentioned that learning effect was not observed in a more recent study of trunk extension using short ROM (Dvir & Keating 2001a). Furthermore, 'learning' or practice-based improvement has not been indicated in all reproducibility studies and hence the above recommendation may not be justified under every protocol.

The findings derived from the above studies indicate that based on relative indices peak moment, work and probably impulse are reproducible within the context of angular motion sagittal tests. This statement may be extended to the peak moment in rotational tests. In both cases it refers, however, to the low/medium end of the velocity spectrum.

REPRODUCIBILITY OF LINEAR MOTION FINDINGS

The reproducibility of findings based on LM testing has been examined using the Cybex Liftask apparatus (Hazard et al 1993). A group of symptom-free women and men were tested twice over a period of 3–30 days. The protocol consisted of practice pulls followed by three maximal pulls to waist height. The linear velocity of the handle was not specified. The ICC of the peak force was 0.96 with a standard error of the mean of 58 N. The latter figure is very agreeable, considering the mean and SD of peak force in the first and second test sessions were 948 and 379, and 926 and 374, respectively. On the evidence of this study, LM test findings may be reproducible. However, it is not possible to specify the range of relevant velocities since the test velocity was not quoted.

PART 4
LUMBAR OFF-SAGITTAL PLANE AND CERVICAL MUSCLE STRENGTH TESTING

AXIAL ROTATION

Axial rotation (AR) testing poses special problems regarding alignment and upper limb placement of subjects. However, all studies adopted the seated position which provides the best stabilization for this particular motion pattern. The first systematic study of AR strength was undertaken by Smith et al (1985). Using the Cybex trunk rotation device, 62 men and 63 women were tested at 30, 60, 90 and 120°/s. The findings were expressed in normalized units, namely (ft-lb/lbbw) × 100. The isometric strength was lower than the corresponding isokinetic scores at all velocities except for 120°/s, in both genders. On the other hand, the concentric relationships were in agreement with the M–ω curve. The maximal normalized peak moment (PM) was reached at 30°/s and was equivalent to 70 and 54% of bodyweight in men and women respectively. A rough estimate of these figures, based on the average weight of the subjects, leads to a PM of some 150 Nm in men and about 85 Nm in women.

Kumar (1997) had carried out a series of studies dedicated to trunk muscle strength. In one of these, concentric AR strength was comprehensively explored using a specially constructed system. The study sample consisted of 42 men and 31 women aged 30–34. Testing was conducted at 10, 20 and 40°/s. Subjects were asked to maximally rotate their trunk to the right and to the left from the neutral position or to bring their trunk to the neutral from a fully prerotated position to the left or to the right. Trunk AR strength was lesser in rotation from the neutral to the asymmetric position than vice versa resulting from the length–tension characteristics of the dominant rotatory muscles. Left–right AR strengths were similar in both men and women. The highest AR strength score was achieved at the low velocity test with a conspicuous dropping off as velocity increased. Mean(SD) PMs for men were 79(25), 58(23) and 39(19) Nm at 10, 20 and 40°/s. The corresponding values for women were 52(19), 40(16) and 25(8) Nm. Thus the women/men AR strength ratio stood at a typical 60%.

Tanaka et al (1997) used the commercially available Cybex Torso Rotation unit in order to compare AR strength in hemiplegic patients (50 men, 15 women) with that of normal subjects (42 men, 38 women). The average age of all participants was 60 years. Tests were carried out at 60, 120 and 150°/s. In normal subjects as well as in the patients there was a striking similarity between the left and right rotation. Noteworthy, there were no significant differences between right and left hemiplegia although patients were generally significantly weaker in AR compared to controls, a finding which was attributed to disuse. The mean(SD) PMs in men were 97(25), 87(20) and 84(25) Nm at 60, 120 and 150°/s while the corresponding figures in women were 54(14), 50(12) and 47(13) Nm. In this case as well, the women/men AR strength ratio ranged from 55 to 60%.

Although in Kumar's study the participants were much younger and the test velocities substantially higher, the AR strength scores were significantly lower than those reported by Tanaka et al. For example, in men the smallest average AR score in the former study was 39 Nm (at 40°/s) whereas in the latter, the score at 60°/s was 97 Nm. Given the moment–velocity relationship and age effect, for the results of these studies to be compatible, the latter score should have been much less than 39 Nm. This very striking incompatibility probably derives from the application of different systems and protocols and serves as reminder for the need to standardize. Interestingly, the male AR strength reported by Smith et al (1985) at 60°/s is estimated at 137 Nm. Although the subjects in this study were much younger than those participating in that of Tanaka et al, the discrepancy (137 versus 97 Nm) is still quite significant.

LATERAL FLEXION

Due to its relatively minor role in the trunk motion repertoire, frontal plane testing of trunk muscles was accorded very little attention. Two well performed studies explored this issue using two distinct test positions. Kumar et al's protocol (1995) consisted of 73 normal subjects (32 women, 41 men) and 10 chronic low back pain (CLBP) patients who were tested in the *seated position* using a specially constructed seat and dynamometer. Subjects were tested concentrically at 30°/s along a range of 60° (30 to each side). Maximal strength was achieved for both genders at 20° of lateral flexion (LF) and exhibited very symmetrical bilateral values. In normal women, PM reached a mean(SD) of 77(23) and 73(33) Nm in right and left LF, respectively. The corresponding figures for men were 105(34) and 100(29) Nm. These scores ranged from 60 to 70% of the strength measured in *isometric* LF. Women were about 60–70% as strong as men. Male patients were about 55% as strong as their normal counterparts.

Huang & Thorstensson (2000) performed LF concentric and eccentric strength testing in 12 healthy men using the *supine position* using an articulated bed (swivel bench). The range of motion was a comparable 50–60° and the angular velocities: 15, 30, 45 and 60°/s. At 15°/s the concentric PM was 140(9) Nm, dropping down to 66(12) at the highest velocity. The eccentric PM reached its maximum mean value at 30°/s: 215(36) and its minimum at 15°/s: 211(43). However, the differences between the PMs at the various eccentric test conditions were less than 4% and insignificant. Interestingly, judging from the findings, the eccentric to concentric strength ratios were quite unusually high ranging approximately between 1.5 and 3.25 at the low and high velocities, respectively. Assuming a 60° range of motion and velocity of 60°/s these input parameters are by no means uncommon. Therefore the associated value of 3.25 cannot be interpreted in terms of comparable test conditions in practically all other muscle groups that have been studied so far.

Since the PM at 30°/s reported by Kumar et al (1995) was quite comparable (mean 105 Nm versus 118 Nm) a possible explanation is based on the very sharp slope of the concentric branch of the $M-\omega$ curve. This may indicate a serious difficulty in overcoming body inertia while in the supine position as well as a possible significant challenge in terms of motor control. Thus although eccentric values in the seated position were not provided in the abovementioned Kumar et al study, it will not come as a surprise to learn from future studies that this outstanding finding could indeed be attributed to the test position. As supine LF is not a typically functional position, and in spite of the errors introduced in the seated or standing position, it seems more relevant to test LF in the upright rather than the horizontal position.

CERVICAL MUSCLE STRENGTH TESTING

Cervical muscle performance is a special issue that falls quite outside the mainstream of lumbar spine isokinetics. Strength measurement of these muscles has been conducted using isometric devices and therefore most of the literature refers to isometric strength. Two recent studies reported the application of isokinetic dynamometers for measuring isometric strength (Garcés et al 2002, Seng et al 2002). Measurements were performed in fixed interval between adjacent head positions and did not include rotation strength. By moving the head in a sequential order it is possible to account in a somewhat better way for the natural variations in the instantaneous axes of rotation (IAR) of the cervical spine. Isokinetic measurement of cervical musculature has been reported in two studies (Portero & Guezennec 1995, Portero et al 2001) using a special attachment for lateral flexion. Lateral flexion may be safer for conducting maximal strength testing compared to the sagittal and transverse planes. Both studies used a protocol consisting of a 30° ROM and the single velocity of 30°/s. Alignment of the lever-arm axis was made with respect to the C7–T1 intervertebral space. Measurements revealed very close bilateral symmetry with an average bilateral difference of less than 1 Nm. Lateral flexion strength ranged on average between 30 ± 5 and 52 ± 6 Nm in normal subjects and in members of the French Olympic bobsleigh team, respectively.

PART 5
REFERENCE VALUES

Considering data from isokinetic AM and LM testing of normal subjects and LBD patients, in terms of population size, only a few studies stand out as adequate sources for a so-called normative database. Indeed, except for the studies by Timm (1988) and Freedson et al (1993), which were based on close to 2700 and 4500 subjects respectively, none of the studies qualifies in the strict statistical sense, for this purpose. This is quite surprising, considering the economic significance of LBD and the specific role strength testing plays in assessment of back function. Thus although 'strength is the most tangible aspect of lumbar spine function' (Saal et al 1990), judgments concerning the functional capacity or degree of impairment are still made on a 'local' basis.

Comparison: types of dynamometer

This situation should be regarded in the context of the major difficulties associated with trunk testing. The use of different dynamometers, protocols and study populations renders the findings of most studies of questionable applicability in individual patients. For example, with respect to type of dynamometer, consider the study of Hupli et al (1997) in which two dynamometers – the Lido Multi-Joint II and the Ariel 5000 – were compared regarding trunk concentric flexion and extension performed at 60 and 120°/s in healthy as well as CLBD patients. The gender-pooled findings revealed 1.7–40% of strength difference between the dynamometers with the main variation attributed to extension. Specifically, when based on the gender, this gap was as much as 50% during extension performed at 60°/s. In flexion, only the test at 60°/s yielded comparable results. In terms of performance both dynamometers have shown very little difference between subjects and patients. Interestingly, whereas the Ariel dynamometer exhibited the expected moment drop-off due to increase in the concentric test velocity, the Lido system has indicated a *rise* in moment. It was argued that the Ariel produced lower absolute scores as it lacked a gravity correction mechanism. Moreover, in both dynamometers there was a sizeable EMG activity, of a different pattern, in lower extremity muscles which due to the test standing position could contribute significantly to the observed variations. Differences in protocols are known to have a dramatic effect on the results and in this respect trunk testing is no exception.

Comparison: experimental conditions

The other major obstacle in trunk testing is the absence of a contralateral segment (in the case of sagittal testing) which deprives users of trunk dynamometry of an essential source of comparison. Unfortunately, axial rotation and lateral flexion strength discrepancy may not provide an adequate filler for this void. Furthermore, only a small number of clinical sites possess dual systems. Consequently in interpreting reference data emphasis should first and foremost be put on those studies that applied the same experimental conditions to normal subjects and to patients alike. Second, clinicians should be aware of the vast diversity in test findings and as a result use the following tables as a general guideline only.

Trunk muscle performance

Tables 9.1–9.7 outline data on trunk muscle performance for *angular* sagittal testing in normal subjects and patients with CLBD. These tables represent by no way an exhaustive attempt. Rather, the guiding principle was inclusion of those papers where the same protocol was tested in normal subjects and in patients or when the database was sufficiently large. Thus there are some well controlled studies that do not appear in the tables since they were limited to either of the subject groups.

Tables 9.1–9.4 outline reference data for flexion and extension (F/E) concentric strength in women and men, healthy and with CLBD, respectively. The following points stand out:

1. a velocity dependent drop-off in strength in both genders and groups
2. a reduction in strength in CLBD compared to normal subjects in both genders and in all test conditions
3. a lesser reduction in strength in male compared to female patients
4. a proportional rise in flexion and extension weakness with increasing velocity
5. an F/E ratio < 1 in healthy subjects (women and men) versus an F/E ratio > 1 in female and male patients

Table 9.1 Concentric flexion and extension strength: normal women

Mode/ velocity	Smith et al* (1985)	Nordin et al** (1987)	Newton et al*** (1993)
	n = 63 standing	*n* = 101 sitting	*n* = 35 standing
Flx 30	68	111	
Ext 30	94 [0.72]	122 [0.91]	
Flx 60	68	107	93 (23)
Ext 60	92 [0.74]	108 [0.99]	95 (31) [0.98]
Flx 90			90 (25)
Ext 90			93 (32) [0.97]
Flx 120	61		80 (27)
Ext 120	79 [0.77]		77 (35) [1.04]

* In %ft-lb/lbbw; ** in Nm; *** in ft-lb; ( ) SD; [ ] estimated ratio: Flx/Ext.

Table 9.2   Concentric flexion and extension strength: women with CLBD

Mode/ velocity	Mayer et al* (1985a)	Newton et al** (1993)	% reduction: Mayer et al***	% reduction: Newton et al
	n = 108 standing	n = 47† standing		
Flx 30	39		43	
Ext 30	36 [1.08]		62	
Flx 60	32	68 (26)	53	27
Ext 60	28 [1.14]	60 (25) [1.13]	70	37
Flx 90		58 (30)		36
Ext 90		50 (30) [1.16]		47
Flx 120	13	49 (33)	79	39
Ext 120	12 [1.08]	33 (26) [1.48]	85	57

* In %ft-lb/lbbw; ** in ft-lb; *** CLBD compared to normal subjects in terms of the mean strength; ( ) SD; [ ] estimated ratio: Flx/Ext; † primary referrals.

Table 9.3   Concentric flexion and extension strength: normal men

Mode/ velocity	Smith et al* (1985)	Newton et al** (1993)	Mayer et al* (1993)	Mandell et al† (1993)
	n = 63 standing	n = 35 standing	n = 160 standing	
Flx 30	94			
Ext 30	124 [0.75]			
Flx 60	94	157 (35)	107 (16)	85
Ext 60	121 [0.77]	175 (52) [0.90]	131 (25) [0.82]	95 [0.89]
Flx 90		152 (35)		
Ext 90		166 (52) [0.92]		
Flx 120	90	146 (34)	94 (19)	69
Ext 120	110 [0.82]	146 (52) [1.00]	106 (26) [0.89]	61 [0.76]

* In %ft-lb/lbbw; ** in ft-lb; ( ) SD; [ ] estimated ratio: Flx/Ext; † estimated from graphic presentation.

6. a trend for increase in the F/E ratio with velocity in both genders and groups.

Tables 9.5 and 9.6 outline data based on the normative study of Freedson et al (1993).

Tables 9.7 and 9.9 are specific to full isokinetic testing of trunk extension. The major points deriving from these tables are:

1. Eccentric strengths are greater than their concentric counterparts irrespective of test protocol, gender or health status.
2. Except for a single instance (Ecc 90°/s) in women (Shirado et al 1995) the higher velocity eccentric strength was smaller than that of the lower velocity, indicating a possible reflexive inhibition.
3. In both women and men the decrease in strength characteristic of CLBD was proportionally more conspicuous under concentric compared to eccentric conditions. Indeed in eccentric strength the differences were not significant. This phenomenon probably reflects the lesser extent of volitional control being particularly significant (Dvir & Keating 2003) at the higher eccentric velocity.

4. For both genders, the eccentric/concentric (Ecc/Con) strength ratio in normal subjects differed significantly between normals and patients.

Table 9.8 relates to comparable testing of the trunk flexors. In terms of the relations between the absolute eccentric and concentric strengths there is a great similarity with the findings of the trunk extensors (point 1 above). There was a conspicuous levelling off of the eccentric strength at the higher compared to the lower velocity. There was no significant reduction in strength in CLBD patients versus normals, particularly as expressed in the male group. In women, the concentric strength was reduced proportionally more than in the eccentric condition. The Ecc/Con ratios were somewhat high compared to the study by Wessel

Table 9.4 Concentric flexion and extension strength: men with CLBD

Mode/ velocity	Mayer et al* (1985a)	Newton et al** (1993)	Mandell et al†† (1993)
	n = 108 standing	n = 47† standing	
Flx 30	55 41%***		
Ext 30	49 [1.12] 60%		
Flx 60	53 44%	132 (47) 16%	63 25%
Ext 60	44 [1.20] 64%	115 (51) [1.15] 34%	63 [1.00] 34%
Flx 90		131 (44) 14%	
Ext 90		107 (54) [1.22] 36%	
Flx 120	28 69%	114 (45) 22%	47 32%
Ext 120	22 [1.27] 80%	87 (49) [1.31] 40%	44 [1.07] 29%

* In %ft-lb/lbbw; ** in ft-lb; *** CLBD compared to normal subjects in terms of the mean strength; ( ) SD; [ ] estimated ratio: Flx/Ext; † primary referrals; †† estimated from graphic presentation.

Table 9.5 Reference values (Nm) for extension in women at 60°/s, based on Freedson et al (1993)

Percentile	Age (years)				
	<21	21–30	31–40	41–50	>50
90	176.3	183.3	199.5	173.6	164.1
70	147.4	155.9	163.1	150.1	116.3
50	130.2	138.3	143.7	137.6	107.1
30	117.0	122.6	124.8	116.5	102.2
10	99.1	104.4	100.3	99.0	84.6

Table 9.6 Reference values (Nm) for extension in men at 60°/s, based on Freedson et al (1993)

Percentile	Age (years)				
	<21	21–30	31–40	41–50	>50
90	320.0	333.6	325.4	330.5	259.9
70	272.3	284.8	280.4	276.6	254.4
50	244.1	254.9	248.1	243.4	222.4
30	212.9	223.7	219.7	211.5	197.2
10	173.6	184.4	183.6	180.3	167.9

Table 9.7 Estimated mean concentric and eccentric trunk extension strength (in Nm/kgbw) in normal subjects vs patients with CLBD, based on graphic data from Shirado et al (1995)

Gender/health status	Con 30°/s	Ecc 30°/s	Con 90°/s	Ecc 90°/s
Women/normal	2.26	3.47 [1.53]	2.08	3.61 [1.73]
Women/CLBD	1.19	2.65 [2.22]	0.62	2.48 [4.0]
Percentage reduction in strength	48	24	70	31
Men/normal	3.13	4.48 [1.43]	2.78	4.38 [1.57]
Men/CLBD	1.96	4.00 [2.04]	1.74	3.96 [2.28]
Percentage reduction in strength	37	7	38	10

Con, concentric; Ecc, eccentric; [ ] Ecc/Con ratio for the same velocity.

et al (1992) who have reported an estimated gender-pooled eccentric/concentric ratio of 1.09 and 1.15 for 30 and 90°/s, respectively. Finally, the F/E ratio was very stable among the normal subjects (women and men). It increased significantly under concentric conditions in CLBD, women and men.

The main source for normal subjects performance of *linear* sagittal activity is the study by Timm (1988, Table 9.10). This study produced some 20 tables relating performance to gender and velocity.

Women performed at a level which was generally about 50% that of men. Table 9.11 combines data from the Kishino et al and Timm studies. The findings for normal subjects in the Kishino study were generally compatible with those of Timm. Differences were somewhat higher scores and a more moderate slope of the force–velocity curve. The same gender performance ratios were indicated. The findings also demonstrated a difference of some 25–30% between normal subjects and LBD patients.

Table 9.8 Estimated mean concentric and eccentric trunk flexion strength (in Nm/kgbw) in normal subjects vs patients with CLBD, based on graphic data from Shirado et al (1995)

Gender/health status	Con 30°/s	Ecc 30°/s	Con 90°/s	Ecc 90°/s
Women/normal	1.15	1.57 [1.36]	1.05	1.59 [1.51]
	0.51*	0.45	0.51	0.44
Women/CLBD	0.87	1.44 [1.65]	0.55	1.45 [2.63]
	0.73	0.54	0.89	0.58
Percentage reduction in strength	24	8	47	9
Men/normal	1.55	2.35 [1.52]	1.43	2.30 [1.61]
	0.50	0.52	0.51	0.53
Men/CLBD	1.44	2.1 [1.46]	1.28	2.1 [1.64]
	0.73	0.52	0.74	0.53
Percentage reduction in strength	7	11	11	11

* Flexion/extension ratio based on findings in Table 9.7; Con, concentric; Ecc, eccentric; [ ] Ecc/Con ratio for the same velocity.

Table 9.9 Concentric and eccentric trunk extension strength (Nm) in normal subjects vs patients with CLBD, based on Dvir & Keating* (2001a), Dvir & Keating (2003)

Gender/health status	Con 10°/s	Ecc 10°/s	Con 40°/s	Ecc 40°/s
Women/normal	185 (43)**	214 (51) [1.16]	156 (30)	190 (35) [1.25]
Women/CLBD	114 (48)	159 (74) [1.43]	100 (51)	172 (75) [1.82]
Percentage reduction in strength	38	26	36	9
Men/normal	296 (57)	333 (78) [1.11]	264 (72)	311 (84) [1.19]
Men/CLBD	208 (70)	277 (83) [1.38]	186 (62)	290 (87) [1.65]
Percentage reduction in strength	30	17	30	7

* Findings of test I; ** mean (SD) rounded to integer; Con, concentric; Ecc, eccentric; [ ] Ecc/Con ratio for the same velocity.

Table 9.10 Isokinetic lifting: across age performance parameters*, based on Timm (1988)

Speed, cm/s	Peak force, newtons	Peak force × 100 / Bodyweight	Average force, newtons	Average force × 100 / Bodyweight	Average power, watts	Total work, joules
15	261 (81)	106 (39)	162 (54)	65 (26)	102 (29)	693 (212)
30	245 (77)	99 (37)	149 (51)	60 (24)	143 (59)	638 (231)
45	227 (74)	92 (35)	129 (46)	52 (22)	185 (79)	558 (205)
60	205 (77)	83 (36)	113 (49)	46 (23)	219 (109)	485 (220)
75	197 (82)	79 (39)	108 (49)	44 (24)	266 (147)	475 (236)
90	181 (79)	73 (37)	95 (47)	38 (25)	307 (118)	421 (217)

* Rounded to integers, mean (SD).

Table 9.11 Mean lifting force in lb/s in normal and LBD subjects. Data in parentheses are normalized units, % lb/lbs bodyweight

	n	Velocity, cm/s		
		45	75	90
Women				
Kishino et al (1985)				
LBD	25	70* (53)	62* (45)	55* (40)
Normal	42	105* (78)	95* (72)	90* (68)
Timm[†] (1988)				
Normal	1001	105 (61)	77 (55)	69 (48)
Men				
Kishino et al (1985)				
LBD	43	140* (68)	130* (63)	120* (57)
Normal	23	210* (115)	200* (110)	195* (107)
Timm[†] (1988)				
Normal	1110	200 (107)	173 (86)	161 (79)

* Figures determined from the graphical data; [†] figures based on the average of the four decade groups 20–59.

PART 6
PERFORMANCE INDICES

Several studies have attempted to incorporate other mechanical parameters such as work and power, in addition to strength, in order to arrive at a composite muscle performance index (Jerome et al 1991, Timm 1992). These indices are said to be:

- more reflective of trunk muscle capacity, as they give equal weight to the peak moment

and average power which are maximal at low and high velocities respectively
- more stable than the peak moment in the sense that they are unaffected by the testing velocity and need not be adjusted for age, height and weight.

The muscle performance index

In order to produce a performance index, test protocols consist of a combination of several velocities. Table 9.12 outlines the original protocol used in the study by Jerome et al (1991).

A muscle performance index (MPI) was defined by Jerome et al (1991) using the following formula:

$$\text{Muscle performance} = 0.125(PM_{L1} + PM_{L2} + AP_{H1} + AP_{H2} + BW_{L1} + BW_{L2} + BW_{H1} + BW_{H2})$$

where: PM, peak moment (torque in the original paper); AP, average power; BW, best work repetition; H_1, H_2, highest and second highest velocity respectively; and L_1, L_2, lowest and second lowest velocity respectively.

Table 9.13 outlines the MPI scores obtained in the study from a group of 160 healthy subjects (83 women, 77 men).

Interpretation of performance index

In interpreting the scores some considerations should be borne in mind.

1. The MPI is based on a combination of parameters which do not share a unified unit. Thus although both peak moment and best work repetition are newton-meters (or in foot-pounds) the former is a moment unit whereas the latter is a unit of work also known as the joule. Moreover, power is given in terms of watts (joules per second). Hence the number obtained from the MPI is meaningless insofar as it is assumed to stand for a single mechanical entity.

2. As no significant differences, within gender, were noted among the MPIs of the three protocols, the selection of the protocol is left to the discretion of the examiner.

3. Currently, this index may only apply to flexion–extension analysis, as its applicability to, for example, axial rotations, has not so far been demonstrated.

4. Similarly, the MPI was derived from a sample of normal subjects, and its value for LBD patients has yet to be proven.

While the full implications of the MPI are not known, its single most important advantage is the simultaneous incorporation of muscle performance indices at different velocities. On the other hand, since trunk performance is often expressed relative to norms, the latter must first be established.

The use of the MPI: an example

A male subject, of 42 years, was tested for trunk extension using protocol II (intermediate velocity, see Table 9.13) and produced the test scores shown in Table 9.14. The MPI was thence calculated:

$$\text{MPI} = 0.125(130 + 120 + 250 + 180 + 120 + 95 + 65 + 50)$$
$$= 126.25$$

If the findings quoted in Jerome et al (1991) represent norms, this score would have translated to about a 42% reduction in performance.

Table 9.12 Test protocol for trunk performance index, based on Jerome et al (1991)

Protocol I: low velocity					
Velocity (°/s)	30	60	90	120	60
Repetitions	5	5	5	5	5
Rest time (s)	30	30	30	30	30
Protocol II: intermediate velocity					
Velocity (°/s)	60	90	120	150	90
Repetitions	5	5	5	5	5
Rest time (s)	30	30	30	30	30
Protocol III: high velocity					
Velocity (°/s)	90	120	150	180	120
Repetitions	5	5	5	5	5
Rest time (s)	30	30	30	30	30

Table 9.13 Mean muscle performance (MP) indices, based on Jerome et al (1991)

Protocol	MP-Flexion	MP-Extension	MP-Flexion*	MP-Extension*
I				
Men	197	240	183	227
Women	110	127	127	147
Pooled	148	177	152	182
II				
Men	202	233	186	218
Women	119	133	137	150
Pooled	163	186	164	186
III				
Men	218	269	190	239
Women	164	197	137	155
Pooled	158	186	162	194

* Adjusted for age, height and weight.

Table 9.14   Scores produced by a 42-year-old man tested for trunk extension, using protocol II (see Table 9.13)

	Velocity (°/s)			
	60	90	120	150
Peak moment (ft-lb)	130	120	110	90
Average power (ft-lb/s)	80	140	180	250
Best work repetition (ft-lb)	120	95	65	50

The average performance deficit

Another performance index, the average performance deficit (APD), incorporates – in addition to peak moment, average power and total work – the endurance ratio which is defined as the work comparison between the first and last half of the set of test repetitions (Timm 1992). Conversion formulae enable the calculation of APD from MPI and vice versa.

Discrimination of normal and LBD subjects

The use of multiple indicators for discriminating normal subjects from LBD patients was demonstrated in an excellent study by Grabiner & Jeziorowski (1992). All subjects were asked to exert maximal extensor effort at three velocities, 60, 120 and 180°/s. A set of non-standard isokinetic parameters were extracted, based on the graphic representation as illustrated in Figure 9.6. A mathematical expression using these parameters correctly discriminated between all control subjects and LBD patients. All the parameters were derived from the two higher velocities, emphasizing the significance of muscle power as a major component in trunk muscle performance.

PART 7
TEST STANDARDIZATION AND INTERPRETATION OF FINDINGS

In variance with the first edition, this edition is very restrictive in interpreting data based on

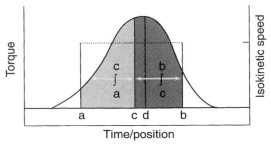

Figure 9.6   Stylized extraction of isokinetic variables; a, onset of isokinetic motion; b, end of isokinetic motion; a–b, isokinetic range; c, midrange moment; d, peak moment; shaded area a–c $^c(\int)_a$, work from onset of isokinetic motion to midrange moment; shaded area c–b $^b(\int)_c$ work from midrange moment to offset of isokinetic motion. Trunk angles are taken from the X-axis, —— moment, –––– isokinetic velocity. X axis refers to the angular position of the lever-arm which is also the displacement of the trunk relative to the initial position. The true isokinetic range is reached past the transient (non-isokinetic) motion. (From Grabiner & Jeziorowski 1992 Clinical Biomechanics 7: 195–200, with permission of Butterworth-Heinemann.)

testing of patients. As mentioned elsewhere in this chapter the diversity of test scores renders any generalization based on these almost irrelevant. Moreover, it is the opinion of this author that in the clinical context, the singular benefit of isokinetic analysis of trunk muscles is the ability to monitor changes and decide when a plateau has been reached. On the other hand, comparison to group 'norms' (whether normal or CLBD) is of little relevance. It is in the particular case of sagittal motion that the absence of a contralateral segment is so crucial.

There is therefore little doubt that standardization of the test is the single most important element which must be resolved before attempting any interpretation. In this context and based on the voluminous data obtained so far, assessment of dynamic performance of trunk muscles in the sagittal plane should consist of 'slow' and 'fast' concentric and eccentric elements. For a comprehensive assessment it may be beneficial to incorporate testing of extension as well as flexion. Thus a patient will have to complete 8 individual test components: 2 (contraction modes) × 2 (velocities) × 2 (movement patterns). For a less rigorous analysis, testing only the extensors should be sufficient, cutting by more than 50% the time and patient effort indicated for the comprehensive assessment. Given the fact that correct lifting involves minimal flexion, the protocol suggested by Dvir & Keating (2001b) is particularly effective as its reproducibility is clinically acceptable, 'learning effect' has been shown not to take place, and is significantly less affected by gravitational effects or by alignment.

From the findings obtained in the various studies mentioned in Part 5 the following principles emerge. In comparison to normal subjects, CLBD patients are likely to exhibit two phenomena: a concentric weakness which is not equalled by the eccentric weakness and an F/E ratio that is very close to unity or even >1. In addition, if the patient is performing at maximal level, the DEC (difference between the eccentric to concentric strength ratio) score should be within the cutoff value (Dvir & Keating 2003). It should be emphasized that appropriate DECs have not yet been defined for all available dynamometers with respect to trunk flexors.

Consequently, if a CLBD patient is judged to be exerting a maximal effort, is exhibiting a reversed F/E ratio and is suffering from what can be described as a particular concentric deficiency in higher velocity testing, this situation may furnish a reasonable baseline relative to which isokinetic analysis can provide an effective platform for clinical decision making. If this patient is undergoing some kind of intervention which addresses strength, sequential monitoring should reveal that the absolute *concentric* extension strength score and probably to a smaller extent that of flexion, increase. This will result in 'normalization' of the F/E ratio although no currently acceptable cutoff value exists with respect to this parameter. Equally, there may be a substantially lesser improvement in the *eccentric* component. Although *endurance* testing could be of great value in monitoring progress, there is a great dearth of knowledge in this respect.

In terms of judging a true improvement the study of Madsen (1996) recommends that not less than 30% of increase in strength, compared to the base level, is required to indicate change (e.g. a real improvement). This study was however confined to healthy subjects, concentric contractions and the fundamental strength variables. It did not address the essential question of the critical CVp in CLBD patients in any of the other relevant parameters. Therefore, this very high cutoff (30%) should be judged using the appropriate scientific and clinical tools. In particular, the relationship between strength improvement and variations in the general functional level should be considered.

PART 8
ISOKINETIC CONDITIONING PROTOCOLS

The question of isokinetic trunk conditioning can be described as terra incognita. Although the principles governing conditioning of muscles in other joint systems may be equally relevant in LBD, almost all clinical literature concerns testing and evaluation rather than treatment.

The indications for trunk muscle conditioning were clearly presented by Mayer and his colleagues in their classical series of papers. Later, in a book on restoration for spinal disorders (Mayer & Gatchel 1988), the authors coined the term the 'deconditioned spine' which referred to measurable deficits in performance, i.e. ROM, strength and endurance, and functional abilities.

As far as muscle capacity is concerned, a significant and selective reduction in extensor performance in maximal effort patients was shown in these studies. Flexion was also compromised in patients performing at a submaximal level, but the main deficit still rested with the extensors. Consequently, the main target in reconditioning of the spine should arguably be the extensors.

A concentric conditioning program

Timm (1987) described the use of concentric isokinetic conditioning of trunk flexors and extensors in the rehabilitation of two back patients. One patient was referred following spinal surgery while the other patient had suffered a right cardiovascular accident. These events had taken place 6 months and 2 years, respectively, before the initiation of the treatment program. Both patients complained of lumbar pain and problems with sitting.

A pyramidal velocity spectrum protocol was used, consisting of 10 repetitions of flexion and extension progressing from 30 to 60, 90, and 120°/s and regressing back down to 30°/s through a ROM of 45°. One minute of rest was allowed between speeds and patients were instructed to perform to personal tolerance while emphasizing the extension component. The ROM was progressively increased to up to 90° of flexion and 10° of hyperextension.

The author quoted consistent improvement in extension and flexion strength during the treatment periods, which typically lasted 2 months, until a complete resolution of the symptoms.

It is, however, difficult to judge the findings of this paper as the strength values quoted by the author were grossly outside the expected capacity of patients, even those who demonstrate outstanding restoration of strength. For instance, one patient whose weight was 179 lb, was reported to reach peak moments of 250 and 291 ft-lb, in flexion and extension respectively, at 30°/s. These numbers translate into 140 and 163 %ft-lb (!), figures attributable to very strong normal males. Though the moments quoted for the other patient were smaller, they too were far from what could reasonably be expected. Thus besides wondering whether the system was properly calibrated one cannot draw any significant conclusion from this study.

However, some elements of the above treatment protocol may be incorporated within a general protocol.

GUIDELINES FOR ISOKINETIC TRUNK CONDITIONING

As far as the isokinetic component of conditioning of low back musculature is concerned, the following considerations should be taken into account:

1. *Assessment of passive compliance following non-isokinetic warm-up*. Most systems are currently equipped with the passive mobility option which requires no effort from the patient to be exerted against the machine. By gradually varying the passive trunk ROM and following the resulting changes in the moment curves one may be able to determine 'failure points'. These may either signify painful sectors of the arc of motion or a disproportionate increase/decrease in soft tissue compliance. These points may consequently serve both as clinical indicators and motion limits.

2. *Proportionately larger emphasis on extension*. The input ratio, in terms of contractile activity, should not be less than 2:1 in favor of extension relative to flexion. Though this is an arbitrary 'rule', the present author believes this to be a more clinically sound proportion. This should be compared with a protocol dictating flexion–extension concentric activity cycles which conform to no particular activities of daily living (ADL) need.

3. *Incorporation of upper force (moment) limits*. Though patients may be their own best judges, it is advisable to set these limits, whenever possible. This option is readily available in all modern systems, and it helps in ensuring that the patient does not inadvertently exceed safety values. Such a limit may be based on the peak moment recorded during prior testing (single exertion).

4. *A spectrum of concentric velocities adjusted to the ROM*. New research is indicating that training within short ROM may induce strength increase outside this ROM (Barak 2003). The velocities used should be compatible with the ROM in a manner described in Chapter 1. For instance, in applying a 30° ROM, the velocities prescribed may be 30, 60 and 90°/s.

5. *Gradual incorporation of eccentric activity*. The stage of incorporation depends on factors which have already been discussed in detail as well as on the patient's tolerance. Prescribing velocities should follow the above guideline. Force or moment limits should be applied throughout.

REFERENCES

Amell T K, Walmsley R P, Narayan Y 2000 The influence of axis placement and subject position on measurement of isokinetic peak moment while using the Lido active back system. Isokinetics and Exercise Science 8: 120–129

Barak Y 2003 The effect of short range of motion muscle conditioning on strength and EMG activity inside and outside the range. Unpublished PhD thesis, Tel-Aviv University, Tel Aviv

Bygott I L, McMeeken J, Carroll S 2001a Gravity correction in trunk dynamometry: is it reliable? Isokinetics and Exercise Science 9: 1–9

Bygott I L, McMeeken J, Carroll S, Story I 2001b A preliminary analysis of the gravity correction procedures applied in trunk dynamometry. Isokinetics and Exercise Science 9: 53–64

Delitto A, Crandell C E, Rose J 1989 Peak torque-to-body weight ratios in the trunk: a critical analysis. Physical Therapy 69: 138–143

Delitto A, Rose S J, Crandell C C, Strube M J 1991 Reliability of isokinetic measurements of trunk muscle performance. Spine 16: 800–803

Diffrient N, Tilley A R, Bardagiy J C 1978 Humanscale 1/2/3. MIT Press, Cambridge, Massachusetts

Dvir Z 1997 Differentiation of submaximal from maximal trunk extension effort: an isokinetic study using a new testing protocol. Spine 22: 2672–2676

Dvir Z, Keating J 2001a The reproducibility of isokinetic trunk extension: a study using very short range of motion. Clinical Biomechanics 16: 627–630

Dvir Z, Keating J 2001b Identification of feigned isokinetic trunk extension effort: an efficiency study of the DEC. Spine 26: 1046–1051

Dvir Z, Keating J 2003 Trunk extension strength and validation of trunk extension effort in chronic low-back dysfunction patients. Spine 28: 685–692

Freedson P S, Gilliam T B, Mahoney T, Maliszewski A F, Kastango K 1993 Industrial torque levels by age group and gender. Isokinetics and Exercise Science 3: 34–42

Gallagher S 1997 Trunk extension strength and muscle activity in standing and kneeling postures. Spine 22: 1864–1872

Garcés G L, Medina D, Milutinovic L, Garavote P, Guerado E 2002 Normative database of isometric cervical strength in a healthy population. Medicine and Science in Sports and Exercise 34: 464–470

Grabiner M D, Jeziorowski J J 1992 Isokinetic trunk extension discriminates uninjured subjects from subjects with previous low back pain. Clinical Biomechanics 7: 195–200

Grabiner M D, Kasprisin J E 1994 Paraspinal precontraction does not enhance isokinetic trunk extension performance. Spine 19: 1950–1955

Grabiner M D, Jeziorowski J J, Divekar A D 1990 Isokinetic measurements of trunk extension and flexion performance collected with the Biodex clinical data station. Journal of Orthopaedic and Sports Physical Therapy 11: 590–598

Hause M, Fujiwara M, Kikuchi S 1980 A new method of quantitative measurement of abdominal and back muscle strength. Spine 9: 171–175

Hazard R G, Reid S, Fenwick J, Reeves V 1988 Isokinetic trunk and lifting strength measurements: variability as an indicator of effort. Spine 13: 54–57

Hazard R G, Reeves V, Fenwick J W, Fleming B C, Pope M H 1993 Test-retest variation in lifting capacity and indices of subject effort. Clinical Biomechanics 8: 20–24

Holm I, Friis A, Brox J I, Gunderson R, Steen H 2000 Minimal influence of facet joint anesthesia on isokinetic performance of patients with chronic degenerative low back disorders. Spine 25: 2091–2094

Huang Q-M, Thorstensson A 2000 Trunk muscle strength in eccentric and concentric lateral flexion. European Journal of Applied Physiology 83: 573–577

Hupli M, Sainio P, Hurri H, Alaranta H 1997 Comparison of trunk strength measurements between two different isokinetic devices used at clinical settings. Journal of Spinal Disorders 10: 391–397

Jerome J A, Hunter K, Gordon P, McKay N 1991 A new robust index for measuring isokinetic trunk flexion and extension: outcome from a regional study. Spine 16: 804–808

Kishino N D, Mayer T G, Gatchel R J et al 1985 Quantification of lumbar function. Part 4: isometric and isokinetic lifting simulation in normal subjects and low-back dysfunction patients. Spine 10: 921–927

Kumar S 1997 Axial rotation strength in seated neutral and prerotated postures of young adults. Spine 22: 2213–2221

Kumar S, Dufresne R M, Van Schoor T 1995 Human trunk strength profile in lateral flexion and axial rotation. Spine 20: 169–177

Langrana N A, Lee C K 1984 Isokinetic testing. Spine 9: 171–175

Langrana N A, Lee C K, Alexander H 1984 Quantitative assessment of back strength under isokinetic testing. Spine 9: 287–290

Madsen O R 1996 Trunk extensor and flexor strength measured by the Cybex 6000 dynamometer. Assessment of short-term and long-term reproducibility of several strength variables. Spine 21: 2770–2776

Mandell P J, Weitz E, Bernstein J I et al 1993 Isokinetic trunk strength and lifting strength measures. Differences and similarities between low-back-injured and noninjured workers. Spine 18: 2491–2501

Marras W S, Mirka G A 1989 Trunk strength during asymmetric trunk motion. Human Factors 31: 238–249

Marras W S, Wongsam P E 1986 Flexibility and velocity of the normal and impaired lumbar spine. Archives of Physical Medicine and Rehabilitation 67: 213–217

Marras W S, King A I, Joynt R L 1984 Measurement of loads on the lumbar spine under isometric and isokinetic conditions. Spine 9: 176–187

Marras W S, Ferguson S A, Simon S R 1990 Three dimensional dynamic motor performance of the normal trunk. International Journal of Industrial Ergonomics 6: 211–224

Mayer T G, Gatchel R J 1988 Functional restoration for spinal disorders: the sports medicine approach. Lea & Febiger, Philadelphia

Mayer T G, Smith S S, Keeley J, Mooney V 1985a Quantification of lumbar function. Part 2: sagittal plane trunk strength in chronic low-back pain patients. Spine 10: 765–772

Mayer T G, Smith S S, Kondraske G et al 1985b Quantification of lumbar function. Part 3: preliminary data on isokinetic torso rotation testing with myoelectric spectral analysis in normal and low-back pain subjects. Spine 10: 912–920

Mayer T G, Gatchel R J, Keeley J, Mayer H 1993 Optimal spinal strength normalization factors among male railroad workers. Spine 18: 239–244

Newton M, Thow M, Somerville D, Henderson I, Waddell G 1993 Trunk strength testing with iso-machines. Part II: experimental evaluation of the Cybex II back testing system in normal subjects and patients with chronic low back pain. Spine 18: 812–824

Nordin M, Kahanovitz N, Verderame R et al 1987 Normal trunk muscle strength and endurance in women and the effect of exercise and electrical stimulation. Part 1: normal endurance and trunk muscle strength in women. Spine 12: 105–111

Parnianpour M, Nordin M, Kahanovitz N, Frankel V 1988 The triaxial coupling of torque generation of trunk muscles during isometric exertions and the effect of fatiguing isoinertial movements on the motor output and movement patterns. Spine 9: 982–992

Porterfield J A, Mostardi R A, King S et al 1987 Simulated lift testing using computerized isokinetics. Spine 12: 683–687

Portero P, Guezennec C-Y 1995 Mise au point d'une méthod d'évaluation de la fonction musculaire du rachis cervical. Annales de Kinéthérapie 22: 31–36

Portero P, Bigard A-X, Gamet D, Flageat J-R, Guezennec C-Y 2001 Effects of resistance training in humans on neck muscle performance and electromyogram power spectrum changes. European Journal of Applied Physiology 84: 540–546

Rantanen P, Airaksinen O, Penttinen E 1994 Paradoxical variation of strength determinants with different rotation axes in trunk flexion and extension strength tests. European Journal of Applied Physiology and Occupational Physiology 68: 322–326

Saal J S, Lerman R M, Keane J P 1990 Objective assessment of lumbar spine function. Critical Reviews in Physical Medicine and Rehabilitation 2: 25–38

Seng K-Y, Lee Peter V-S, Lam P-M 2002 Neck muscles strength across the sagittal and coronal planes: an isometric study. Clinical Biomechanics 17: 545–547

Shirado O, Kaneda K, Ito K 1992 Trunk-muscle strength during concentric and eccentric contraction: a comparison between healthy subjects and patients with chronic low-back pain. Journal of Spinal Disorders 5: 175–182

Shirado O, Ito K, Kaneda K, Strax T E 1995 Concentric and eccentric strength of trunk muscles: influence of test

postures on strength and characteristics of patients with chronic low-back pain. Archives of Physical Medicine and Rehabilitation 76: 604–611

Smidt G L, Amundsen L R, Dostal W F 1980 Muscle strength at the trunk. Journal of Orthopaedic and Sports Physical Therapy 1: 165–170

Smidt G L, Hering T, Amundsen L et al 1983 Assessment of abdominal and back extensor function: a quantitative approach and results for chronic low-back patients. Spine 8: 211–219

Smidt G L, Blanpied P R, White R W 1989 Exploration of mechanical and electromyographic responses of trunk muscles to high-intensity resistive exercises. Spine 14: 815–830

Smith S S, Mayer T G, Gatchel R J, Becker T J 1985 Quantification of lumbar function. Part 1: isometric and multispeed isokinetic trunk strength measurements in sagittal and axial planes in normal subjects. Spine 10: 757–764

Stokes I A F 1987 Axis for dynamic measurement of flexion and extension torques about the lumbar spine: a computer simulation. Physical Therapy 67: 1230–1233

Tanaka S, Hachisuka K, Ogata H 1997 Trunk rotatory muscle performance in post-stroke hemiplegic patients. American Journal of Physical Medicine and Rehabilitation 76: 366–369

Thorstensson A, Arvidson A 1982 Trunk muscle strength and low back pain. Scandinavian Journal of Rehabilitation Medicine 14: 69–75

Thorstensson A, Nilsson J 1982 Trunk muscle strength during constant velocity movements. Scandinavian Journal of Rehabilitation Medicine 14: 61–68

Timm K E 1987 Case studies: use of the Cybex extension flexion unit in the rehabilitation of back patients. Journal of Orthopaedic and Sports Physical Therapy 8: 578–581

Timm K E 1988 Isokinetic lifting simulation: a normative data study. Journal of Orthopaedic and Sports Physical Therapy 9: 156–166

Timm K E 1991 Effect of different kinetic chain states on the isokinetic performance of the lumbar muscles. Isokinetics and Exercise Science 1: 153–160

Timm K E 1992 Lumbar spine testing and rehabilitation. In: Davies G E (ed) A compendium of isokinetics in clinical usage. S & S Publishers, Onalaska, Wisconsin, pp 497–532

Wessel J, Ford D, van Drietsum D 1992 Measurement of torque of trunk flexors at different velocities. Scandinavian Journal of Rehabilitation Medicine 24: 175–180

10 Isokinetics of the shoulder muscles

CHAPTER CONTENTS

Since the publication of the first edition, a relatively large number of studies dedicated to various aspects of shoulder isokinetics have appeared. Many of these related to measuring clinical outcomes following surgical procedures and will not be reviewed in this chapter. On the other hand, some developments took place with respect to the actual testing of shoulder musculature and understanding of the reciprocal contraction mode ratios, also known as the dynamic control (DCR) or functional ratios. Both issues will be discussed in this chapter.

PART 1
GENERAL PRINCIPLES OF SHOULDER ISOKINETICS AND TESTING PROCEDURES

GENERAL PRINCIPLES

The most striking feature of the shoulder complex is the extensive range of movement it affords the arm and hand. Arm motion may be described in terms of three independent movements: swing, elevation and axial rotation. Swing is defined in terms of the angle spanned by the arm as it moves within a plane defined at a given angle of arm elevation and relative to an initial position. For instance if the angle of arm elevation is 90° and its initial position is that of maximal horizontal adduction, a maximal swing of the arm would result in a position of maximal horizontal abduction.

Elevation and scapation

Elevation is probably the most complex among the three movements. It is the movement of the arm away from the body along a plane described by the swing angle(s), and therefore its classification according to the usual anatomical planes seems to have no kinematical merit.

On the other hand, elevation in the scapular plane, also known as scapation (Townsend et al 1991) is of particular significance. Performed at a swing angle of about 20–30° relative to the coronal plane, scapation is characterized by a relatively smooth rotation of the scapula over the rib cage. If no axial rotation of the arm is present, the juxtaposition of the articular surfaces of the humeral head and the glenoid is better than in any other plane. Moreover, the joint capsule is exposed to a minimal amount of stretch. Therefore, evaluation of shoulder muscle performance is best carried out in this plane, especially in patients who suffer from disorders of the rotatory mechanism and/or the capsule (Greenfield et al 1990, Warner et al 1990). This test position has now become very common among practitioners of shoulder testing.

Axes misalignment during isokinetic testing of shoulder elevation

During elevation, the position of the glenohumeral joint proper is not fixed and actually changes quite dramatically. Since for a valid measurement of muscle moment, the biological and motor axes must be maintained in alignment (collinearity); deviation of the bioaxis introduces an error. In one of the original works of this problem (Walmsley 1993a,b) it was estimated that in order to account for this misalignment, the peak moment recorded by the dynamometer during abduction and flexion of the arm should be reduced by some 12.5%.

Mandalidis et al (2001a,b) have assessed the error introduced in measuring the moment during concentric scapation in 20 healthy subjects using isokinetic dynamometry at velocities of 30, 60 and 120°/s. Kinematic planar measurements were recorded using a motion analysis system. Measurements were taken at steps of 12° along a range of motion (ROM) of 60° (from 30 to 90° of

scapation) and the displacement of the center of glenohumaral joint rotation (CGR) was estimated using trigonometric techniques. It was revealed that the CGR did not migrate more than 25 mm and 12 mm proximally and superiorly, respectively. These translate into a maximal misalignment of about 3 cm. Based on the protocol applied the dynamometric recordings *underestimated* the true moment by no more than 6.2%. Velocity did not affect the results or error.

It is therefore suggested that shoulder scapation strength be measured according to this protocol which has also been shown to possess very acceptable reproducibility (Mandalidis et al 2001a,b). This protocol features robust stabilization and the use of an elbow splint which prevents undue flexion in this joint as well as the complex effect of the biceps. It is also clear that testing at the standing position should be avoided unless special circumstances dictate otherwise.

Relationship of arm elevators and shoulder girdle elevators

The importance of the relationship between the muscles responsible for elevating the arm and those which elevate the shoulder girdle is generally overlooked in isokinetic studies (Dvir & Berme 1978). The latter, principally the trapezius (particularly in elevations up to 90–100°) and serratus anterior, rotate the girdle and ensure the stabilization of the acromion. The rotation of the girdle, particularly the scapula, greatly increases humeral ROM, while acromial stabilization prevents the loss of effective deltoid length. The force couple created by the simultaneous activity of these muscles is essential to elevation, since the mass of the upper limb exceeds by a large margin that of the girdle. In the absence of this couple the scapula could override the humerus and no elevation would be possible. Therefore, isokinetic examination of the glenohumeral elevators is to a large extent an examination of the entire mechanism of elevation.

The present author could find no study investigating the separate contributions to elevation of the two muscle groups. Such information could cast light on the mechanism of elevation.

Given the theoretical importance of muscle balance (e.g. the internal versus the external rotators of the glenohumeral joint), imbalance of girdle rotators and humeral elevators might explain phenomena such as deltoid insufficiency, limited ROM and even impingement due to overriding. Measurement of the concentric activity of the girdle elevators against a superiorly positioned isokinetic resistance might provide information about this.

ISOKINETIC TESTING OF SHOULDER MUSCLES

PREPARATION

Because of the risk of injury to the complex shoulder mechanisms, the safety and comfort of the patient must be the prime consideration. Following trauma, surgical intervention or rotator cuff dysfunction, maximal effort testing should not be attempted before submaximal efforts are well tolerated; normally not less than 1 month after the injury or procedure (Albert & Wooden 1991). Moreover, after the first dislocation of a shoulder, there should be a much longer period before any isokinetic testing because of the need for strict immobilization (Reid et al 1991).

Where joint motion must be limited, for instance, because of instability or pain, the mechanical stops should be placed with great care, either manually or using the software.

Warm-up

Warm-up is an essential part of maximal effort isokinetic testing. It should consist preferably of upper limb repetitive low-load isotonics (Albert &

Wooden 1991) or submaximal aerobics lasting up to 5 minutes, so that the test scores are not adversely affected by fatigue. Preparatory submaximal repetitions on the dynamometer could then be performed, at a comfortable lever-arm nominal movement time (see Chapter 2) of 0.5–1 s/movement cycle. For instance, if the ROM is 90° the speed could be adjusted to between 90 and 180°/s irrespective of whether the general movement is one of arm elevation or rotation.

In considering the various input parameters, the movement pattern is a major element. These parameters obviously include: the test ROM; patient positioning and stabilization; alignment of the biological and mechanical axes; plane-specific versus diagonal movements; test angular velocities, and the types of muscle contraction involved.

TEST ROM

Irrespective of all other considerations, the clinical status of the patient is an overriding principle. For instance, if an assessment of elevation performance is sought, the ROM for a patient with impingement should not extend above shoulder level. Furthermore, if the measured parameter is strength, a ROM may be used outside of which strength does not vary unpredictably, as far as is known.

In an isokinetic study of shoulder musculature, Shklar & Dvir (1995) examined the moment–angular position (MAP) curves for concentric and eccentric contractions. Testing was carried out with the subjects seated and the findings are outlined in Table 10.1. There were two basic curve shapes: 'inverted-U' and 'flat'. For muscle groups presenting with the former curve shape, identification of the peak moment angle and hence isokinetic ROM

Table 10.1 Angle of peak moment for shoulder muscles, measured in degrees from the neutral position, based on Shklar & Dvir (1995)

	Mode	Flexors	Extensors	Abductors	Adductors	Internal rotators	External rotators
Women	Concentric	0–120*	0–105	0–105	0–105	45	0–105
	Eccentric	45	90	60	30	60	0–105
Men	Concentric	0–105	75	75	0–105	60	0–105
	Eccentric	60	60	75	45	75	0–105

* Flat curve; values refer to the tested range.

is straightforward. Obviously for the 'flat' curves the strength was practically the same throughout the range. In this case the test angular velocity would be taken into account as a greater ROM is required in higher velocities.

Long and short ROMs

To analyze the effect of ROM on strength, a later study of concentric and eccentric shoulder flexion compared testing at two angular sectors: 80 and 16°, namely a five-fold reduction in ROM (Dvir et al 2002, see also Chapter 2). In attempting to control the movement time of the lever-arm as much as possible, the velocities used in the longer ROM (40 and 160°/s) were reduced proportionately to 8 and 32°/s, respectively. The shorter ROM occupied the middle section of the longer ROM which extended from 50 to 130° of elevation. Thus the shorter ROM coincided generally with a horizontal arm position. It was revealed that testing the shoulder flexors at a substantially reduced ROM led to flattening of the sigmoid M–ω curve, namely *lower* eccentric and *higher* concentric strength scores compared to the respective scores derived from the longer ROM. However, due to the symmetric nature of the flattening this has resulted in comparable isometric strength obtained using interpolation of lower concentric and eccentric velocities.

As this particular short ROM protocol has not yet been applied to clinical situations, the extent to which bilateral differences will be equivalent upon using either short or longer ROM cannot be answered at the moment. However, testing at properly located short ROMs (within the full ROM of the shoulder) may be significantly less threatening to vulnerable and/or painful shoulder structures while still portraying muscle performance. The principle of short ROM testing may be equally applicable to the testing of other shoulder muscles (e.g. internal and external rotators) and is a concept that awaits further research.

POSITIONING AND STABILIZATION

Shoulder test positions, primarily for evaluation of the rotator musculature, have been described in terms of whole body and upper limb postures. The elbow joint was maintained at 90° of flexion in all studies. The positions used have been:

1. Standing with the arm at a slight elevation. This position is also known as the standing/ neutral.
2. Seated with the arm in either slight elevation (seated/neutral) or in any other combination of swing and elevation.
3. Supine with either extended or partly flexed hip and knee joints, with the shoulder in 90° abduction.
4. Prone with the arm hanging freely below the supporting surface.

Movements other than humeral rotation, i.e. elevation or the more complex diagonal motions, are preferably tested using the supine or seated positions.

Effect of posture on rotator performance

The effect of posture on the performance of the rotator mechanism has been the subject of a number of studies.

Soderberg & Blaschak (1987)

These authors used three angular velocities – 60, 180 and 300°/s – to test subjects in six different seated examination positions. In the neutral position, the arm hung freely with 0° abduction or flexion. The arm positions at 45°, and then 90°, of abduction were defined as the 'midabduction' and 'full abduction' positions. The corresponding positions, at 45 and 90° of flexion were termed 'midflexion' and 'full flexion' positions. The arm position at 45° of flexion and abduction was termed midposition. Stabilization was provided only for the forearm, using a V-shaped padded trough to support the elbow. Gravity correction was not performed.

The differences in the mean peak moment between the six positions were found to be significant. The order of positions for decreasing strength for the internal rotators was: neutral, full flexion, full abduction, midabduction, midposition and midflexion. For the external rotators it was: full abduction, neutral, midposition, midabduction, full flexion and midflexion.

The authors suggested that the differences were caused by: gravitational factors, which were not accounted for; variations in the length–tension relationships of the rotator cuff and other muscles, and variations in the ligament and capsule structures which provide the fulcrum. They did not explain why the highest internal rotation moment was produced in the neutral position; the muscles involved are not necessarily at their optimal length in this position.

On the other hand the fact that full abduction led to the maximal external rotation moment agreed with the length pattern of teres minor and infraspinatus. It was concluded that the neutral position for both internal and external rotators was optimal.

Hageman et al (1989)

Hagemen et al (1989) compared the 45° abduction and 45° flexion positions in both concentric and eccentric test conditions. No stabilization other than elbow support was used. They found that the 45° abduction position resulted in significantly higher concentric and eccentric strength values for external rotation for both women and men, and generally comparable results in internal rotation.

Walmsley & Szybbo (1987), Hinton (1988) and Reid et al (1989)

Walmsley & Szybbo (1987) compared the concentric internal and external rotatory strength in three positions: standing with the arm at 15° abduction (neutral), seated with the arm flexed at 90° and supine with the arm at 90° abduction. While the elbow was supported in all positions there seems to have been no stabilization in the standing position, but straps were used in the supine position. Their findings indicated that the preferred positions for internal and external rotation were standing/neutral and seated/flexed respectively.

A study by Hinton (1988) supported the findings with respect to testing internal rotators but

indicated that the supine/90° abduction position was significantly better for external rotation.

Using basically the same test positions, Reid et al (1989) failed to support these observations, finding that peak concentric moments did not differ significantly between standing and supine positions.

Greenfield et al (1990), Hellwig & Perrin (1991)

The effect on rotator strength of two variants of the standing position, i.e. the arm elevated at 45° in the frontal or the scapular plane, and without proper stabilization, was investigated by Greenfield et al (1990). It was concluded that the scapular plane was the more suitable as, in this plane, the joint was in a loose-packed position, allowing unrestricted motion during rotation. It was therefore better suited for patients with various dysfunctions of the shoulder joint, such as rotator cuff impingement or chronic dislocations.

Another study compared rotator performance in the scapular and frontal planes (Hellwig & Perrin 1991). Using the seated, stabilized, 90° abducted arm position, and also evaluating eccentric performance, the authors failed to demonstrate significant differences between the two planes although they recommended testing in the scapular plane.

Smith et al (2001)

In a meticulously described study, Smith et al (2001) focused on developing a standardized technique for measuring rotational strength with the scapula in a protracted position. This position is common to a range of daily and occupational activities. For testing, the subject was seated and the dynamometer seat was rotated 45° relative to the sagittal. The elbow was maintained at 90° flexion using a plastic brace whereas wrist movement was prevented using a wrist pad (Figs 10.1 and 10.2). Stabilization of the subject was accomplished using pelvic and thoracic straps. In order to create scapular protraction (anterior movement relative to the rib cage) the seat was backward along the plane formed by the arm and forearm. This 7–8 cm movement resulted in about 3–4 cm

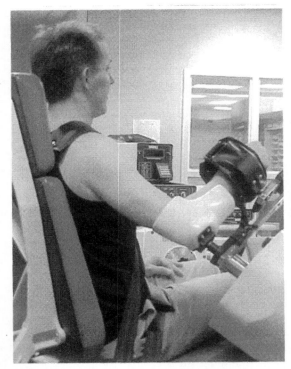

Figure 10.1   Test position of 45° scapation and scapula in the neutral position. (From Smith et al 2001.)

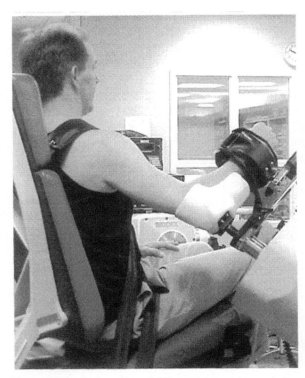

Figure 10.2   Test position of 45° scapation and scapula in the protracted position. (From Smith et al 2001.)

of scapular protraction. Rotational motion took place along a ROM of 75° and a single velocity of 90°, using an isometric preactivation bias of 25 N.

A test-retest design revealed almost perfect intraclass correlation coefficients (3,1) ranging from 0.97 to 0.99 for both internal and external rotations. Significantly, the standard errors of measurement were between 2 and 3% for internal rotation and about 3–6% in external rotation leading to an overall excellent reproducibility. In consequence, this protocol is highly recommended for testing rotational movement in normal subjects. Its applicability for patients has yet to be determined.

Test position and activity pattern

Particular positions may be more suitable for specific subjects, as has been indicated in a study which examined rotator testing in prone and supine positions in a group of swimmers (Falkel et al 1987). It was shown that rotator strength in the prone position was significantly higher than in the supine, by 20–40%. These findings reflect the importance of the correspondence between the test position and the general activity pattern of the joint under consideration.

Stabilization

Like alignment, stabilization is particularly important because of the large number of muscles involved in the execution of even simple movements. Clearly, there is a direct association between the magnitude of the moment developed by the muscle(s) and the degree of stabilization required; submaximal, compared with maximal contractions may not require very rigorous stabilizing.

As mentioned earlier stabilization has two purposes: to portray, as faithfully as possible, the length–tension relationships of the muscles under consideration; and to maintain at a minimal level, or even to exclude, contributions from other muscles. Thus, prone positioning for rotator cuff testing calls for minimal stabilization as friction and gravity limit postural demands. On the other hand, the upright position, when used for rotator cuff testing, requires stabilization at nearly all the major joint systems, particularly at the spine and pelvis.

Methods of stabilization

Various methods of stabilization have been described. The least rigorous consists of supporting the elbow only. At the other extreme, Wilk et al (1991) describe stabilization of the trunk, while the subject is in the seated position, using a combination of a pelvic strap and a pair of straps which cross each other diagonally at mid-sternal level. Other studies, using the supine position, describe the application of two straps, at mid-thoracic and pelvic levels.

Conclusions

In view of the foregoing discussion, there does not seem to be an acceptable formula concerning the selection of position and method of stabilization. The use of diagonal patterns may not be ideal for evaluating the rotator cuff, however appealing this method in terms of expediency or functionality. Also there is for instance no indication as to whether the same extent of stabilization is needed in treatment sessions as in testing. Since most shoulder activities are performed with the trunk vertical, functionality is not served by horizontal positioning, although the latter improves stabilization. On the other hand, testing/treating the shoulder while the patient stands means that, because of the design of most isokinetic dynamometers, shoulder movement other than rotations cannot be assessed. Also, this position almost precludes effective stabilization and may not be comfortable for longer periods of conditioning.

Consequently, considering all of the commonly tested/treated shoulder motions, as well as the increasing number of studies using such stabilization it seems that the optimal position is in sitting. The trunk should remain upright or very slightly inclined, and stabilized, mainly during testing, according to the method described by Smith et al (2001). This calls for chest as well as pelvic straps to be applied where the previous may cross each other at mid-sternal level or remain parallel.

Therefore, for testing humeral (internal/external) rotations the arm should be positioned in the scapular plane, between 30 and 45° anterior to the frontal plane and elevated to approximately 45°, with the elbow flexed at 90° and supported. Supporting the elbow and ensuring that it remains at 90° of flexion is probably vital to the reproducibility and hence should be followed when criterion (follow-up) measurements are performed. The forearm should remain in neutral position, i.e. neither pronated nor supinated. Based on this specific arm position, alignment should be made relative to the humeral shaft, i.e. the shaft and the motor axis should be collinear.

Elevation and/or depression in the scapula as off-scapular plane motion patterns may be tested similarly but the swing angle determines the orientation of the subject vis-à-vis the plane of lever-arm motion. In variance with humeral rotation measurements where the elbow is kept in 90° of flexion, in this case the elbow should be braced in full or nearly full extension and the forearm maintained in pronation with respect to alignment. For testing scapation as well as elevation/depression in the sagittal and frontal planes, the common practice is to position the axis of the actuator against a point which is roughly 2–3 cm below the inferior lip of the acromial arch.

DIAGONAL MOVEMENTS

Since evaluation of rotator function is carried out in positions which are not optimal for elevation and vice versa, diagonal patterns of arm motion have been recommended as a general testing position (Albert & Wooden 1991, Fig. 10.3). These movements are performed in the supine or seated position, either on the supporting surface of the system or on a special apparatus like the Cybex UBXT. The actuator is placed at an angle relative to the coronal and sagittal planes of the subject, so that the full potential of the arm ROM may be realized.

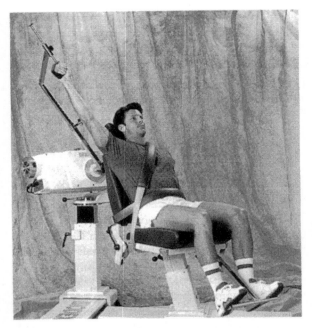

Figure 10.3 Diagonal movements testing attachment. The plane of motion is determined using rotation/tilt of the dynamometer head and plinth. A supine position is also very commonly used.

These patterns have two variants. The first diagonal, also known as D1, consists of the simultaneous combination of flexion, adduction and external rotation and its opposite sequence extension, abduction and internal rotation. The second diagonal, D2, corresponds to flexion, abduction, external rotation and its opposite, extension, adduction and internal rotation.

Since a comprehensive isokinetic evaluation is a time-consuming process and hence also an expensive one, the idea of using diagonal movements as a single combined replacement for all major glenohumeral movements has been forcefully advocated by Albert & Wooden (1991). The reasons given were enhanced functionality, incorporation of shoulder complex joints other than the glenohumeral, loading of a larger number of muscles and a shorter testing time. These are important considerations and one would not hesitate to recommend the use of diagonal movements particularly for treating patients with strength deficits.

However, diagonal motion testing may not be as clinically relevant since the findings are not specific, and hence cannot assist in revealing the source of a problem. Moreover, due to the complexity of the motion pattern, the reproducibility of findings based on diagonal pattern testing, performed either in the seated or supine position, might prove to be particularly unsatisfactory. To date, no study could be located that has looked into this issue. Therefore, at this juncture, diagonal activities remain a general *training* option rather than a recommended method of testing.

TEST ANGULAR VELOCITIES
Arbitrary choice of velocities

This topic is of central importance to the assessment of the shoulder but has received surprisingly little attention. Although modern isokinetic systems allow fine control of the actuator's angular velocity, research into shoulder muscle performance has popularized the use of 60°/s and/or its multiples. Although this practice certainly helps to standardize the tests, no study has ever demonstrated its biomechanical or clinical rationale. Also, kinematic analysis of the arm during isokinetic motion would reveal that the component angular velocities, those of swing, elevation and rotation are rarely equal. Hence, to use the same velocities for assessing muscle performance in, say, rotation and elevation, may be erroneous. Clearly, the current choice of velocities is still arbitrary rather than scientific.

Very high functional velocities

The shoulder joint angular velocities attained during certain sporting activities, such as pitching in baseball, have been reported to reach thousands of degrees per second (Pappas et al 1985). This figure, besides being an order of magnitude above the maximal velocity of all dynamometers in clinical usage, relates to the velocity of the *long axis of the arm*, and is therefore irrelevant as far as rotatory velocity components are concerned. It should also be pointed out that these extremely high velocities occur through a very limited arc of motion. Hence even if a suitable dynamometer were to become available, the chance of recording a reproducible force of any significant magnitude would be low.

Obviously the problem facing the athlete is that of accelerating the segments of the upper limb, requiring a system of strong, rapidly recruitable and highly coordinated muscles. Measurement of some of these factors may be achieved satisfactorily with existing systems.

Velocities used in research

Though in a few instances only one test velocity has been used for measuring performance (Reid et al 1989, Otis et al 1990, Greenfield et al 1990, Magnusson et al 1990) most studies have employed a protocol using either two (Ivey et al 1985, Cook et al 1987, Walker et al 1987, Connelly Maddux et al 1989, Hageman et al 1989, Warner et al 1990, McMaster et al 1991) or three (Soderberg & Blaschak 1987, Walmsley & Szybbo 1987, Brown et al 1988, Ellenbecker 1991, Schexneider et al 1991, Walmsley & Hartsell 1992) distinct velocities. The velocities most often used were 60, 180 and 300°/s.

High speed test

The question of whether a high speed test, 300°/s or above, should be incorporated, has been addressed incidentally by Cook et al (1987) who studied the moment ratios of extensors/flexors and internal/external rotators in baseball pitchers and non-pitchers. The test velocities were 180 and 300°/s. It was assumed that strength imbalances would be more conspicuous in the faster test since pitchers were accustomed to moving their arm at higher speeds. However, it was found that 300°/s was too fast for both groups, supporting another study (Wallace et al 1984) which suggested that the optimal speed for testing of flexion and extension was 120°/s.

Recommended test velocities

In trying to answer this question, reference should be made separately to rotational movements and long humeral motions (elevation/depression). *Also, the combination of concentric and eccentric tests must be taken for granted.* Since the main purpose of isokinetic testing is to assess bilateral differences and monitor change, any velocity that is well tolerated by patients may serve for this particular purpose. Indeed, if there are velocity-specific deficiencies, expressed particularly with respect to elevation/depression, these should be carefully monitored when the patient is an athlete or a professional whose work poses specific high speed demands. From a quite different perspective and incorporating previous results (Dvir et al 2002), the use of velocity as an independent parameter may not be essential as results based on a short test ROM may be as effective while reflecting totally different absolute velocity figures.

However, if rotational strength is to be assessed using a single velocity, this may be chosen between 90 and 120°/s. This recommendation is based on an effective internal and external rotation ROM of 60–90° resulting in motion duration of between 0.5 and 1 s. Such duration allows a reasonable build-up of muscular force and an isokinetic motion through a viable sector. Alternatively one could use a two-angular-velocities protocol, in which case a gradient of 1:4 consisting of 30:120°/s would be recommended.

The situation is slightly different regarding long humeral motions where one should consider the much higher angular velocities that may develop. Consequently for spanning the $M–\omega$ curve, a three-velocity protocol, consisting for instance of 45, 90 and 180°/s, could effectively serve a test ROM of 120°/s.

PART 2
REPRESENTATIVE VALUES IN SHOULDER ISOKINETICS

GENERAL CONSIDERATIONS

The range of options involved in testing the shoulder is an obstacle to establishing normative values. Though the database has increased in recent years, a standard procedure is notably lacking leading to incompatible data. Moreover, the number of subjects in the studies quoted in this chapter, except for that of Freedson et al (1993), was small, rarely exceeding 30 in one homogeneous group. Findings derived from such groups can hardly serve as a basis for generalization. An attempt will be made here to put these findings into an acceptable perspective. As with other joint systems, reference values for shoulder isokinetic performance should normally be based on three factors: gender, age and general activity level.

Gender differences

Concerning gender, the usual difference in muscle strength is maintained and is highly significant. However, normalization to bodyweight tends to diminish the factor by which men are stronger than women. Thus for instance, calculations based on the peak moment, derived from concentric testing at 60°/s (Ivey et al 1985) show that on average women have about 55% the strength of men. When normalized to bodyweight this figure is about 72%. Shklar & Dvir (1995) have reported that female strength scores for concentric testing at 60°/s were 53 and 66% compared with those of males for the absolute and normalized ratios respectively. This study also investigated eccentric muscle performance and the ratios at 60°/s were 55 and 72% respectively.

Age range

The age range in all the studies was typically adolescence to the middle of the fourth decade and therefore any large variations in measured strength would not be a result of this factor.

Activity level and the effect on dominance

Participation in athletic activities, specifically those that incorporate forceful arm motions, does account for significant bilateral performance differences. Among these activities, asymmetrical sports have a particular significance, highlighting the issue of side dominance and its effect on bilateral ratios of muscle strength. Shoulder muscles of the dominant side in baseball pitchers

(Cook et al 1987, Brown et al 1988, Hinton 1988) and water polo players (McMaster et al 1991) were found to be significantly stronger than their nondominant counterparts. Moreover, although dominance was examined with particular emphasis on the rotator cuff, at least two studies (Ellenbecker et al 1988, McMaster et al 1991) indicated that in athletes the dominance effect also encompassed other major muscle groups. Consequently, care should be taken when interpreting bilateral strength ratios of athletes who use their upper limbs in an asymmetrical manner.

Findings based on normal subjects (Ivey et al 1985, Connelly Maddux et al 1989, Reid et al 1989, Otis et al 1990, Shklar & Dvir 1995) did not indicate any effect of dominance. On the other hand, two studies (Warner et al 1990, Cahalan et al 1991) did indicate a significant dominance effect regarding a number of selected movement planes and test velocities. It should, however, be noted that poor stabilization and positioning in the former study and splinting of the elbow at 90° of flexion (overstabilization) in the latter could account for the findings. Therefore, whether the same degree of caution in interpreting bilateral differences is warranted with respect to the healthy non-athletic population is debatable.

ORDER AND MAGNITUDE IN SHOULDER MUSCLE STRENGTH

The strength order of shoulder muscles has been investigated using concentric testing at 60 and 180°/s (Ivey et al 1985) and at 60, 180 and 300°/s (Cahalan et al 1991). In the former study it was indicated that the strongest muscle group was the adductors followed by the extensors, flexors, abductors, internal rotators and external rotators (ERs). In the latter study this order was changed in only one respect, namely the extensors were found to be stronger than the adductors. The same strength order was later indicated by Shklar & Dvir (1995, see below). These findings were supported by other studies of concentric performance which, however, did not include all six groups of muscles. Adductors were stronger than abductors (Reid et al 1989, McMaster et al 1991), extensors were stronger than flexors and flexors were stronger than abductors (Otis et al 1990). These muscle groups were in turn stronger than the rotators, for which all studies to date have shown the internal rotators to be stronger than the external rotators.

CONCENTRIC AND ECCENTRIC PERFORMANCE VALUES

In a comprehensive analysis (Shklar & Dvir 1995) of the shoulder the concentric and eccentric performance parameters of the major muscle groups were measured. The order mentioned above was true for all velocities, for the two contraction modes and for women and men alike. Differences in positioning and stabilization and, particularly, the application of a gravity correction procedure in this study could account for the change in order. Indeed, in a study by Perrin et al (1992), gravity correction exerted a highly significant effect on the strength findings of the rotator group. It was argued that the internal rotators were assisted by gravity whereas the opposite was true for the external rotators. Adopting the same line of reasoning, in the above studies, the adductors were reinforced by gravity more than

the extensors, leading to the reversal in the strength order when a gravity correction was applied.

Tables 10.2–10.7 show findings from the Ivey et al (1985), Cahalan et al (1991) and Shklar & Dvir (1995) studies which were based on mixed samples of 31, 50 and 30 normal non-athletic subjects, respectively. The systems used were Cybex UBXT (Ivey et al 1985), Cybex II (Cahalan et al 1991) and KinCom II (Shklar & Dvir 1995). Attention is drawn to the fact that Cahalan et al (1991) have used an orthoplast splint for stabilizing the elbow, whose weight could be one of the reasons for the limited compatibility of their findings with those derived from the other two studies. Comparison of the figures derived from these studies show a close agreement in flexor, extensor and abductor strength, a fair agreement for internal and external rotators and up to a 47% difference in adductor strength.

A recent study (Mandalidis et al 2001b) tested a group of 22 male subjects performing concentric scapation at two angular velocities: 60 and 120°/s. Scapation was recorded between 30 and 90° of elevation. One of the study's objectives was to examine the effect of the transient moment oscillations on the reproducibility of strength findings.

Table 10.2 Reference values for abductor group concentric and eccentric strength (in Nm). The data are based on Ivey et al (1985), Cahalan et al (1991)* and Shklar & Dvir (1995) using 31, 50 and 30 non-athletic subjects respectively. In Tables 10.2–10.7 data from Cahalan et al 1991 are reproduced by permission of J.B. Lippincott Co.

	60°/s			120°/s	180°/s			300°/s
	Ivey	Caln	S&D	S&D	Ivey	Caln	S&D	Caln
Concentric								
Men								
Mean	56.6	52.9	50.5	50.5	42.4	44.7	43.6	36.6
SD	15.5	12.2	13.0	13.0	14.0	12.2	11.9	10.8
Women								
Mean	29.4	27.1	28.4	26.6	21.1	17.6	24.8	10.9
SD	9.0	5.4	4.6	11.9	6.9	5.4	3.5	4.1
Eccentric								
Men								
Mean			64.8	67.9			73.1	
SD			18.2	17.3			18.3	
Women								
Mean			37.3	38.9			41.8	
SD			6.1	7.5			7.2	

* Dominant side; Ivey, Ivey et al; Caln, Cahalan et al; S&D, Shklar & Dvir.

Table 10.3 Reference values for adductor group concentric and eccentric strength (in Nm). The data are based on Ivey et al (1985), Cahalan et al (1991)* and Shklar & Dvir (1995) using 31, 50 and 30 non-athletic subjects respectively

	60°/s			120°/s	180°/s			300°/s
	Ivey	Caln	S&D	S&D	Ivey	Caln	S&D	Caln
Concentric								
Men								
Mean	89.6	108.5	72.9	69.8	74.8	99.0	66.1	88.1
SD	22.3	21.7	19.6	15.2	23.1	19.0	17.4	19.0
Women								
Mean	50.4	52.9	34.4	31.0	41.6	46.1	29.4	38.0
SD	9.1	8.1	6.9	5.3	7.5	9.5	4.4	10.8
Eccentric								
Men								
Mean			95.2	92.7			97.5	
SD			28.0	27.8			22.3	
Women								
Mean			46.7	47.5			50.2	
SD			8.9	9.0			8.2	

* Dominant side; Ivey, Ivey et al; Caln, Cahalan et al; S&D, Shklar & Dvir.

Table 10.4 Reference values for external rotator group concentric and eccentric strength (in Nm). The data are based on Ivey et al (1985), Cahalan et al (1991)* and Shklar & Dvir (1995) using 31, 50 and 30 non-athletic subjects respectively

	60°/s			120°/s	180°/s			300°/s
	Ivey	Caln	S&D	S&D	Ivey	Caln	S&D	Caln
Concentric								
Men								
Mean	32.4	35.3	25.6	22.9	28.7	25.8	21.2	19.0
SD	7.9	6.8	7.9	6.4	9.2	5.4	5.7	5.4
Women								
Mean	18.9	19.0	16.3	14.1	15.2	9.5	13.5	5.4
SD	4.1	8.1	2.5	2.6	3.1	4.1	3.2	2.7
Eccentric								
Men								
Mean			32.0	30.9			31.3	
SD			8.1	8.5			7.8	
Women								
Mean			19.9	19.8			19.6	
SD			4.6	4.6			4.4	

* Dominant side; Ivey, Ivey et al; Caln, Cahalan et al; S&D, Shklar & Dvir.

Table 10.8 outlines the peak moment data. Worth mentioning, the figures reported in this study are higher by some 10% than those reported for shoulder flexors by either Ivey et al (1985) or by Shklar & Dvir (1995) who used the same dynamometer and test velocity. Furthermore, they are significantly higher than the values reported for abduction strength. Thus measurement error, dynamometer type and study population notwithstanding, this study points to scapation being indeed an optimal plane for testing elevation strength.

Freedson et al (1993) reported testing 4541 women and men. Shoulder flexor and extensor

Table 10.5   Reference values for internal rotator group concentric and eccentric strength (in Nm). The data are based on Ivey et al (1985), Cahalan et al (1991)* and Shklar & Dvir (1995) using 31, 50 and 30 non-athletic subjects respectively

	60°/s			120°/s	180°/s			300°/s
	Ivey	Caln	S&D	S&D	Ivey	Caln	S&D	Caln
Concentric								
Men								
Mean	49.5	62.4	42.7	38.2	44.5	54.2	37.1	46.1
SD	16.6	19.0	13.4	11.9	15.0	17.6	11.4	17.6
Women								
Mean	26.7	29.8	27.4	26.1	23.3	23.1	26.3	19.0
SD	3.9	5.4	6.2	6.4	4.1	5.4	6.6	5.4
Eccentric								
Men								
Mean			47.4	46.5			45.2	
SD			14.8	15.1			15.8	
Women								
Mean			27.4	26.1			26.2	
SD			6.2	6.4			6.6	

* Dominant side; Ivey, Ivey et al; Caln, Cahalan et al; S&D, Shklar & Dvir.

Table 10.6   Reference values for extensor group concentric and eccentric strength (in Nm). The data are based on Ivey et al (1985), Cahalan et al (1991)* and Shklar & Dvir (1995) using 31, 50 and 30 non-athletic subjects respectively

	60°/s			120°/s	180°/s			300°/s
	Ivey	Caln	S&D	S&D	Ivey	Caln	S&D	Caln
Concentric								
Men								
Mean	80.4	118.0	84.9	82.4	64.8	103.1	73.3	86.8
SD	20.1	24.4	20.5	21.1	17.7	23.1	19.0	20.3
Women								
Mean	43.0	54.2	38.7	38.0	33.7	43.4	35.5	25.8
SD	9.5	5.4	9.1	6.9	7.5	9.5	7.5	8.1
Eccentric								
Men								
Mean			112.2	113.5			113.8	
SD			30.0	33.1			30.2	
Women								
Mean			56.3	58.1			59.8	
SD			8.2	9.6			8.2	

* Dominant side; Ivey, Ivey et al; Caln, Cahalan et al; S&D, Shklar & Dvir.

strength was measured in two velocities, using the seated position. No gravity correction was apparently performed. These findings provided probably the only normative database and are presented in terms of percentiles, age and gender, as outlined in Tables 10.9 and 10.10.

Shoulder protraction and retraction

Although shoulder muscle testing was explored exclusively using angular motion patterns, linear patterns are not outside the realm of the shoulder complex. Activities like sawing require that the hand assume a linear trajectory which is brought

Table 10.7 Reference values for flexor group concentric and eccentric strength (in Nm). The data are based on Ivey et al (1985), Cahalan et al* (1991) and Shklar & Dvir (1995) using 31, 50 and 30 non-athletic subjects respectively

	60°/s			120°/s	180°/s			300°/s
	Ivey	Caln	S&D	S&D	Ivey	Caln	S&D	Caln
Concentric								
Men								
Mean	62.3	67.8	61.2	57.1	51.0	59.7	53.8	48.8
SD	12.5	16.3	13.3	9.8	11.4	16.3	10.3	14.9
Women								
Mean	35.6	29.8	36.5	35.5	39.1	23.1	32.3	16.3
SD	8.7	6.8	6.1	6.4	7.5	8.1	5.8	6.8
Eccentric								
Men								
Mean			72.4	75.2			77.1	
SD			18.0	18.4			18.1	
Women								
Mean			43.1	45.7			47.7	
SD			7.7	8.8			8.7	

* Dominant side; Ivey, Ivey et al; Caln, Cahalan et al; S&D, Shklar & Dvir.

Table 10.8 Reference values of non-free and free of transient moment oscillations (TMO) isokinetic peak moment (in Nm) during scapation for the dominant and non-dominant (non-dom) sides (From Mandalidis et al 2001b)

Session	Side	Non-free of TMO		Free of TMO	
		60°/s	120°/s	60°/s	120°/s
1	Dominant	69.7(12.8)[†]	67.3(14.4)	68.9(13.2)	62.7(13.8)*
2	Dominant	68.8(13.6)	69.1(14.4)	67.2(13.1)	63.1(13.9)*
1	Non-dom	69.4(16.1)	66.5(14.4)	68.5(15.20)	62.4(13.6)*
2	Non-dom	71.1(16.9)	68.4(16.9)	70.0(15.8)	62.7(14.6)*

[†] Mean (SD) * $p < 0.01$ between free and non-free TMO data.

Table 10.9 Reference values (Nm) for flexion (F) and extension (E) in men. From Freedson et al (1993) Isokinetics and Exercise Science 3: 34–42, with permission of Butterworth-Heinemann

	Percentile	<21 years		21–30 years		31–40 years		41–50 years		>50 years	
		F	E	F	E	F	E	F	E	F	E
60°/s	90	75.4	117.3	81.4	123.4	77.3	119.7	78.0	115.7	67.7	108.1
	70	63.7	102.4	69.2	107.1	66.4	104.4	65.8	104.4	57.0	94.6
	50	57.6	92.9	61.7	98.3	59.7	95.6	59.0	96.3	51.5	84.8
	30	50.2	84.8	54.2	88.8	52.3	86.8	52.9	85.3	46.8	78.5
	10	41.4	73.2	46.1	75.9	45.4	75.9	44.6	72.5	39.7	62.1
180°/s	90	61.0	95.6	65.1	101.0	61.0	97.6	60.3	94.6	52.5	90.9
	70	48.8	82.7	52.9	86.8	50.2	84.1	49.5	84.6	42.0	74.6
	50	42.7	73.9	46.1	78.0	44.1	75.9	44.1	76.6	38.0	68.5
	30	37.3	65.8	40.7	69.2	38.6	68.6	38.6	67.8	32.1	63.1
	10	29.8	55.6	32.5	57.6	31.2	57.8	29.8	54.1	29.2	48.4

Table 10.10 Reference values (Nm) for flexion (F) and extension (E) in women. From Freedson et al (1993) Isokinetics and Exercise Science 3: 34–42, with permission of Butterworth-Heinemann

	Percentile	<21 years		21–30 years		31–40 years		41–50 years		>50 years	
		F	E	F	E	F	E	F	E	F	E
60°/s	90	38.0	63.1	40.7	65.1	43.4	67.0	40.0	63.6	34.2	54.4
	70	32.5	54.9	33.9	56.0	36.6	58.3	34.6	55.5	30.1	51.0
	50	28.5	49.5	30.5	51.6	32.3	52.2	29.8	50.2	26.4	46.6
	30	25.4	45.0	27.8	46.6	28.5	46.8	26.4	45.7	22.0	40.8
	10	21.7	38.8	23.1	41.4	22.4	40.0	21.2	40.8	18.2	34.6
180°/s	90	28.5	48.8	30.5	52.9	32.5	53.6	28.5	48.1	23.5	42.6
	70	23.6	42.0	25.8	47.7	26.4	45.4	24.4	41.3	20.3	35.0
	50	20.3	38.0	22.4	40.0	23.1	40.7	20.3	38.0	15.5	32.5
	30	17.2	33.2	19.0	35.9	19.0	32.3	17.1	32.1	12.2	27.0
	10	13.6	27.3	14.9	29.8	13.6	28.5	13.6	30.5	4.5	19.4

about by coordinated angular motions taking place at the various joints of the shoulder complex, notably the scapulothoracic, the elbow and the wrist. Isokinetic measurement of the forces exerted by the hand necessitate a linear motion attachment that is available in certain dynamometers. A study of this motion pattern has been undertaken by Cools et al (2002) who have expanded the measurements in order to allow reproducibility analysis.

The experimental set-up consisted of a Biodex 3 dynamometer which has a special linear attachment. Female and male subjects were tested while seated and stabilized using pelvic and contralateral chest straps (Fig. 10.4). Concentric testing was conducted at 12.2 and 36.6 cm/s using an individually based linear ROM corresponding to maximal protraction and retraction. As the findings reported in this paper were mixed for women and men they are not presented in this book. However worth noting is a protraction/retraction strength ratio of about 1.

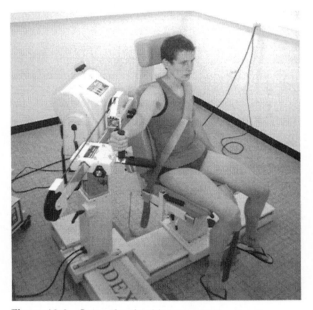

Figure 10.4 Set-up for shoulder protraction–retraction. (From Cools et al 2002 Isokinetics and Exercise Science 10: 129–136, with permission of IOS Press.)

PART 3
MUSCLE STRENGTH RATIOS

The issue of antagonistic muscle strength ratios has gained growing interest in recent years particularly with respect to the rotational components: the internal and external. This attraction stems from the notion that glenohumeral joint (GHJ) instability or excessive laxity derives, at

least in part, from muscle strength imbalance. These pathologies are often seen in some overhead sporting activities (throwing events, swimming, tennis, etc.) where the GHJ experiences a transition from an elevated and externally rotated position (initial phase) towards a depressed and internally rotated position (terminal phase). This forceful depression is brought about by *concentric* (con) action of the GHJ depressors (e.g. pectoralis major and latissimus dorsi) as well as the internal rotators (Glousman et al 1988) and is obviously reinforced by any additional inertia contributed by an external object held by the hand.

Given the inherent instability of the GHJ, such powerful activities may jeopardize the integrity of the joint. A dynamic solution to this problem is offered by *eccentric* (ecc) contraction of the antagonistic muscles that operate to slow down the rotational movement of the humeral head. The accumulated recognition among students of shoulder muscle performance caused a transition from the application of same contraction mode ratios to the use of reciprocal contraction mode ratios.

External (ER) and internal (IR) ratios

Previous research and practice looked into ratios like ER_{con}/IR_{con} or ER_{ecc}/IR_{ecc} or their reciprocals. In a clinical study of rotator performance, three groups (healthy individuals and patients with either instability or impingement syndrome) were concentrically tested at 90 and 180°/s (Warner et al 1990). In the healthy group, the IR strength of the dominant side was approximately 30% higher than on the other side, leading to a parallel difference in the peak moment-based IR/ER ratios. Patients were divided into those who had involvement of the dominant side (the dominant group) and those whose involved side was non-dominant (the non-dominant group). Findings from both groups were then compared with those derived from the dominant and non-dominant sides of the control subjects.

In the dominant group, significant differences in the IR/ER ratios were demonstrated between patients with instability and patients with impingement. Whereas the former had a ratio close to 100%, for the latter it was nearly 200%. In the non-dominant group there was a parallel but a non-significant trend. Analysis of the absolute IR and ER strength failed to reveal weaknesses in either of these groups.

The authors suggested that the relatively low IR/ER ratio in the instability group indicated an 'association between relative imbalance of IR and ER strength and anterior instability'. On the other hand, the relatively high value of this ratio in the

impingement group could not be interpreted in terms of the available data. The authors nevertheless suggested that a relative weakness of the external rotators was an important factor in impingement.

Further studies followed, focusing on athletes and on the ER/IR ratio. For instance, it was indicated that the concentric ER/IR ratio was around 0.75 in control subjects versus 0.64 in swimmers, emphasizing the relative weakness of the external rotation apparatus. Except for two studies, research indicated that the range of this ratio was consistently 0.6–0.7 with apparently no significant velocity effect. On the other hand, if confidence intervals were to be set this range could grow to between 0.4 and 0.9. The proportions for eccentric contractions stayed within this range.

Ratios relating abductor and adductor, as well as flexor and extensor strength, have also been computed and representative scores are given in Table 10.11. However, unlike the rotational strength ratios (see below) which may well possess some discriminatory power, such has never been, nor is it likely to be, the case with the general ratio: elevators/depressors, be it either in the frontal or the sagittal plane. The reason for that lies in their function which is for moving the upper extremity rather than preserving the joint.

Dynamic control ratio

A different approach to shoulder muscle strength ratios has been offered by Bak & Magnusson (1997). Using the dynamic control ratio (DCR), suggested originally by the Dvir et al (1989) model for differentiating the chronic anterior cruciate ligament deficient knee from uninvolved knee: H_{ecc}/Q_{con} (see Chapter 7) these authors have looked into the reciprocal ratio: ER_{ecc}/IR_{con}.

Two matched groups of athletes, one with unilateral shoulder pain (Neer & Welsh phase I and II) and a control group were compared. The test was carried out in sitting, arm positioned at the scapular plane, elbows maintained at 90° with a single angular velocity of 30°/s. Table 10.12 outlines the conventional (ER_{con}/IR_{con}) ratio and the functional ratio (the DCR) which indicates that in symptomatic shoulders the conventional and

Table 10.11 Shoulder muscles peak moment ratios

Source	Gender	Mode	Ordinary/athletic	n	Abductors/adductors	Flexors/extensors	External rotators/internal rotators
Alderink & Kuck (1986) 90, 120, 210, 300°/s	M	Concentric	Athletic	24	0.50–0.70	0.48–0.55	0.68–0.76
Brown et al (1988) 180, 240, 300°/s	M	Concentric	Athletic	41	–	–	0.61–0.72
Connelly Maddux et al (1989) 60, 180°/s	F, M	Concentric	Ordinary	17, 20	–	–	0.67, F, 0.62, M
Cook et al (1987) 180, 300°/s	M	Concentric	Ordinary, athletic	19	–	0.70–0.99	0.70–0.87
Ellenbecker et al (1988) 90, 210, 300°/s	M	Concentric	Athletic	22	–	0.76–0.82	0.65–0.72
Hinton (1988) 90, 240°/s	M	Concentric	Athletic	26	–	–	0.55–0.63
McMaster et al (1991) 30, 180°/s	M	Concentric	Ordinary, athletic	25	0.48–0.69	–	0.55–0.78
Reid et al (1989) 60°/s	M	Concentric	Ordinary, athletic	80	0.50 (ordinary only)	–	0.53–0.66
Shklar & Dvir (1995) 60, 120, 180°/s	F, M	Concentric Concentric Eccentric Eccentric	Ordinary	30	0.85–0.90, F 0.68–0.71, M 0.81–0.85, F 0.71–0.77, M	0.92–0.97, F 0.71–0.75, M 0.77–0.80, F 0.67–0.69, M	0.67–0.74, F 0.59–0.62, M 0.75–0.79, F 0.69–0.74, M
Soderberg & Blaschak (1987) 60, 180, 300°/s	M	Concentric	Ordinary	20			0.57–0.69

Table 10.12 Shoulder rotational strength ratios
(From Bak & Magnusson 1997)

Ratio	Injured side	Uninvolved side	Control group
ER_{con}/IR_{con}	0.83 (0.11)[a]	0.78 (0.18)	0.66 (0.11)[b]
ER_{ecc}/IR_{ecc}	0.71 (0.12)	0.78 (0.15)	0.67 (0.07)[c]
ER_{ecc}/IR_{con}	1.08 (0.18)[d]	0.89 (0.15)	0.86 (0.09)[b]

[a] Mean(SD); [b] $p = 0.02$; [c] $p = 0.01$; [d] $p = 0.04$.
ER, external rotation; IR, internal rotation;
con, concentric; ecc, eccentric.

frontal ratios were significantly higher compared to their matched controls pointing to IR insufficiency. However, using conventional ratios, neither the 'con-con' nor 'ecc-ecc' ratios were able to differentiate between the involved and uninvolved sides. This capability was indicated only with respect to the DCR.

It should be borne in mind that this study referred specifically to swimmers where the overhead activity profile is rather limited. This may have also been the reason for the inversion of the ER/IR ratio across the three variants. Unfortunately, no absolute strength values were provided and therefore whether the high DCR in the involved side is an outcome of the eccentric (ER) or the concentric (IR) components is impossible to delineate. Moreover, a more recent study indicated that the dominant side was associated with a greater DCR compared to the non-dominant side (Gulick et al 2001). Obviously further research is needed with a special emphasis on defining cutoff scores for select patient populations. However, the fact that the shoulder-related DCR may operate in a comparable fashion to its knee counterpart is on its own of decisive theoretical and applied value and will certainly continue to be at the focus of isokinetic research.

PART 4
ISOKINETIC CONDITIONING

In principle, the rationale of treatment protocols for the shoulder should not differ from that for other major joint systems. It is based on velocity dependent muscle overloading. Under isokinetic conditions, concentric and eccentric alike, the available, sometimes the maximal, muscle tension is accommodated by the resistance of the system. The physiological load imposed on the joint is equally important. This load is expressed in newton-meter seconds (Nms), corresponding to the time for which the moment is acting, or the contraction impulse (Sale 1991). A large number of shoulder problems require attention to the possible impact of glenohumeral (or other) joint loading and thus the impulse is a cardinal factor in protocol design.

It should also be mentioned that all factors concerned with the safety of the patient in isokinetic testing also hold for isokinetic conditioning.

Principles of rehabilitation

The published literature on the general use of isokinetic treatment procedures for the shoulder has not been significantly enriched since the publication of the first edition. Most of the papers are based on case studies and their findings may not be generalized. However, from its initiation and through its progression, shoulder rehabilitation follows two principles (Davies 1992) in initiation and progression:

1. Arm motion is initially very limited, i.e. contractions are performed at fixed angles; this followed by short arc motion, and then movements spanning the full ROM.
2. The shoulder muscle contraction mode is initially isometric, followed by concentric and then eccentric. The magnitude of these contractions varies from submaximal to maximal.

Velocities in rehabilitation

The choice of speeds used in treatment sessions depends primarily on the patient's tolerance. If tolerance is assured, the speed(s) in which significant deficits are indicated require particular attention.

It should be emphasized that lower speeds mean higher impulse, and therefore an increase of joint loading and, frequently, pain. Consequently higher speeds are better as a conditioning input. On the other hand these speeds involve higher accelerations which may lead to significant inertial forces. The solution in this case is to employ the damping procedure, an option the present author has used quite liberally in isokinetic conditioning. Limiting the arc of motion is another method of containing pain but this applies generally.

Albert & Wooden (1991) suggest another guideline for speed selection, the '25% rule': if strength deficit at the low testing speed of 60°/s is greater than 25%, rehabilitation at this speed is indicated; otherwise it should be at the medium/high speed of 180°/s.

Velocity spectrum rehabilitation protocols

The use of velocity spectrum rehabilitation protocols (VSRPs) has been advocated for other joints, and the shoulder is no exception. Because of the high angular velocities attainable by the arm, the 'velocities pyramid' may shift to the right, i.e. the lowest velocity is 60°/s or even higher, whereas the apex of the pyramid, the highest speed, may reach hundreds of degrees per second.

In a case study of a functional subluxation of the shoulder joint, the VSRP for the internal and external rotators started at 180°/s and proceeded up to 450°/s at 30°/s intervals (Engle 1991). Ten repetitions at each of these speeds with 20 s of interset rest were performed. No upper limit to the number of repetitions at the highest speed was set, and the patient was directed to reach fatigue.

However, in view of the guideline set by Wallace et al (1984) it seems that the value of very high speeds is questionable. Moreover, the present author doubts if such high speeds induce a genuine isokinetic effort. Thus in a more relevant VSRP, the peak would be set at velocities around 200°/s.

Concentric and eccentric conditioning

The use of concentric and eccentric conditioning protocols, in the case of chronic anterior shoulder instability, has been advocated in an excellent paper by Glousman et al (1988). This study centered on dynamic electromyography of shoulder muscles, comparing baseball pitchers with chronic instability to a control group. It was demonstrated how muscle imbalance, because of weak internal rotators (subscapularis, pectoralis major and latissimus dorsi) and scapular protractors (serratus anterior) on one hand, and their sound antagonists on the other, may cause or aggravate the instability.

The authors pointed out that: 'during a muscle strengthening program, improper synchrony and decreased muscle activity must be corrected. Often, asymmetrical or subtle differences cannot be appreciated'. The last sentence almost prescribes the use of isokinetic testing since this is the only method through which such differences may be discovered. Moreover, with the emerging knowledge that was discussed before the incorporation of an eccentric component in due course is quite an imperative.

This incorporation raises the questions 'when' and 'how?' A possible protocol which is fairly functional could consist of submaximal D1 and D2 patterns, attempted relatively late in the rehabilitation process. The present author would recommend using, at this stage, low/medium eccentric speeds, 90–120°/s, and probably higher concentric speeds. At the very last stage, high speed concentric and eccentric motions may be attempted, providing the safety of the patient is ensured.

REFERENCES

Albert M S, Wooden M J 1991 Isokinetic evaluation and treatment of the shoulder. In: Donatelli R (ed) Physical therapy of the shoulder, 2nd edn. Churchill Livingstone, Edinburgh

Alderink G J, Kuck D J 1986 Isokinetic shoulder strength of high school and college-aged pitchers. Journal of Orthopaedic and Sports Physical Therapy 7: 163–172

Bak K, Magnusson P 1997 Shoulder strength and range of notion in symptomatic and pain-free elite swimmers. American Journal of Sports Medicine 25: 454–459

Brown L P, Niehues S L, Harrah A, Yavorsky P, Hirschman H P 1988 Upper extremity range of motion and isokinetic strength of the internal and external rotators in major league baseball players. American Journal of Sports Medicine 16: 577–585

Cahalan T D, Johnson M E, Chao E Y S 1991 Shoulder strength analysis using the Cybex II isokinetic dynamometer. Clinical Orthopaedics and Related Research 271: 249–257

Connelly Maddux R E, Kibler W B, Uhl T 1989 Isokinetic peak torque and work values for the shoulder. Journal of Orthopaedic and Sports Physical Therapy 10: 264–269

Cook E E, Gray V L, Savinar-Nogue E, Medeiros J 1987 Shoulder antagonistic strength ratios: a comparison between college level baseball pitchers and nonpitchers. Journal of Orthopaedic and Sports Physical Therapy 8: 451–461

Cools A M, Witvrouw E E, Danneels L A, Vanderstraeten G G, Cambier D C 2002 Test-retest reproducibility of concentric strength values for shoulder girdle protraction and retraction using the Biodex isokinetic dynamometer. Isokinetics and Exercise Science 10: 129–136

Davies G J 1992 Compendium of isokinetics in clinical usage. S & S Publications, La Crosse, Wisconsin

Dvir Z, Berme N 1978 Elevation of the arm in the scapular plane: a mechanism approach. Journal of Biomechanics 11: 98–103

Dvir Z, Eger G, Halperin N, Shklar A 1989 Thigh muscle activity and anterior cruciate ligament insufficiency. Clinical Biomechanics 4: 87–91

Dvir Z, Steinfeld-Cohen Y, Peretz C 2002 The identification of feigned isokinetic shoulder flexion weakness in normal subjects. American Journal of Physical Medicine and Rehabilitation 81: 178–183

Ellenbecker T S 1991 A total arm strength isokinetic profile of highly skilled tennis players. Isokinetics and Exercise Science 1: 9–22

Ellenbecker T S, Davies G E, Rowinski M J 1988 Concentric versus eccentric isokinetic strengthening of the rotator cuff: objective data versus functional test. American Journal of Sports Medicine 16: 64–69

Engle R P 1991 Isokinetic analysis in acromioclavicular joint rehabilitation: a case study. Isokinetics and Exercise Science 1: 49–55

Falkel J E, Murphy T C, Murray T F 1987 Prone positioning for testing shoulder internal and external rotation on the Cybex isokinetic dynamometer. Journal of Orthopaedic and Sports Physical Therapy 8: 368–370

Freedson P S, Gilliam T B, Mahoney T, Maliszeski A F, Kastango K 1993 Industrial torque levels by age group and gender. Isokinetics and Exercise Science 3: 34–42

Glousman R E, Jobe F W, Tibone J E et al 1988 Dynamic electromyographic analysis of the throwing shoulder with glenohumeral instability. Journal of Bone and Joint Surgery 70A: 220–226

Greenfield B H, Donatelli R, Wooden M J, Wilkes J 1990 Isokinetic evaluation of shoulder rotational strength between the plane of the scapula and the frontal plane. American Journal of Sports Medicine 18: 124–128

Gulick D T, Dustman C, Ossowski L T et al 2001 Side dominance does not affect dynamic control strength ratios in the shoulder. Isokinetics and Exercise Science 9: 79–84

Hageman P A, Mason D J, Rydlund K W, Humpal S A 1989 Effect of position and speed on eccentric and concentric isokinetic testing of the shoulder rotators. Journal of Orthopaedic and Sports Physical Therapy 11: 64–69

Hellwig E V, Perrin D H 1991 A comparison of two positions for assessing shoulder rotator peak torque: the traditional

frontal plane versus the plane of the scapula. Isokinetics and Exercise Science 1: 202–206

Hinton R Y 1988 Isokinetic evaluation of shoulder rotational strength in high school baseball pitchers. American Journal of Sports Medicine 16: 274–279

Ivey F M, Calhoun J H, Rusche K, Bierschenk J 1985 Isokinetic testing of shoulder strength: normal values. Archives of Physical Medicine and Rehabilitation 66: 384–386

Magnusson S P, Gleim G G, Nicholas J A 1990 Subject variability of shoulder abduction strength testing. American Journal of Sports Medicine 18: 349–353

Mandalidis D G, Florides P, O'Brien M 2001a Scapular plane isokinetic shoulder elevation: effect of shoulder and motor centers of rotation transient misalignment on moment data. Isokinetics and Exercise Science 9: 91–99

Mandalidis D G, Donne B, O'Reagn M, O'Brien M 2001b Effect of transient moment oscillations on the reliability of isokinetic shoulder elevation in the scapular plane. Isokinetics and Exercise Science 9: 100–109

McMaster W C, Long S C, Caiozzo V J 1991 Isokinetic torque imbalances in the rotator cuff of elite water polo players. American Journal of Sports Medicine 19: 72–75

Otis J C, Warren R F, Backus S I, Santner T J, Mabrey J D 1990 Torque production in the shoulder of the normal young adult male: the interaction of function, dominance, joint angle and angular velocity. American Journal of Sports Medicine 18: 119–123

Pappas A M, Zawacki R M, Sullivan T J 1985 Biomechanics of baseball pitching: a preliminary report. American Journal of Sports Medicine 13: 223–235

Perrin D H, Helwig E V, Tis L L, Shenk B S 1992 Effect of gravity correction on shoulder rotation isokinetic average force and reciprocal group ratios. Isokinetics and Exercise Science 2: 30–33

Reid D C, Oedekoven G, Kramer J F, Saboe L A 1989 Isokinetic muscle strength parameters for shoulder movements. Clinical Biomechanics 4: 97–104

Reid D C, Saboe L A, Burnham R 1991 Common shoulder problems in the athlete. In: Donatelli R (ed) Physical therapy of the shoulder, 2nd edn. Churchill Livingstone, Edinburgh

Sale D G 1991 Testing strength and power. In: MacDougall J D, Wenger H A, Green H J (eds) Physiological testing of the high performance athlete, 2nd edn. Human Kinetics Books, Champaign, Illinois

Schexneider M A, Catlin P A, Davies G J, Mattson P A 1991 An isokinetic estimation of total arm strength. Isokinetics and Exercise Science 1: 117–121

Shklar A, Dvir Z 1995 Isokinetic strength relationships in shoulder muscles. Clinical Biomechanics 10: 369–373

Smith J, Padgett D J, Kotajarvi B R, Eischen J J 2001 Isokinetic and isometric shoulder rotation strength in the protracted position: a reliability study. Isokinetics and Exercise Science 9: 119–127

Soderberg G L, Blaschak M J 1987 Shoulder internal and external rotation peak torque production through a velocity spectrum in differing positions. Journal of Orthopaedic and Sports Physical Therapy 8: 518–524

Townsend H, Jobe F W, Pink M, Perry J 1991 Electromyographic analysis of the glenohumeral muscles during a baseball rehabilitation program. American Journal of Sports Medicine 19: 264–272

Walker S W, Couch W H, Boester G A, Sprowl D W 1987 Isokinetic strength of the shoulder after repair of a torn rotator cuff. Journal of Bone and Joint Surgery 69A: 1041–1044

Wallace W A, Barton M J, Murray W A 1984 The power available during movement of the shoulder. In: Bateman J, Welsh C (eds) Surgery of the shoulder. B C Decker, Philadelphia

Walmsley R 1993a Movement of the axis of rotation of the glenohumeral joint while working on the Cybex II dynamometer. Part I: flexion/extension. Isokinetics and Exercise Science 3: 16–20

Walmsley R 1993b Movement of the axis of rotation of the glenohumeral joint while working on the Cybex II dynamometer. Part II: abduction/adduction. Isokinetics and Exercise Science 3: 21–26

Walmsley R P, Hartsell H 1992 Shoulder strength following surgical rotator cuff repair: a comprehensive analysis using isokinetic testing. Journal of Orthopaedic and Sports Physical Therapy 15: 215–222

Walmsley R P, Szybbo C 1987 A comparative study of the torque generated by the shoulder internal and external rotator muscles in different positions and at varying speeds. Journal of Orthopaedic and Sports Physical Therapy 9: 217–222

Warner J P, Micheli L J, Arslanian L E, Kennedy J, Kennedy R 1990 Patterns of flexibility, laxity and shoulder strength in normal shoulders and shoulders with instability and impingement. American Journal of Sports Therapy 18: 366–375

Wilk K E, Arrigo C A, Andrews J R 1991 Standardized isokinetic testing protocol for the throwing shoulder: the throwers' series. Isokinetics and Exercise Science 1: 63–71

Isokinetics of elbow, forearm, wrist and hand muscles

The first edition of this book did not include a chapter dedicated to the isokinetics of elbow, wrist and hand (grip) muscles. It was felt that the reference material was in many ways lacking. Admittedly not much has changed since, although judging from computerized searches there is a conspicuous interest in the relationship between elbow surgery and clinical outcome measures (Fuchs & Chylarecki 1999, Karunakar et al 1999, Ambacher et al 2000, Bell et al 2000, Hildebrand et al 2000, Musmayer et al 2000).

There are a few possible reasons for this relative dearth. As far as the elbow is concerned injuries to this joint and its associated structures are less prevalent than those affecting the shoulder. Hence the surgical–rehabilitation input is much smaller. Moreover, the critical dependence of the highly mobile shoulder joints on a balanced and meticulously coordinated activity of the muscles comprising the shoulder complex, particularly the rotator cuff, necessitates a profound analysis of their performance profiles. This situation has no parallel in the elbow. Moreover, from the methodological viewpoint, testing of the flexors and extensors of the elbow often requires special configuration as the more common test position calls for a horizontal forearm placement. In most dynamometers this is quite difficult to achieve without the use of an external seat or plinth.

Moving more distally, wrist and hand muscles are even less researched. In this case an added reason is the fact that as far as the surgical and general clinical aspects are concerned, both joint systems are within the realm of hand surgery/therapy.

Interestingly, hand specialists have for some 50 years used dynamometry as a standard tool (Mathiowetz et al 1984) for assessing grip and pinch functions. Simple, cheap, portable and widely available instruments like the Jamar grip dynamometer rendered the use of sophisticated, expensive and heavy isokinetic dynamometers almost irrelevant. This may have distanced hand clinicians from isokinetic testing even though *wrist* strength cannot be measured using the above simple devices.

In spite of these considerations, the few isokinetic studies of the distal joint systems of the upper extremity add new and important information regarding the performance of several key muscle groups. In the light of the findings it is clear that further research is acutely needed.

ISOKINETICS OF ELBOW AND FOREARM MUSCLES

The elbow provides the major connection between the shoulder complex and the hand. Its main function, via its flexors, is the approximation of objects with respect to the axial skeleton, once the shoulder has been placed in a position that enables such action. As its activity is closely coordinated with that of the shoulder joints the elbow works as a hand–body distance actuator and controller. On the other hand, elbow–forearm muscles permit rotation of the hand about the longitudinal axis of the forearm, a movement that is anatomically known as pronation and supination. This section describes therefore the test protocols and reference figures for the flexors, extensors, pronators and supinators.

Control parameters

Testing flexion and extension

Two distinct subject positions are in use when testing this motion pattern. One is the supine position where the subject's arm rests on the support surface (plinth) and the forearm is free to move along the full range of motion (ROM). This position has been described in several studies (Sale & MacDougall 1984, Griffin 1987). Although

the stabilization provided while testing in the supine position is very acceptable, its main problem lies in its applicability in terms of providing a large enough support for any subject as well as the ability to align the motor and biological axes. In the majority of cases the supine position necessitates the use of an independent plinth. The alternative and most common test position is in sitting. The basic requirement of proximal stabilization is satisfied by ensuring that the arm is supported horizontally or is prevented from moving if it hangs freely. Three different test positions of the arm have been described:

1. The arm is flexed 90° and is supported horizontally. Movement of the elbow takes place in a substantially sagittal plane (Mandalidis & O'Brien 2001).
2. The arm is abducted 90° and is supported horizontally. Movement of the elbow takes place in a substantially transverse (horizontal) plane (Gallagher et al 1997).
3. The arm is flexed 90° and abducted 30°. Movement of the elbow takes place in a substantially sagittal plane (Alfredson et al 1998).

Placing the arm at an elevated position has an effect on the long head of the triceps (elongation) but may also influence the bicipital heads. In terms of gravitational effect, position 2 is the most favourable since the forearm moves horizontally. Such protocol requires that the dynamometer head is tilted 90°, an option that is not available in all of the commercial dynamometers. Stabilization of the trunk is essential in all seated positions as the resistive force vectors are substantial. Performance of extension is better controlled than flexion since the resistive vector (against a possible movement of the trunk backward) will be provided by the seat's backrest. On the other hand, elbow flexion (either concentric or eccentric) will tend to move the trunk forward. This movement should be controlled by two straps: one across the chest at mid–lower sternal level and one vertically around the shoulder and proximal to the acromion. Alignment is made with reference to the lateral epicondyle (Morrey & Chao 1976). The trunk should remain upright throughout the test. Unless otherwise indicated, the forearm should remain in the neutral (thumb-up) position. The force resistance pad should be placed as distally as possible, just proximal to the styloid process.

The reported range of motion and velocities vary from study to study. For example Madsen (1996) tested the elbow flexors and extensors along an arch of 120°, from full extension (designated as 0°) using 30, 120 and 240°/s. Mandalidis & O'Brien (2001) tested elbow flexion over a range of 60°, from 20 to 80° of flexion at 60 and 120°/s. The magnitude of the isometric preactivation bias (IPB) if ever applied, was not reported in any of these studies. The differences between these test protocols are reflected in the diversity of the associated strength values.

Testing pronation and supination

Pronation and supination result from a relative rolling of the long shafts of the radius and ulna. This specific movement is expressed in turning of the palm of the hand from the volar side-up position (supinated) to dorsal side-up position (pronated). It is basically an axial motion and therefore requires that the hand holds the resistance handle while rotating it. In order to prevent co-movement of shoulder internal and external rotation, measurement of axial rotation of the forearm must be conducted with the elbow flexed, preferably at 90° (Fig. 11.1). Testing is performed

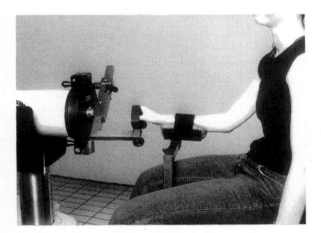

Figure 11.1   Set-up for pronation–supination. (From Forthomme et al 2003 Isokinetics and Exercise Science, in press, with permission of IOS Press.)

with the subject seated and stabilized at trunk level but especially at the arm as this is the proximal segment relative to the forearm. A special handle attachment is provided with the dynamometer. The range of motion reported in previous studies ranged from full pronation to full supination (Hartsell et al 1995) to 160° (Forthomme et al 2003). The velocities differed equally.

Reference values

Tables 11.1–11.5 outline reference values for elbow flexion, extension, pronation and supination. The number of studies allowing full referencing is very small. With respect to elbow flexors, four of the six studies referred to male and three to female groups. Comparison of the scores at the low and high velocity ends reveals some uniformity regarding the male scores. The highest and lowest concentric strength scores at 30 and 60°/s range from 45 to 62 Nm. It should be emphasized that the findings by Housh et al are quite outstandingly high, particularly in the high velocities. At 180°/s, and notably with the elbow supinated, flexion strength drops to 30–46 Nm. For women, the scores obtained by Frontera et al (1993) and Alfredson et al (1998) showed concentric strength at the low velocity end of around 20 Nm. Except for two conflicting studies (Gallagher et al 1997, Alfredson et al 1998) extension strength is comparable to flexion strength. In terms of absolute moment, pronation and supination strength scores are much lower than the corresponding flexion/extension scores ranging from 5 to 15 Nm. As for the pronation/supination strength ratio, the majority of studies report a value greater than 1, although not by a high margin (except for VanSwearingen 1983 who quoted a difference of about 50%).

ISOKINETICS OF WRIST MUSCLES

The wrist constitutes the major distal link between the upper extremity and the hand. It is this most complex of joints that is responsible for placing the hand in the most optimal position for object grasp and manipulation and hence its singular importance. The wrist enables flexion, extension,

Table 11.1 Elbow flexors: peak moment (mean ± SD, in Nm)

Study	Sex (N)	Test position	ROM (°)	Contraction	Velocity (°/s)	D	ND
Knapik & Ramos (1980)	M (352)	Sitting	Not specified	CON	30	50[a]	
				CON	90	35[a]	
				CON	180	27[a]	
Griffin (1987)	W (30)	Supine	80 (40–120)	CON	30	34.1 ± 6.7	
				CON	120	30.1 ± 5.2	
				CON	210	26.9 ± 4.7	
				ECC	30	38.0 ± 8.3	
				ECC	120	39.1 ± 8.9	
				ECC	210	35.6 ± 7.8	
Frontera et al (1993)	W (107) 45–78[b]	Supine	Not specified	CON	60	21 ± 6.5[d]	
				CON	180	13.5 ± 5.5[d]	
	M (71) 45–78[b]			CON	60	45 ± 11.5[d]	
				CON	180	31.5 ± 9[d]	
Housh et al (1993)	M (10)	Sitting	Not specified	CON	60	61.6 ± 12.9	
				CON	120	55.2 ± 12.7	
				CON	180	46.8 ± 12.8	
				CON	240	41.4 ± 10.8	
				CON	300	33.5 ± 9.4	
Alfredson et al (1998)	W (11)	Sitting	Not specified	CON	60	23.6 ± 4.0	25.4 ± 3.4*
				CON	180	21.2 ± 3.6	23.5 ± 4.1*
				ECC	60	30.7 ± 4.6	34.0 ± 7.6*
Mandalidis & O'Brien (2001)	M (30)	Sitting	80	CON	60	52.1 ± 13.7 7.8[c]	50.8 ± 10.9 15.6[c]
				CON	120	48.7 ± 12.7 4.1[c]	45.7 ± 9.5 12.3[c]

CON, concentric; ECC, eccentric; D, dominant; ND, non-dominant; [a] approximate figure derived from graphic illustration, data based on 319/352 right-handed subjects; [b] age range; [c] 95% standard error of measurement; [d] value is the average of the mean and SD scores of the test and retest; * ND > D ($p < 0.05$).

radial and ulnar deviation of the hand. The movements of pronation and supination are shared by the elbow and wrist and are therefore described under isokinetics of elbow muscles. Among the four wrist motions – flexion, extension, ulnar and radial deviation – the first two have been more comprehensively explored (Forthomme et al 2003). Only one study using isokinetic dynamometry related to radial and ulnar deviation strength (Kauranen et al 1997).

Control parameters

Testing is conducted with the subject in the seated position, the forearm in a pronated position, resting on a horizontal surface and the elbow flexed at 60°. Axes alignment is made with respect to the distal head of the ulna. The hand holds the lever-arm handle so that test conditions remain similar for both flexion and extension (Fig. 11.2). The ROM is adjusted according to the subject's (patient) pain-free arc. In the study by Forthomme et al (2003) which focused on normal subjects, this arc covered 140°, 70° in flexion and 70° in extension. It should however be noted that such a large ROM may not be essential, particularly where pain is present.

Reference values

Tables 11.6–11.8 outline the peak moment scores derived from three studies (Kauranen et al 1997, Friedman 1998 & Forthomme et al 2003). The study by Stonecipher & Catlin (1984) was not

Table 11.2   Elbow extensors: peak moment (mean ± SD, in Nm)

Study	Sex (N)	Test position	ROM (°)	Contraction	Velocity (°/s)	D	ND
Sale & MacDougall (1984)	M (25)	Supine	Not specified	CON CON	30 180	53 ± 2.5[c] 43.9 ± 2.6[c]	
Knapik & Ramos (1980)	M (352)	Sitting	Not specified	CON CON CON	30 90 180	43[a] 37[a] 30[a]	
Frontera et al (1993)	W (107) 45–78[b] M (71) 45–78[b]	Supine	Not specified	CON CON CON CON	60 180 60 180	22 ± 8.5[d] 15 ± 6.5[d] 42 ± 13[d] 31 ± 10[d]	
Housh et al (1993)	M (10)	Sitting	Not specified	CON CON CON CON CON		62.2 ± 14.1 51.7 ± 13.8 43.7 ± 10.4 37.7 ± 9.4 33.0 ± 6.9	
Alfredson et al (1998)	W (11)	Sitting	Not specified	CON CON ECC	60 180 60	36.1 ± 7.3 28.4 ± 5.6 51.8 ± 10.7	35.8 ± 6.6 29.4 ± 4.8 48.4 ± 9.8

CON, concentric; ECC, eccentric; D, dominant; ND, non-dominant; [a] approximate figure derived from graphic illustration, data based on 319/352 right-handed subjects; [b] age range; [c] values quoted for right extremity only; [d] value is the average of the mean and SD scores of the test and retest.

Table 11.3   Forearm pronators: peak moment (mean ± SD, in Nm)

Study	ROM (°)	Sex (N)	Test	PM (D)[a]	Normalized PM (D)[b]
Hartsell et al (1995)	Full pronation to full supination	W (20) M (20)	CON 60 CON 120 CON 180 CON 60 CON 120 CON 180	8.3 ± 1.6 7.1 ± 1.2 6.2 ± 1.0 13.6 ± 4.1 12.1 ± 3.7 11.3 ± 3.4	
Friedman (1998)	Not specified	W (25)	CON 120	4.7 ± 1.3	
Forthomme et al (2003)	160° (80° pronation to 80° supination)	W (20) M (20)	CON 30 CON 90 ECC 60 CON 30 CON 90 ECC 60	7.0 ± 2.0 5.5 ± 1.3 8.4 ± 2.3 11.0 ± 4.0 10.5 ± 3.6 15.0 ± 5.2	0.11 ± 0.02 0.09 ± 0.01 0.14 ± 0.03 0.15 ± 0.03 0.14 ± 0.03 0.21 ± 0.04

CON, concentric; ECC, eccentric; PM, peak moment; D, dominant, [a] in Nm, [b] in Nm/kgbw.

included since strength scores of women and men were pooled together. The study by Forthomme et al (2003) is by far the most comprehensive as distinct groups of women and men were tested and measurements related to concentric as well as eccentric exertions.

In addition to the strength values, the reproducibility of the findings was assessed based on a group of 10 subjects that were tested twice, 10 days apart. The reproducibility index of choice was the coefficient of variation (CVp) used before Madsen (1996).

Table 11.4 Forearm supinators: peak moment (mean ± SD, in Nm)

Study	ROM (°)	Sex (N)	Test	PM (D)[a]	Normalized PM (D)[b]
Hartsell et al (1995)	Full pronation to full supination	W (20)	CON 60	5.4 ± 1.3	
			CON 120	9.4 ± 1.8*	
			CON 180	5.0 ± 1.1	
		M (20)	CON 60	11.3 ± 2.8	
			CON 120	10.1 ± 2.3	
			CON 180	9.1 ± 2.2	
Friedman (1998)	Not specified	W (25)	CON 120	6.0 ± 1.3	
Forthomme et al (2003)	160° (80° pronation to 80° supination)	W (20)	CON 30	6.6 ± 1.4	0.11 ± 0.02
			CON 90	6.2 ± 1.2	0.10 ± 0.02
			ECC 60	9.0 ± 1.5	0.15 ± 0.03
		M (20)	CON 30	10.9 ± 2.3	0.15 ± 0.02
			CON 90	9.6 ± 1.1	0.14 ± 0.01
			ECC 60	15.6 ± 5.1	0.20 ± 0.04

CON, concentric; ECC, eccentric; PM, peak moment; D, dominant; [a]in Nm, [b]in Nm/kgbw, * probably a mistaken figure.

Table 11.5 Pronation/supination strength ratio (From Forthomme et al 2003)

Gender	Test	D	ND
Men	CON 30	1.05 ± 0.16	1.33 ± 0.33*
	CON 90	1.04 ± 0.25	1.12 ± 0.36
	ECC 60	1.04 ± 0.16	1.08 ± 0.36
Women	CON 30	1.08 ± 0.42	1.22 ± 0.25
	CON 90	0.94 ± 0.23	1.45 ± 0.42*
	ECC 60	0.92 ± 0.18	1.07 ± 0.18

CON, concentric; ECC, eccentric; D, dominant; ND, non-dominant, * difference significant at 0.05 level.

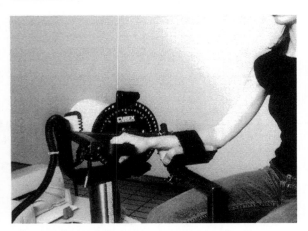

Figure 11.2 Set-up for wrist flexion–extension. (From Forthomme et al 2003 Isokinetics and Exercise Science, in press, with permission of IOS Press.)

Kauranen et al (1997) used a different dynamometer and recorded peak moments in a group which consisted predominantly of women. The results were slightly lower but compatible with those derived by Forthomme et al (2003), both in terms of the absolute values and the concentric flexion/extension strength ratio which was around 2. Collectively, these findings indicate that the wrist flexors are significantly and substantially stronger than the extensors, in agreement with the mass and role of the flexor apparatus. A significant dominance effect of this ratio was revealed (Forthomme et al 2003) but apart from the male flexors group, dominance does not seem to have an effect on either of the muscle groups. With respect to the flexors in the male group, bilateral differences of more than 20% have been recorded, rendering this specific muscle group an exception. In terms of reproducibility the smallest and largest CVp scores refer to flexion (4.9%) and extension (9.4%) strength tested concentrically at 30°/s (Forthomme et al 2003). These figures mean that as little as 13% and more than 25% increase is required in flexion and extension, respectively, to indicate a true improvement.

Measurement of the radial and ulnar deviation strength of the wrist has also been conducted (Kauranen et al 1997). The peak moments at 60 and 180°/s for the ulnar deviators were 9.1(2.7) and

Table 11.6 Wrist flexors: peak moment (mean ± SD, in Nm)

Study	ROM (°)	Sex (N)	Test	PM (D)	Normalized PM (D)[a]
Kauranen et al (1997)	Not specified	W (12)	CON 60	12.9 ± 4.1	
		M (2)	CON 180	11.0 ± 3.4	
Friedman (1998)	Not specified	W (25)	CON 120	3.2 ± 1.4	
Forthomme et al (2003)	140° (70° flexion to 70° extension)	W (20)	CON 30	15.7 ± 4.3	0.28 ± 0.08
			CON 90	14.6 ± 3.4	0.26 ± 0.06
			ECC 60	19.3 ± 5.7	0.35 ± 0.11
		M (20)	CON 30	26.1 ± 2.8	0.35 ± 0.05
			CON 90	26.7 ± 4.5	0.35 ± 0.04
			ECC 60	33.4 ± 4.9	0.44 ± 0.06

CON, concentric; ECC, eccentric; PM, peak moment; D, dominant; [a] in Nm/kgbw.

Table 11.7 Wrist extensors: peak moment (mean ± SD, in Nm)

Study	ROM (°)	Sex (N)	Test	PM (D)	Normalized PM (D)[a]
Kauranen et al (1997)	Not specified	W (12)	CON 60	5.9 ± 2.2	
		M (2)	CON 180	4.8 ± 2.1	
Friedman (1998)	Not specified	W (25)	CON 120	3.0 ± 1.0	
Forthomme et al (2003)	140° (70° flexion to 70° extension)	W (20)	CON 30	7.6 ± 1.6	0.13 ± 0.02
			CON 90	6.9 ± 1.8	0.12 ± 0.03
			ECC 60	15.4 ± 3.6	0.26 ± 0.06
		M (20)	CON 30	11.3 ± 2.3	0.15 ± 0.03
			CON 90	10.5 ± 1.8	0.14 ± 0.02
			ECC 60	17.1 ± 4.2	0.23 ± 0.08

CON, concentric; ECC, eccentric; PM, peak moment; D, dominant; [a] in Nm/kgbw.

Table 11.8 Wrist flexion/extension strength ratio (From Forthomme et al 2003)

Gender	Test	D	ND
Men	CON 30	2.38 ± 0.43	1.77 ± 0.52*
	CON 90	2.55 ± 0.29	1.99 ± 0.40*
	ECC 60	2.02 ± 0.53	1.59 ± 0.39*
Women	CON 30	2.25 ± 0.77	1.80 ± 0.51*
	CON 90	2.16 ± 0.63	1.93 ± 0.90
	ECC 60	1.23 ± 0.28	1.27 ± 0.28

CON, concentric; ECC, eccentric; D, dominant; ND, non-dominant; * difference significant at 0.05 level.

strength of these muscles were given. It should be emphasized that relative to the neutral position, the maximal ROM in ulnar deviation is substantially larger than in radial deviation and hence applying the same velocities to both may be disadvantageous with respect to the radial deviators.

ISOKINETICS OF GRIP MUSCLES

Among the typical functions of the hand, for example power grip and precision handling, the former is particularly suitable for isokinetic studies although these have not been seriously undertaken among students and practitioners of this technology. Dynamic grip strength measurement is a very unusual application of isokinetic dynamometry. This highly specialized hand function is characterized predominantly by *static* muscle

8.5(2.2) Nm, respectively whereas the corresponding values for the radial deviators were 12.2(3.2) and 11.2(2.4) Nm. Unfortunately no details regarding the protocol employed in measuring the

contraction, once the thumb and finger joints have assumed the specific configuration dictated by the shape of the object and the intended purpose of manipulating it. Thus although reaching this final configuration involves typically low magnitude dynamic contraction of quite a large number of muscles, the actual grip is realized by exerting static forces on the object. On the other hand, isokinetic measurements of maximal grip force portray continuously the muscular capacity focusing to a much lesser extent on the static component. It is therefore constructive to start this section with a short discussion of the common isometric method for measuring grip strength.

Measuring grip strength

The standard instrument for this purpose is the Jamar (Preston) dynamometer. This apparatus is designed to measure grip at five different flexion positions (rungs) of the fingers, from the most extended to the most flexed with respect to the metacarpophalangeal (MCP) and interphalangeal (IP) joints. A hydraulic system, in conjunction with a force dial, measures the force exerted by the finger muscles against a stable handle (see Fig. 11.4). Typically the measurement is performed at each of the five rungs resulting in five distinct force values. In subjects without hand pathology, the force–position (rung) curve takes the shape of an inverted U at either rung 2 or 3 and tapering-off towards rungs 1 and 5 (Fig. 11.3). Reference

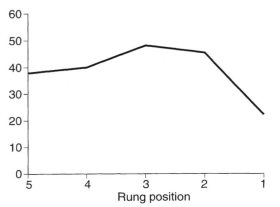

Figure 11.3 Jamar grip strength curve. X axis, rung; Y axis, strength in kgf. Note maximal strength at rung 3: 48 kgf.

isometric strength values have been recorded among women and men with respect to age decades (Mathiowetz et al 1984).

Forceful dynamic grip is not a common activity. It may be exemplified by cutting of hard material using special scissors or during powerful squeezing. This is a typical concentric muscle action in terms, for example, of the long flexors of fingers 2–5. Electromyographic studies have indicated that concurrently with the agonistic flexors, the antagonistic extensor apparatus is acting in order to maintain optimal length–tension of the agonists. Hence the extensors are undergoing a simultaneous eccentric contraction. Thus, dynamic (as well as static) measurement of grip strength shows in fact the net moment: flexor–extensor.

What distinguishes grip is that it is an inherently multiple joint configuration performed in a so-called close kinetic chain activity. In the absence of a 'single axis' of rotation, characterizing the more proximal wrist and elbow joints, the measured intrinsic strength should be expressed in force (N) rather than moment (Nm) units although as far as the dynamometer is concerned, the extrinsic result is the generation of moment about the motor axis. Thus, while from the pure mechanical point of view it is possible to express the results in Nm, it would be a mistake to assign the moment value to a specific joint.

Grip force attachment

A special attachment for measuring grip force has been described by Dvir (1997). It consists of the following components: frame, stable thumb handle and fingers piece (Fig. 11.4). The frame itself consists of a stable part which connects to the dynamometer's seat frame (not shown) and an adjustable surface that can move forward or backward using a regulating screw. This movement ensures that large as well as small palms can be accommodated and is quite critical for recording the full range of available motion.

Force sensor placement and range of motion

The moving fingers handle is located exactly opposite the thumb handle. In order for the trajectory of the fingers handle to be substantially linear while covering a ROM which would allow effective control of velocity, it was experimentally verified that this handle should be placed 30 cm below the motor axis, approximating, piecewise, the situation in the Jamar dynamometer. This length of lever-arm translates into about 5.5 cm of linear mobile (fingers) handle motion which accommodates the palm size of the vast majority of adult subjects. At this lever-arm length the corresponding angular sector of motion is 8°. It must be emphasized that this angular ROM should not be interpreted in terms of either MCP or IP joint motion. Indeed, the MCP joint may move along an arc of 90° during the test. For subjects with particularly large or small palms this range may be increased to 9° or 7°, respectively. In addition, the stage in lever-arm motion where the fingers handle points directly downward (270°) should coincide with the middle of the range of biological motion (half way between full extension and full flexion of the finger joints) so that the small error introduced by the non-orthogonality of the force vector and force pad is maximally reduced.

Stabilization and subject positioning

Due to the multiple joint closed configuration, isokinetic grip testing is probably the only instance in which full stabilization of the proximal segment is realized. This is enabled by the stable thumb handle which operates as a solid buttress against any unnecessary movement. The test is conducted with the subject seated, back supported, arm flexed 10–15° and forearm resting comfortably on the adjustable frame. Foot support is recommended for subject comfort.

Contraction modes, test velocities and isometric preactivation bias

Concentric as well as eccentric testing is recommended. Although eccentric contraction of the flexors is a true rarity, simulated by attempting to grip an inflating balloon (lengthening of the flexors), it appears that this mode of contraction is essential in the verification of grip effort (see Chapter 5). Using 8° ROM, the velocities used in both the concentric and eccentric tests were 4, 8 and 16°/s (Dvir 1997). With respect to the isometric preactivation bias (IPB), it was revealed that the application of either a low or a high value, 25 and 75% respectively of the lowest static score recorded at either rung 1 or 5 of the Jamar, did not affect the peak moment. As a certain level of IPB is essential for the initial feel of resistance, an IPB of 100 N for men and 50–75 N for women is recommended unless the individual's strength is extremely low. In most patients, 25% of the recorded strength at either rung 1 (most flexed) or rung 5 (most extended) should be effective. Clearly, due to the test position and negligible weight of the fingers, no gravity correction procedure is indicated.

Reference values

The study by Dvir (1997) consisted of 16 women aged 19–52. This age range may render the

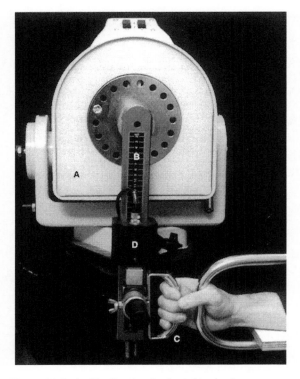

Figure 11.4 Isokinetic grip attachment and set-up. A, motor; B, lever-arm; C, fingers piece; D, load cell. (From Dvir 1997.)

Table 11.9 Grip strength: peak and average force values (N) for low IPB

Contraction mode and velocity (°/s)	Peak force: mean (SD)	Average mean (SD)
CON 4	207.9 (38.2)	163.2 (28.2)
CON 8	170.0 (42.9)	139.4 (34.4)
CON 16	152.0 (42.9)	129.8 (35.8)
ECC 4	319.5 (58.9)	238.2 (40.7)
ECC 8	315.8 (54.9)	247.7 (43.1)
ECC 16	327.5 (61.7)	260.5 (51.2)

CON, concentric; ECC, eccentric.

following strength scores slightly non-specific due to some age-related reduction in strength. Table 11.9 outlines the results in terms of the low IPB protocol. The force–velocity relationship derived from this study is depicted in Figure 1.12. As is clearly evident, the shape of the curve which consists of the average force values is substantially sigmoidal. It also crosses the isometric condition (the y axis, 0° velocity) very close to the peak maximal isometric strength, calculated from the Jamar-based measurements. This is possibly the only instance where such correspondence has been indicated. At the time of writing up of this edition, no parallel male reference values were available.

Clinical application of isokinetic grip testing has recently been described (Dvir 2002). Although the main objective was analysis of effort, the isokinetic findings were compared with isometric test results. Unlike the absence of relationship between the two modes of testing revealed in a previous study of healthy subjects (Dvir 1997), in patients the correlation between isometric and isokinetic (peak moment) strength scores was 0.65. On the other hand no current study indicates which of the two modalities is more indicative in terms of function or predictability.

REFERENCES

Alfredson H, Pietilä T, Lorentzon R 1998 Concentric and eccentric shoulder and elbow muscle strength in female volleyball players and non-active females. Scandinavian Journal of Medicine and Science in Sports 8: 265–270

Ambacher T, Winter E, Piert M, Mayer F, Weise K 2000 Functional results after suture repair in ruptures of the long biceps tendon with special consideration of subacromial impingement. Unfallchirurgie 103: 761–768

Amundsen L 1990 Muscle strength measurements: instrumented and non-instrumented. Churchill Livingstone, Edinburgh

Bell R H, Wiley W B, Noble J S, Kuczynski D J 2000 Repair of distal biceps brachii tendon ruptures. Journal of Shoulder and Elbow Surgery 9: 223–226

Dvir Z 1997 The measurement of isokinetic fingers flexion strength. Clinical Biomechanics 12: 472–481

Dvir Z 2002 Clinical application of the DEC parameter in assessing optimality of muscular effort: a report of 34 patients. American Journal of Physical Medicine and Rehabilitation 81: 178–183

Forthomme B, Croisier J-L, Foidart-Dessalle M, Crielaard J M 2003 Isokinetic assessment of the forearm and wrist muscles. Isokinetics and Exercise Science. In press.

Friedman P J 1998 Isokinetic peak torque in women with unilateral cumulative trauma disorders and healthy control subjects. Archives of Physical Medicine and Rehabilitation 79: 816–819

Frontera W R, Hughes V A, Dallal G E, Evans W J 1993 Reliability of isokinetic muscle strength testing in 45- to 78-year-old men and women. Archives of Physical Medicine and Rehabilitation 74: 1181–1185

Fuchs S, Chylarecki C 1999 Do functional deficits result from radial head resection? Journal of Shoulder and Elbow Surgery 8: 247–251

Gallagher M A, Cuomo F, Polonsky L, Berliner K, Zuckerman J D 1997 Effects of age, testing speed and arm dominance on isokinetic strength of the elbow. Journal of Shoulder and Elbow Surgery 6: 340–346

Griffin J W 1987 Differences in elbow flexion torque measured concentrically, eccentrically and isometrically. Physical Therapy 8: 1205–1208

Hartsell H D, Hubbard M, Van Os M 1995 Isokinetic strength evaluation of wrist pronators and supinators: implications for clinicians. Physiotherapy Canada 47: 252–257

Hildebrand K A, Patterson S D, Regan W D, MacDermid J C, King G J 2000 Functional outcome of semiconstrained total elbow arthroplasty. Journal of Bone and Joint Surgery 82A: 1379–1386

Housh D J, Housh T J, Johnson G O, Wei-Kom C 1993 The relationship between isokinetic peak torque and cross sectional area of the forearm flexors and extensors. Isokinetics and Exercise Science 3: 133–138

Karunakar M A, Cha P, Stern P J 1999 Distal biceps ruptures. A follow up of Boyd and Anderson repair. Clinical Orthopaedics and Related Research 363: 100–107

Kauranen K, Siira P, Vanharanta H 1997 The effect of strapping on the motor performance of the ankle and wrist joints. Scandinavian Journal of Medicine and Science in Sports 7: 238–243

Knapik J L, Ramos M U 1980 Isokinetic and isometric torque relationships in the human body. Archives of Physical Medicine and Rehabilitation 61: 64–67

Madsen O R 1996 Torque, total work, power and torque acceleration energy assessed on a dynamometer: reliability of knee and elbow extensor and flexor strength measurements. European Journal of Applied Physiology 74: 206–210

Mandalidis D G, O'Brien M O 2001 Isokinetic strength of the elbow flexors with the arm in supination and in the neutral position. Isokinetics and Exercise Science 9: 111–118

Mathiowetz V, Weber K, Volland G, Kashman N 1984 Reliability and validity of grip and pinch strength. Journal of Hand Surgery 9A: 222–226

Morrey B F, Chao E Y S 1976 Passive motion of the elbow joint. A biomechanical analysis. Journal of Bone and Joint Surgery 58A: 501–508

Musmayer S, Odinsson A, Holm I 2000 Distal biceps tendon rupture operated on with the Boyd and Anderson technique: follow-up of 9 patients with isokinetic examination after 1 year. Acta Orthopaedica Scandinavica 71: 399–402

Sale D G, MacDougall J D 1984 Isokinetic strength in weight trainers. European Journal of Applied Physiology 53: 128–132

Stonecipher D R, Catlin P A 1984 The effect of forearm strap on wrist extensor strength. Journal of Orthopaedic and Sports Physical Therapy 6: 184–189

VanSwearingen J M 1983 Measuring wrist muscle strength. Journal of Orthopaedic and Sports Physical Therapy 4: 217–228

Index